Stanley A. Goldberg
San Francisco State University

CLINICAL INTERVENTION
A Philosophy and Methodology for Clinical Practice

Merrill, an imprint of
Macmillan Publishing Company
New York

Maxwell Macmillan Canada
Toronto

Maxwell Macmillan International
New York   Oxford   Singapore   Sydney

Cover art: © Kathy Hickey, Southeast School, F.C.B.M.R./D.D.
Editor: Ann Castel
Production Editor: Mary Harlan
Text Designer: Anne Flanagan
Cover Designer: Thomas Mack
Production Buyer: Patricia A. Tonneman
Illustrations: Carlisle Communications, Ltd.

This book was set in New Baskerville by Carlisle Communications, Ltd. and was printed and bound by Book Press, Inc., a Quebecor America Book Group Company. The cover was printed by Lehigh Press, Inc.

Copyright © 1993 by Macmillan Publishing Company, a division of Macmillan, Inc. Merrill is an imprint of Macmillan Publishing Company.

Printed in the United States of America.

All rights reserved. No part of this book may be reproduced or transmitted in any form or by any means, electronic or mechanical, including photocopy, recording, or any information storage and retrieval system, without permission in writing from the Publisher.

Macmillan Publishing Company
866 Third Avenue
New York, NY 10022

Macmillan Publishing Company is part of the
Maxwell Communication Group of Companies.

Maxwell Macmillan Canada, Inc.
1200 Eglinton Avenue East, Suite 200
Don Mills, Ontario M3C 3N1

Library of Congress Cataloging-in-Publication Data
Goldberg, Stanley A.
    Clinical intervention : a philosophy and methodology for clinical
  practice / Stanley A. Goldberg.
       p.   cm.
    Includes bibliographical references and index.
    ISBN 0-675-22160-9 (casebound)
    1. Speech therapy. I. Title.
RC423.G63 1993
616.85′5061—dc20   92-32416
                                                      CIP

Printing: 1 2 3 4 5 6 7 8 9   Year: 3 4 5 6 7

*To the clinical artistry of Audrey Holland
and Herbert Rubin*

To the patience of my family—Wendy, Jessica and Justin

To the friendship and understanding of Henry Chung

Preface

Becoming a master clinician involves not only completing courses and field experiences successfully, but also knowing how to apply theories within a clinical setting. Strategies for applying theoretical constructs are usually in the form of clinical models. Without a clinical model, students can find themselves thrust into a maze of theory and practice with few guideposts or methods of organizing the diverse areas into a usable approach. The resulting confusion often results in anxiety, a feeling that every experienced clinician can remember. Fromm-Reichmann's (1963) description of anxiety is one that most clinicians can relate to: Anxiety is described as "a most unpleasant interference with thinking processes and concentration, as a diffuse, vague and frequently objectless feeling of apprehension or as a discomforting feeling of uncertainty and helplessness" (p. 129). Clinician anxiety can lead to difficulty in understanding interactions or responding appropriately to clients. One clinician described it as an inability to be "in tune" with her client. Another clinician, in attempting to explain a disastrous session to his supervisor, said, "It was like I was standing outside of myself, watching me saying stupid things. I knew I didn't make any sense, but I couldn't do anything else. I was frozen."

Although all clinical educators would agree that a student's feeling of panic serves no useful function, they disagree on the extent to which directed instruction should be used with inexperienced clinicians. The debate is between self-discovery and guided instruction.

SELF-DISCOVERY VS. GUIDED INSTRUCTION

Educators differ on the roles they believe self-discovery and guided instruction should play in the acquisition of knowledge and clinical skills. Many believe that providing answers to students denies those students an opportunity to problem solve, which is a critical component in the development of clinical competency. Others maintain that the service provided to clients should not be compromised for the sake of clinical training. Rather, guided instruction can protect the client while not sacrificing the development of problem-solving skills.

Self-Discovery

Some psychologists believe that anxiety can be a source of growth, since it requires the person experiencing the feeling to react against its causes (Whitaker & Malone, 1953). According to this type of reasoning, new clinicians reduce their anxiety by determining the most appropriate methods of helping their clients. The reduction of anxiety functions as an incentive for the clinician to acquire academic and practical knowledge.

Some clinical educators believe this type of self-discovery is a more appropriate way of learning than directly providing the information to the clinician. However, some evidence suggests that the self-discovery form of learning is not necessarily as effective or beneficial as guided instruction (Ausubel, 1968; Dreyfus & Dreyfus, 1986). Without adequate knowledge, self-discovery learning is less likely to lead to the development of clinical skills and is more likely to result in unnecessary anxiety. Many people in instructional technology maintain that before someone can be creative, they need something to think about (Gagné, 1970). The negative effects of anxiety on learning were known over 40 years ago (May, 1961). For example, anxious clinicians have difficulty understanding events as they are occurring, and as a result, may not learn from their mistakes. The loss of confidence and self-esteem not only is felt by the clinician but is also experienced by the client. Clients come for help because they are experiencing communicative failure, not as a goodwill gesture to facilitate clinical training. One may ask if it is ethical to allow clients to continue to view themselves as failures for the sake of training new clinicians. Although how one achieves a balance between training requirements and service is an issue rarely discussed in the literature, it continues to concern clinical educators. An approach that many believe allows for the training of clinicians while providing ethical, quality service is the guided instruction model of supervision.

Guided Instruction

How can skills be developed so that the clinician's "artistry" is fulfilled while not jeopardizing the interests of the client? It is not sufficient to provide only content knowledge of each disorder. This would be similar to teaching language by presenting lists of words to a nonverbal child and hoping that complete sentences would be eventually produced without further instruction. An analogous situation exists with the acquisition of clinical competencies. In the training of speech-language pathologists, the melding of theory and practice occurs in the clinical practicum, which becomes the real life laboratory for testing theories and intervention strategies. To the horror of many new clinicians, they find that the gap between the ideal and the real is monumental. The language impaired child described in their seminar is nowhere to be found. The aphasic client who should respond to an accepted form of therapy is uncooperative. The stutterer is presenting a pattern of stuttering that is not even mentioned in the textbooks. Some new students may decide, unwisely, that much of the academic material covered in their seminars is of little value with real clients.

Dreyfus and Dreyfus (1986) maintained that the transition from academic knowledge to practical knowledge involves several steps. They found that the brilliant student did not automatically become a competent teacher. Their research with classroom teachers indicated that new teachers needed a strategy for applying academic knowledge within a classroom setting. In the absence of such a strategy, new teachers were ineffective and often developed teaching styles that were antithetical to learning. Many teachers who were left on their own did eventually develop appropriate teaching methods, but only after several years of frustration on the part of their students and themselves. Their research indicated that few teachers were considered to be "highly skilled" by their peers prior to completing five years of teaching. They concluded that during this apprentice period, teachers needed to be provided with strategies or even scripts for teaching.

Speech pathologists are also teachers. They are responsible for teaching a client how to effect communicative and attitudinal changes. If it requires five years of practice for a classroom teacher to be considered highly skilled, how long does it take for someone in the area of speech pathology to be considered a "master clinician"? Presumably longer, since the amount of knowledge to be acquired and applied is greater. An application strategy is needed if the interests of clients are to be protected and if clinicians are to be provided with support in the development of their clinical skills. An application strategy is a model, or set of procedures, for modifying the constructs taught in the classroom into a form that is compatible with the diversity of client personalities and problems. It is the tailoring necessary to make the suit fit. The Cultural Communication Model (CCM) is designed for this purpose. This model, which is presented in Chapter 1, becomes the template on which subsequent chapters are framed.

❏ ❏ ❏ *TEXT ORGANIZATION*

The acquisition of new behaviors can occur randomly, with some structure, or in a carefully planned manner. Clinical skills are very complex entities that usually depend on successive acquisition of precursor skills. The teaching and learning of these skills should be as well planned and sequential as any new linguistic behavior taught to a client. The chapters are divided into three parts: (a) Clinical Foundations; (b) Clinical Behaviors; and (c) Clinical Intervention. The chapters are sequentially ordered so that new clinicians can gradually acquire the fundamental knowledge necessary to develop clinical competency. Each chapter should be viewed as an independent unit of knowledge that is necessary to acquire the material that follows in subsequent chapters.

The sequence of material covered in each chapter is identical. At the beginning of each chapter, important orienting questions are given to direct the student to the chapter's main focus. At the end of each chapter, suggested readings and specific assignments related to the chapter's text are provided. Most of these assignments are appropriate for meeting the American Speech-Language-Hearing Association's clinical observation requirement. The suggested sequence of events is (a) reading, (b) lecture and discussion, and (c) observation. A brief synopsis of each chapter follows.

Chapter 1. The model of communication presented in this chapter views clients as complex individuals whose communicative problem constitutes only one aspect of their behavior and personality. Their problems and behaviors must be understood in relation to their culture, experiences, cognition, and needs.

Chapter 2. This chapter presents a model for understanding the role of the clinician. The clinician is viewed as a compassionate scientist whose overwhelming concern for the client's growth requires the constant validation of clinical procedures.

Chapter 3. The importance of measuring behaviors and collecting data is presented. Types of objective and subjective data are explained along with procedures used for their collection.

Chapter 4. This chapter explains the methods for observing the specific speech, and vocalic behaviors that are the domain of speech-language pathologists.

Chapter 5. The chapter focuses on linguistic and metalinguistic analysis of both children and adults.

Chapter 6. The chapter contains descriptions of nonverbal behaviors that are vocalic and those associated with body movements. Methods for analyzing self- and other-directed behaviors are discussed. Body movements are classified in terms of identifiable visual units, such as face, arms/hands, and posture.

Chapter 7. This chapter presents a discussion of the principles of learning, based on educational research. These principles have been shown to facilitate the remediation of communicative disorders and to enhance cognitive development.

Chapter 8. Basic counseling techniques and dynamics of group process as it relates to speech pathology are presented. Both clinical and school settings are covered. Leader qualities necessary for effective group therapy are discussed.

Chapter 9. A generic intervention model is presented. The model is competency-based, criterion-referenced, and features a lattice structure that is based on successive approximations of target behaviors. The emphasis of the chapter is on providing the inexperienced clinician with an appropriate clinical interaction model.

Chapter 10. The chapter contains a completed template that new students can use for their first clients. It presents a format for interacting with clients and their families from initial contact through termination.

ACKNOWLEDGMENTS

A number of outside readers reviewed various drafts of the manuscript. I thank the following individuals for their comments and suggestions:

- Darlene G. Davies, San Diego State University
- Pam Dutcher, Andrews University
- Robin Wright Fromherz, Mt. Angel College and Seminary
- Mary Anne Hanner, Eastern Illinois University
- Betsy P. Vinson, University of Florida Speech and Hearing Clinic

In addition, I thank the staff at Macmillan Publishing for their assistance: Ann Castel, Editor; Mary Harlan, Production Editor; Anne Flanagan, Text Designer; and Cindy Peck, copy editor.

Contents

PART I
Clinical Foundations — 1

CHAPTER 1
The Communicative Disorder — 3

THE CLIENT AS A COMMUNICATOR — 4
FUNCTION OF MODELS — 5
MODELS OF COMMUNICATION AND DISRUPTION — 5
   Fairbanks Model ❑ Wepman's Operational Levels of CNS
CULTURAL COMMUNICATIONS MODEL (CCM) — 10
   Culture ❑ Microcultures ❑ Combining Macro and Microcultures ❑ Language as the Expression of Culture ❑ Cognition ❑ Experience
SUMMARY — 28
SUGGESTED READINGS — 29
❑ *Activity 1.1:* Microcultural Values — 30

CHAPTER 2
The Clinician as a Caring Scientist — 31

THE SCIENTIFIC APPROACH — 32
   Types of Scientific Knowledge ❑ Contexts of Knowledge Acquisition ❑ Clinical Experimentation
THE CARING APPROACH — 39
   Personality Traits of the Clinician ❑ Values

COMBINING SCIENCE AND COMPASSION	49
SUMMARY	51
SUGGESTED READINGS	51
❑ *Activity 2.1:* A Clinical Experiment—ABA Design	52
❑ *Activity 2.2:* A Self-Evaluation of Values and Ethics	53

❑ ❑ ❑ PART II
Clinical Behaviors   57

CHAPTER 3
Observation and Measurement   59

REASONS FOR DATA COLLECTION	60
Assessment ❑ Accountability ❑ Motivation	
PRINCIPLES OF OBSERVATION	61
A Multidimensional Process ❑ A Nonjudgmental Process ❑ Contexts for Observing ❑ Number and Length of Observations ❑ Observer Roles	
DATA COLLECTION DEVICES	65
Videotapes ❑ Audiotapes ❑ Counters ❑ Written Forms	
SAMPLING PROCEDURES	67
Timed Segments Throughout the Session ❑ Designated Segment	
UNITS OF MEASUREMENT	68
Simple Enumeration ❑ Number of Correct Responses ❑ Percentage of Correct Responses ❑ Learning Curve ❑ Type Token Ratio ❑ Latency of Response ❑ Amplitude of Response ❑ Rating Scales	
SUMMARY	77
SUGGESTED READINGS	77
❑ *Activity 3.1:* Simple Enumeration	78
❑ *Activity 3.2:* Type Token Ratio	80
❑ *Activity 3.3:* Rating Scales	84

CHAPTER 4
Speech Behaviors   85

PHONOLOGY AND ARTICULATION	86
Phonemes ❑ Types of Disorders ❑ Vowels ❑ Diphthongs ❑ Consonants	

CONTENTS

STUTTERING	98
Covert Behaviors ❑ Overt Behaviors ❑ Listener Reactions	
VOICE	105
Disorders of Pitch ❑ Disorders of Loudness ❑ Disorders of Duration ❑ Disorders of Quality ❑ Disorders of Resonance	
CLEFT PALATE SPEECH	110
Hypernasality ❑ Articulation ❑ Nasal Fricative	
SUMMARY	111
SUGGESTED READINGS	112
❑ *Activity 4.1:* Phonological and articulatory disorders	113
❑ *Activity 4.2:* Fluency	115
❑ *Activity 4.3:* Voice	117

CHAPTER 5
Verbal Behaviors — 119

CHILD AND ADOLESCENT LANGUAGE DISORDERS	120
Language Disorders	
ADULT LANGUAGE DISORDERS	128
Aphasia ❑ Traumatic Brain Injury	
METALINGUISTIC ANALYSIS	133
Children's Metalinguistic Analysis ❑ Adult Metalinguistic Analysis	
SUMMARY	140
SUGGESTED READINGS	140
❑ *Activity 5.1:* Language Observation	141
❑ *Activity 5.2:* Aphasia Observation	145
❑ *Activity 5.3:* Metalinguistic Analysis	146

CHAPTER 6
Nonverbal Observation — 153

LEVELS OF ANALYSIS	154
Prekinesics ❑ Microkinesics ❑ Social Kinesics	
CONTEXT	158
Linear-Temporal Context ❑ Multidimensional Behavior Context ❑ Individual Behavior Repertoires ❑ Environmental Context ❑ Cultural Context	

CONTENTS

FUNCTIONS OF NONVERBAL BEHAVIORS	160
Amplify the Message ❑ Contradict the Message ❑ Qualify the Message ❑ Sending an Unrelated Message	
CLINICAL IMPLICATIONS	161
Sending Ability and Rank Order ❑ Factors Affecting the Sender	
SUMMARY	163
SUGGESTED READINGS	163
❑ *Activity 6.1:* Individual Behavioral Repertoires	164
❑ *Activity 6.2:* Linear-Temporal Context	166
❑ *Activity 6.3:* Observation of Environmental Context	167

❑ ❑ ❑ ## PART III
Clinical Intervention   **169**

CHAPTER 7
Principles of Learning   ***171***

LEARNING CONTINUA	172
Stages in Learning and Retrieval ❑ Levels of Learning	
COGNITION AND LEARNING STYLES	177
OPERANT CONDITIONING	178
History ❑ Ethical and Moral Conditions of Behavior Change ❑ Mediation ❑ Basic Concepts ❑ Positive and Aversive Stimuli ❑ Reinforcement Schedules ❑ Response Differentiation ❑ Operant Principles of Therapeutic Intervention	
SUMMARY	203
SUGGESTED READINGS	204
❑ *Activity 7.1:* Identification of Learning Continua	204
❑ *Activity 7.2:* Operant Procedures	205

CHAPTER 8
Principles of Group Therapy   ***207***

SETTING REQUIREMENTS	208
Public Schools ❑ Senior Centers ❑ Preschools ❑ Community Centers	

CONTENTS

FUNCTION OF GROUPS — 210
Changing Speech and Language Behaviors ❑ Generalization of Behaviors ❑ Discussion Groups ❑ Baseline Data Through Group Observation

QUALITIES OF THE GROUP LEADER — 219
General Competency ❑ Empathic ❑ Multidimensional ❑ Age-Specific Characteristics

CULTURAL VARIABLES — 221
Misunderstandings Between Cultures in Group Settings ❑ Group and Ethnic Cultures

SUPPORT GROUPS — 222
Functions of Support Groups ❑ View of the Profession

SUMMARY — 223
SUGGESTED READINGS — 223
❑ *Activity 8.1:* Group Time Management — 224
❑ *Activity 8.2:* Group Control — 225
❑ *Activity 8.3:* Group Functions — 226

CHAPTER 9
Clinical Strategies — *229*

STRATEGIES OF IMPLEMENTATION — 231
Cognitive Psychology Scaffolding ❑ Competency-Based Clinical Intervention Format (CBCIF) ❑ Computer-Assisted Instruction

STRATEGIES — 242
Memory ❑ Retrieval ❑ Generalization ❑ Selection of Strategies

SUMMARY — 245
SUGGESTED READINGS — 247
❑ *Activity 9.1:* Skill and Strategy Observation — 248

CHAPTER 10
The First Client — *249*

PREPARING FOR THE FIRST SESSION — 250
Clinical Records ❑ Pre-Clinical Telephone Interview

GOALS FOR THE FIRST SESSION — 258
Establishing the Purpose of Therapy ❑ Role Expectations ❑ Trust ❑ Diagnostic Therapy

ANALYZING THE FIRST SESSION	260
SUMMARY	266
SUGGESTED READINGS	266

❑❑❑ APPENDIXES

Appendix A ASHA Observation Supplement	267
Appendix B American Speech-Language-Hearing Association's Code of Ethics	269
Appendix C Multicultural/Bilingual Assessment Materials	273
Appendix D Phonological and Articulation Diagnostic Tests	275
Appendix E Language Diagnostic Tests	277
Appendix F Stuttering Tests	283
Appendix G Voice Tests	285
Appendix H Neurogenic Cognitive Tests	287
Appendix I Selected Publishers' Addresses for Listed Diagnostic Tests	291
Appendix J Language Therapy and Parent Involvement	295
Appendix K Articulation Therapy and Parent Involvement	297
Appendix L Voice Therapy and Parent Involvement	299
Appendix M Stuttering Therapy and Parent Involvement	301
References	303
Index	313

PART I
Clinical Foundations

Therapy is a temporary or finite process in which clients come for support and guidance as they contemplate changing about themselves something they don't like. It is unlike any other interpersonal relationship they may have experienced in that both members of the dyad concern themselves primarily with one member. It is the needs, feelings, thoughts, attitudes, and actions of the client that predominate. For the client, therapy means always being in the hot seat; for the therapist it means always responding in terms of the client (p. 261).

Shames and Rubin's (1986) description of the clinical dyad forcefully articulated the importance of understanding the roles of the participants. The situation is unique, requiring clinicians to understand both themselves and their clients in a way that is rarely necessary in day-to-day interactions. Plato's famous observation that the unexamined life is not worth living is also applicable to clinical situations. For the clinician, it becomes paramount not only to identify specific communicative behaviors of clients, but also to be sensitive to the underlying causes of those behaviors. The clinician must also appreciate the centrality of the speech-language pathologist's role.

In this section some of the basic foundations necessary for developing clinical sensitivity will be explored. In Chapter 1 various models of understanding clients and their behaviors will be discussed. In Chapter 2 the focus is on the characteristics of the ideal clinician, one who is both scientific and compassionate.

Chapter 1
The Communicative Disorder

STUDY GUIDE

- What is the function of models?
- Describe the major components of the Fairbanks model of communication.
- How does Wepman's model of the central nervous system provide clinicians with a framework for understanding specific communicative disorders?
- What are the major components of a Cultural Communication Model (CCM)? How does each component contribute to our understanding of the client?
- What is the relationship between the macroculture and microcultures?
- What is the relationship between language and culture?
- How does cognition affect language usage?
- How does experience affect language usage?

Like it or not, most of our best therapies, like medical therapies for diseases for which causes are unknown, are most likely to be provided by intuitive, caring clinicians attuned to specific needs of specific persons with specific problems who respond to a particular clinician's artistry.

William Perkins (1986, p. 33)

Perkins' eloquent statement describes what many believe are the characteristics of the ideal clinician, a combination of scientific thought and compassion, expressed in a manner that is embraced by the client. These skillful practitioners do not come to the field fully equipped to provide quality service. The skills of a master clinician develop not only as the result of the successful completion of many courses but also after the clinician has had a wide variety of experiences and has applied theories within a clinical setting.

The clinical science of speech-language pathology offers the practitioner a unique opportunity to combine theory and practical techniques for the benefit of communicatively impaired individuals. The study of speech-language pathology begins with knowledge of physical and behavioral sciences that is then applied in dynamic practical settings. The application requires not only intelligence but also the sensitivity and compassion that is vital to any helping profession. To accomplish this, the clinician should understand the relationship between clients and their disorders. To develop this understanding, one must explore the nature of communication and the variables that affect it. In this chapter, both will be examined.

THE CLIENT AS A COMMUNICATOR

Many people believe that labels are useful in quickly identifying and conveying information about clients and their disorders. In an era when data overload is prevalent, this shortcut method of lumping information functions as an organizational tool. Terms such as *stutterer, aphasic, mentally disabled,* and *orthopedically disabled* provide visual and intellectual descriptions of clients without the need to list specific behaviors associated with the condition. However, problems result when we apply labels to clients. Clearly, a person with disfluencies possesses more characteristics than those associated with the label *stutterer*. The condition of someone with cerebral palsy is more complex than that of a person who has impaired motor responses. The client with a functional vocal disorder requires more therapy than someone who loses her voice three times each month. The need for going beyond labels was addressed by Holland (1977). In her aphasia assessment instrument, Communicative Ability in Daily Living (CADL), she maintained that clients with aphasia should be viewed as impaired communicators, not just as people with specific types of brain damage. It is impossible to avoid the use of labels. However, the clinician should realize that the client is not the label, but rather an individual whose communicative competence is impaired.

If clients are viewed as impaired communicators rather than as people whose personalities are defined by their disorders, the clinician's approach to intervention becomes multidimensional. The clinician must consider not only the basic communication needs of clients but also their values, needs, and the changes they expect in their lives as a result of success or failure of therapy. Although all of these areas are important in treatment, the communicative needs of clients should still be considered as the primary focus of therapy. Examining communication models can help us understand how specific impairments may affect clients.

FUNCTION OF MODELS

Unlike the clean and unvarying laws of the physical sciences, the laws of human interaction and development often become obscured by unknown variables that cannot be controlled. Few aphasics fit neatly into a specific category; all children with Down syndrome do not function identically; not all stutterers can be fluent when they prolong their speech. Because of the great variability we find in our clients, it is often difficult to apply a "textbook procedure" directly to a specific clinical situation. Modifications, therefore, are not only acceptable but desirable.

These differences between theories and reality were emphasized by the linguist Korzybski (1958) who wrote that the map is not the territory. By this he meant that to explore any aspect of human experience, one needs to have a way of orienting oneself, a way of developing a semblance of order. However, if one assumes that the map, or theory, is identical to reality, one can become as disoriented as if the map or theory was not available. The techniques presented in this book are maps for understanding the principles of communicative restructuring. They, too, are modifiable procedures for creatively and effectively dealing with the liquidity of human behavior. The importance of viewing theories and rationales as permeable structures was noted by Perkins (1986) when he wrote, "We will be well-advised to proceed pragmatically, using clinical sessions experimentally to determine the effectiveness of our procedures, irrespective of whether they fit a particular rationale" (p. 33). According to Perkins, when disparities exist between our models and our successful therapy procedures, revisions should be made in the model, not in the effective procedure. With poetic license, one might say, "If the model fits, use it." If it does not, alter it.

Speech-language pathology students should be familiar with two general types of clinical models. The first are models of communication and disruption. These models present a theory of how messages are sent, received, and disrupted. Communication models allow the student to understand how normal communication can be disrupted. The second type of model is that of intervention. Intervention models are protocols for treatment and will be presented in Part III of this text.

MODELS OF COMMUNICATION AND DISRUPTION

Fairbanks Model

Fairbanks (1954) proposed one of the first useful theories of how communication is disrupted. Although the model is almost 40 years old, it still provides a relevant description of communication failure. The system has been applied to both machine and human communication. His *General Communication System* (Figure 1.1) contains two major components, a transmitter and a receiver. If we apply the theory to human beings, the information source is the "talker" and the destination is the "listener." To send a message, the talker must code it using appropriate linguistic rules. The message is then sent by way of an oral signal. The listener receives the signal through the use of the auditory mechanism and then decodes it using knowledge of linguistic rules, thereby understanding the message that was sent by the talker. In the model, if a noise is introduced between the sending of the signal and its reception, the message may become distorted or eliminated.

In the Fairbanks model, "noise" is analogous to a communicative disorder. Noise therefore disrupts the communicative process and affects both the speaker and the listener. Understanding that a communicative disorder affects both the speaker and the listener enables the clinician to construct an appropriate intervention program. Intervention programs must account for the reaction of the persons who will be interacting with clients and will be affected by their impaired communicative ability. Both normal and impaired communication are synergistic. That is, the speaker and listener affect each other. Intervention programs that treat only the disorder are incomplete because listener reactions to an impaired communicator may further complicate the disorder. For example, a child with a severe phonological disorder may reduce his verbal output to avoid constantly being asked to repeat an utterance. A language disordered child who cannot verbally convey her feelings may express them in socially unacceptable nonverbal behaviors. A stutterer who feels pain whenever he observes a listener's reaction to his facial grimaces may minimize his contact with other people. And an aphasic who is treated as if he is mentally incompetent may choose to become passive.

Wepman's Operational Levels of CNS

If "noise" can be anything that distorts the sending or reception of a message, then it can be found anywhere in the system. Wepman, Jones, Bock, and Van Pelt (1960) developed a much more sophisticated version of communicative functioning with a model of operational levels of function in the central nervous system (Figure 1.2). In this model, the functioning of a single person is examined. If we look at the normal operations of the central nervous system that are related to hearing and speaking, we can better understand how various communicative disorders with a physiological etiology can affect a person's ability to communicate.

Let us first use the model to analyze a simple greeting in which communication is normal. One individual meets another on the street. The first person says, "Hello. How's the family?" The second responds, "Fine. Thanks for asking." The analysis starts with the listener. At the reflex level, the normal sensory apparatus of the hearing mechanism allows the individual to receive auditory signals. Sound waves generated from the speaker's voice vibrate the tympanic membrane, which moves the ossicles, causing the oval window to move, setting

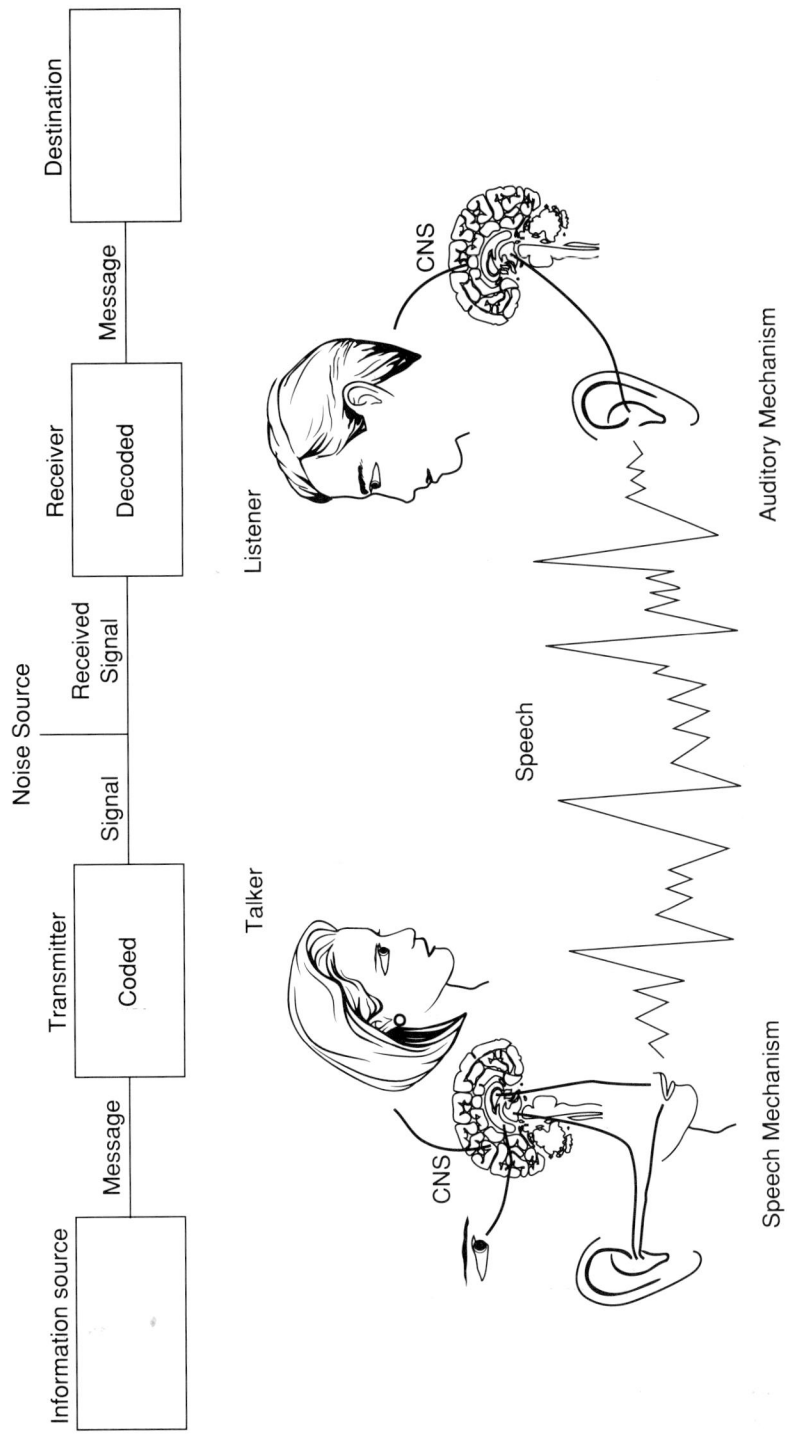

Figure 1.1
Fairbanks general communication system

Source: From "A Theory of the Speech Organism as a Servosystem," by G. Fairbanks, 1954, *Journal of Speech and Hearing Disorders, 19*, pp. 133–139. Copyright 1954 by the *Journal of Speech and Hearing Disorders.* Reprinted by permission.

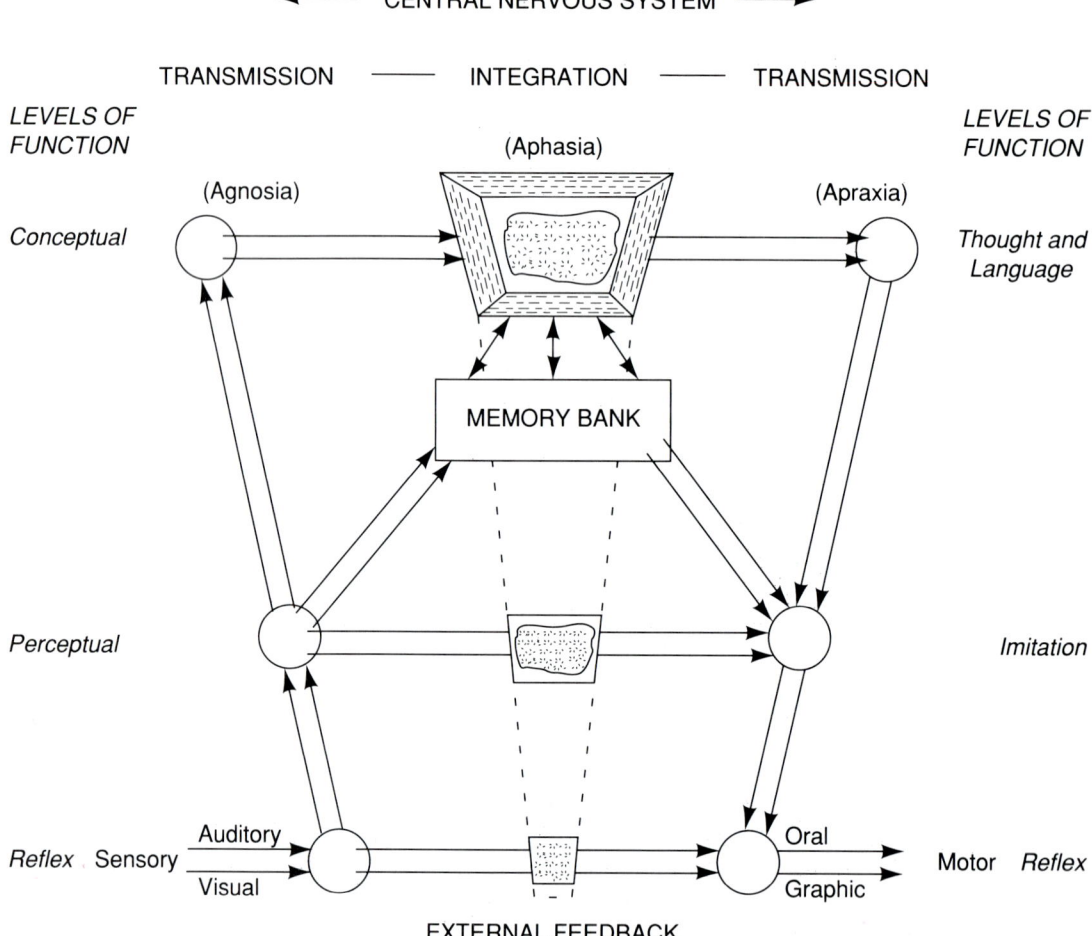

Figure 1.2
Wepman's operational levels of the central nervous system
Source: From "Studies in Aphasia: Background and Theoretical Formulations" by J. Wepman, L. V. Jones, R. D. Bock, and D. Van Pelt, 1960, *Journal of Speech and Hearing Disorders, 25,* pp. 323–332. Copyright 1960 by the *Journal of Speech and Hearing Disorders.* Reprinted by permission.

the cilia of the inner ear in motion, and leading to the generation of an electrical signal into the eighth cranial nerve. Then, at the perceptual level, these signals are transmitted along the eighth cranial nerve where they are recognized by certain areas of the brain as speech signals. Each of the words spoken is recognized as a meaningful unit of speech. At the conceptual level, the words are then matched with similar signal configurations in the memory bank and are identified as speech and language units having specific meanings. Each word is matched with its stored meaning, and the receiver must decode the linguistic rule used by the speaker to place the words into a meaningful order.

With the message successfully received and decoded, the listener decides to respond with a phrase of appreciation. To produce a meaningful utterance, the person must now retrieve the appropriate sounds, words, and linguistic rules for word assembly from within the memory bank. This occurs at the thought and language level. After the words and rules for their order of production have been retrieved, the person must innervate the larynx and muscles of articulation to say, "Fine. Thanks for asking." What just took over 100 words to describe occurs in fractions of a second, without the slightest awareness on the part of the individual whose reception and production of speech and language was just described. Actually, as you are reading this material, you are constantly performing a similar decoding procedure.

We now have a model of how communication relates to the normal operation of the central nervous system. If the model is correct and useful, it can provide us with a way of identifying what happens when "noise" is introduced into the system. The noise in Wepman's model is a physical pathology. Let us again use the greeting example and introduce an impairment at each level of the model. If a pathology such as an immobile stapes or physical deterioration of the cilia is introduced at the reflex level, our individual will be unable to hear the signal or hear it only at a diminished level. This would be identified as a hearing impairment. He might be able to hear only part of the greeting or hear it at a reduced volume level. If a pathology affected the transmission of a normally received signal, such as a tumor on the eighth cranial nerve, the signal would be distorted, resulting in the person's inability to perceive the signal as an identifiable unit of speech or language. This would be an example of a perceptual disorder. The distortion may affect only the perception of specific words or possibly the entire transmission. It would be analogous to listening to a radio station and having a second radio signal "bleed" into the first, causing the words spoken or sung to become unintelligible. This type of disorder is known as *auditory agnosia,* the inability to attach meaning to the words that are heard because of signal distortion. If the signal has not been distorted but the individual is unable to match it for meaning with previously learned information, it is a conceptual integration disorder, or *aphasia.* Although each word was accurately received, the individual may not remember the meaning of one or more words. Even if he understands the meaning of each word, the utterance will not be understandable unless the linguistic rule for ordering the placement of the words is retrieved. Aphasia can occur in various forms and severity. The person may not be able to retrieve the names of objects, events, or feeling states, or the grammar of the person's speech may be affected. A problem with the transmission of a signal away from the brain at the conceptual level is known as *apraxia.* It involves difficulties in retrieving the specific phonemes that are required to produce certain words. In the greeting example, the person wishes to say, "Fine. Thanks for asking." For each phoneme, he must retrieve the instructions for how to place the articulatory structures. For example, to produce an /f/ phoneme, the upper teeth must be placed on top of the lower lip and air must be let out in a steady stream through the front of the mouth. Although no one thinks about how to produce sounds, the process of matching and retrieval is always in operation whenever we speak. The individual

Table 1.1
Etiologies attributed to various disorders

	Disorders						
Possible Etiologies	**Stuttering**	**Voice**	**Articulation**	**Child Language**	**Aphasia**	**Apraxia**	**Dysarthria**
Neurological	x	x	x	x	x	x	x
Anatomical	x						
Physiological	x	x	x				
Functional	x	x	x	x			
Unknown	x			x			

with apraxia has difficulty with this retrieval. Similar phonemes are substituted for the targets, producing utterances such as, "Jesus is a shoving leopard" instead of "Jesus is a loving shepherd." If problems exist in innervating the musculature, the disorder is located at the transmission reflex level. This form of muscular weakness is known as *dysarthria*. The individual with dysarthria can easily retrieve the correct notations of where to place the articulators. The problem occurs when the muscles are innervated to produce the movement. The speech of individuals with dysarthria is labored and often distorted. The speech of individuals with cerebral palsy is typical of dysarthria.

Wepman's elegant model of communication and its disorders has proved to be a useful physiological model of communicative disorders. However, not all of these disorders are physiologically based. The etiology may be functional, anatomical, unknown, or a combination of these factors. Table 1.1 shows etiologies that have been attributed to other communicative disorders. As the table indicates, more than one etiology for a communicative disorder may exist. Wepman's model also does not account for nonphysiological variables that affect both the presentation of the disorder and its treatment. To understand our clients' needs and to determine the most efficient and ethical way to meet them, a comprehensive communication model is needed, one that considers not only the specific speech or language disorder but also the client's culture, cognitive abilities, experiences, and needs. The following model is an attempt to do just that.

CULTURAL COMMUNICATIONS MODEL (CCM)

Communication is a complex process for both the sender and the receiver. A message is more than just the operation of the central nervous system and the appropriate use of linguistic forms to express ideas. A message is a communication containing elements of the person's past history, current values and beliefs, and future expectations. It cannot be understood merely by understanding a dictionary meaning of the words or having knowledge of the linguistic rules used for its conveyance. A client's communications must be understood within a broader context. A full understanding of clients' needs requires clinicians to be cognizant of their culture, experiences, cognitive functioning, and values.

Figure 1.3 illustrates the relationship each of these areas has to the production of communicative utterances. The overriding parameter of meaning is the individual's cultural environment. Within this environment, the cognitive abilities and the experiential knowledge of the individual each contribute to the meaning and understanding of verbal messages. How these messages are produced and understood depends on the individual's needs and personal values.

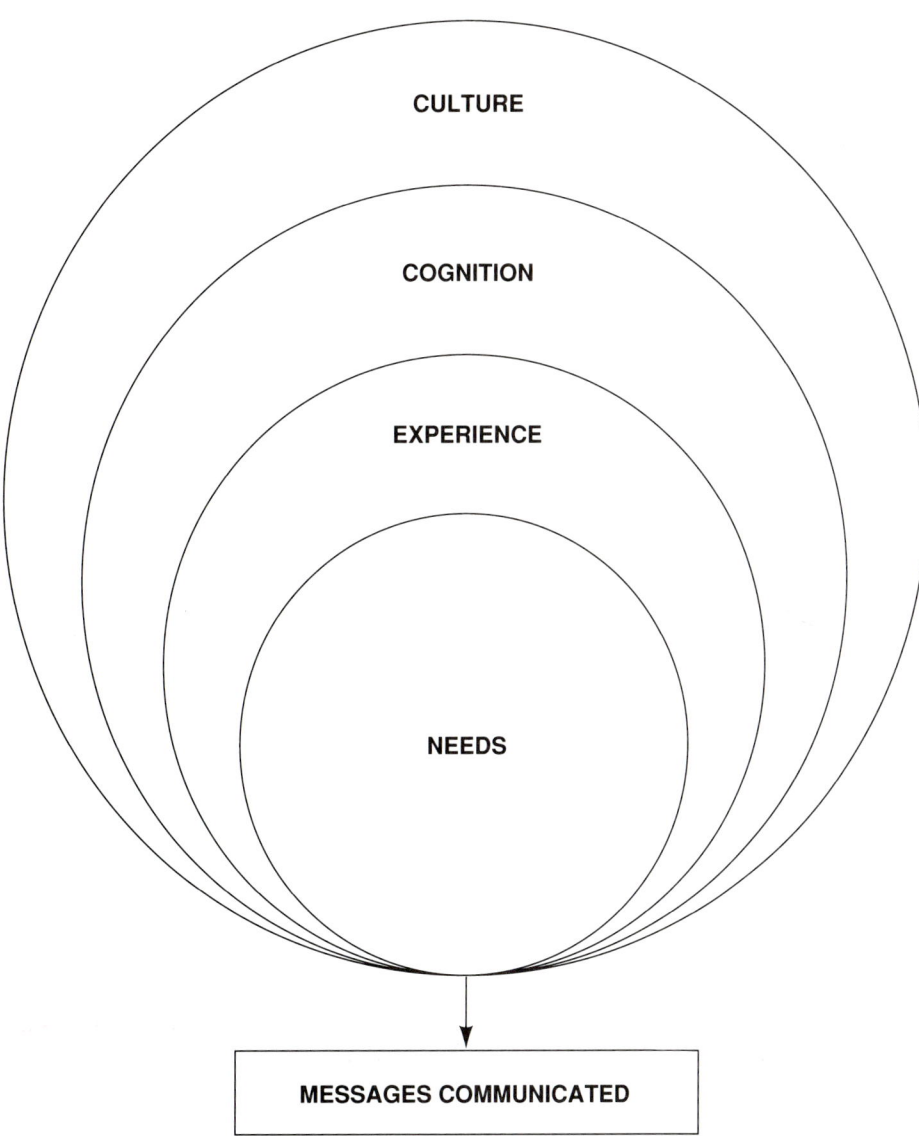

Figure 1.3
Cultural communication model (CCM)

Culture

We live in a multicultural and ethnically diverse society in which individuals develop and often act in accordance with culturally related values. With changing population demographics and the recent influx of immigrants from Southeast Asia, Central America, and the Caribbean, professionals in the helping sciences have had to learn new ways of interacting with their clients. The importance of acknowledging the effects of culture on all clinical interactions has been emphasized by various authors (Cole, 1989; Culatta & Goldberg, in press; Shames, 1989). Current appeals for cultural sensitivity in the area of communicative disorders result from a long-standing undervaluation of the ethnic diversity of clients. Although critically important, ethnicity is only one of many cultural categories. According to the anthropologist Goodenough (1987), *culture* is a shared way of perceiving, believing, evaluating, and behaving. When culture is viewed in this manner, it becomes apparent that culture is not limited only to ethnicity but also occurs as a result of different sources of shared values and methods of communication. A useful model was developed by two educators who have written extensively on cultural diversity. Gollnick and Chinn's (1990) approach to understanding cultures can serve as an important foundation for developing clinical sensitivity. They maintain that a macroculture and many microcultures exist within the United States. The macroculture of the United States and all other countries consists of values on which most political and social institutions are based. For example, these are 10 values they believe are inherent in the macroculture of the United States (Gollnick & Chinn, 1990, p. 13):

1. Status based on occupation, education, and financial worth
2. Achievement valued above inheritance
3. Work ethic
4. Comforts and rights to such amenities
5. Cleanliness as an absolute value
6. Achievement and success measured by the quantity of material goods purchased
7. Egalitarianism as shown in the demand for political, economic, and social equality
8. Inalienable and God-given rights for every individual that include an equal right to self-governance or choice of representatives
9. Humanitarianism that is usually highly organized and often impersonal
10. New and modern perceived as better than old and traditional

Microcultures

Although macrocultural values bind the population together as a whole, they are not sufficient for understanding individual value systems. Each individual is a member of a macroculture, but also shares values with members of subcultures known as *microcultures*. Each microculture is differentiated from others by specific values, speech and linguistic patterns, learning styles, and behavioral patterns. Gollnick and Chinn list eight types of microcultures:

1. Ethnic or national origin
2. Religion

3. Gender/Sex
4. Age
5. Exceptionality
6. Urban-Suburban-Rural
7. Geographic Region
8. Class

From these microcultures, values emerge, and from values, styles of communication and interactions develop. Cultural identification for most Americans involves a blending of various microcultures. To illustrate the concept of blending, imagine the value system of a 35-year-old African American with a Ph.D. from Stanford, who is employed as a computer expert by a large corporation in San Francisco. He grew up in New York City and was the only son of parents who were physicians. Although he might share many of the same ethnic values as a 65-year-old religious African American woman with a grade-school education living in a rural area of Alabama, vast differences in other values would also exist. Their values, styles of interaction, and methods of communication have developed from many different experiences. The background that clients bring into the clinic is no less complex than our examples of the computer expert and religious woman. Clients come to the clinic with an amalgam of values, beliefs, and behaviors from the macroculture and their various microcultures. Although cultural identification with one microculture may dominate the values and behavioral patterns of an individual, it is rarely sufficient for understanding that person. Therefore, it is imperative that the clinician be sensitive to how various cultural components affect the communicative disorder, the client, and the clinical interaction.

In many situations, a lack of sensitivity to an individual's microcultural values may result in little more than an annoyance on the part of the offended person. The orthodox Jew who is invited to a dinner and is then served pork may be offended by his host's ignorance or religious insensitivity, but the event will probably be shortly forgotten or even become the centerpiece of a humorous story he will relate to his friends. The clinical situation, however, is very different. Clients enter the clinic as vulnerable individuals. They not only have a communication problem, but they have failed to find its solution. They also give permission to the clinician to probe feelings they may not have previously shared with anyone. Even more threatening, they may allow the clinician to place them in embarrassing situations or guide them into changing the way they perceive themselves and others. Because of the very intrusive and highly personal nature of the clinical interaction, insensitivity to the client's culture can have serious consequences. At the very least, the client may become defensive, refusing to allow himself to be vulnerable with an individual who does not respect or understand his values. At worst, the client may begin to evaluate his values as inappropriate, unacceptable, or worse, deviant.

One important determinant in the success of therapy is the client's perception of the clinician. The client evaluates not only the clinician's professional competence but also her worth as a caring, protective, and supportive individual. Many of these judgments are made on the basis of the clinician's nonverbal and verbal behaviors, some of which are very obvious and direct, whereas others are extremely subtle. The client interprets the meaning of these behaviors from their own referent culture. Eye contact avoidance, for example, which is a sign of respect for authority within the Japanese culture, could be interpreted as being disrespectful within the American macroculture. The integral relationship between values and behaviors is one that is often unseen by the individual exhibiting them (Hall, 1959). The culturally sensitive clinician must have a general awareness of her client's cultural values and understand how her verbal and nonverbal behaviors will be interpreted by that client.

Cultural differences also become apparent when examining a society's philosophy and values. The cultural patterns of various regions of the world dictate specific kinds of social interaction patterns that may be confusing to some professionals and result in information being misinterpreted. For example, politeness in some Asian cultures may be inappropriately identified as agreement, as in the case of the Laotian father who nodded his head when asked to do an unacceptable activity with his daughter. It is imperative that speech pathologists and audiologists familiarize themselves with the cultural values and rules of social interchange of the populations they serve.

Speech-language pathologists cannot be expected to be experts in anthropology. Nor can they be expected to be intimately aware of all the microcultural variables of each cultural subgroup in our country. It may, however, be appropriate to adapt some of the concepts and methods used by cultural anthropologists (Miller, 1979). Anthropologists study the culture before beginning the field study to acquire a basic understanding of the communication and interaction patterns of the inhabitants. When the study begins, anthropologists make it clear to the individuals they are interacting with that there is much they do not understand and will probably say or do some things that may offend. Their errors are made out of ignorance, not disrespect. And they would appreciate being corrected so that they will not repeat the mistakes. In addition to the general disclaimer, anthropologists also try to identify individuals who may serve as resources in the learning process. Procedures similar to these have helped anthropologists such as Margaret Mead (1930), who became accepted by societies whose cultures were very different from her own.

Speech-language pathologists can use a similar strategy for developing clinical sensitivity. The culture of the population being served should be studied. Of particular interest are greeting patterns, the communicative intent of nonverbal behaviors, how the culture views the communicative disorders, usual interaction patterns between children and parents, and role expectations of professionals. This information can provide a basis for clinical interactions. Many clinics and training programs identify individuals who can serve as resource persons. These can be people from the community, the clinic staff, or faculty from departments in schools of ethnic studies.

Ethnic or National Origin. Ethnic identity for many individuals constitutes their dominant microculture. It ties them to other individuals with a common history, values, attitudes and behaviors (Yetman, 1985). The commonality may involve physical characteristics, behaviors, language, values, or place of residence.

Within the United States, the term *race* is often used interchangeably for ethnicity, especially in identifying African Americans, whites, Asians, and Native Americans. *Race* is a term used by physical anthropologists to describe groups of people by their physical attributes. Its simplification of cultural values led UNESCO in 1950 to recommend that the term no longer be used to describe groups of people (Montagu, 1972).

It would be difficult for speech-language pathologists to become knowledgeable of all ethnic cultures. They should however, become familiar with the basic behavioral patterns of the ethnic cultures from which their clients will most likely come. The east, west, and southern coastal areas and large cities throughout the country have the most diverse ethnic cultures. For example, on the West Coast it is very likely that clients will come from various Asian, South Pacific, Central American, South American, Far Eastern, European, and African American ethnic cultures. In San Francisco, for example, the New Comer High School has students from over 27 ethnic cultures. The Southwest has large Native American Indian and Latino populations. Chicago has been a center for eastern Europeans for many years. In the eastern part of Pennsylvania, the Pennsylvania Dutch constitute an important and large microculture. New York is home to many people from the Caribbean. Miami has the largest Cuban population outside of Havana.

Population demographics are constantly changing. Speech-language pathologists practicing in a small midwestern town may find that the insular nature of their location is only a temporary phenomenon. The task of assembling culturally relevant assessment and therapy material is an ongoing process. A general source of information appears in Appendix A of this text, which is the American Speech-Language-Hearing Association's resource guide to multicultural tests and materials.

Clients do not necessarily expect the clinician to be familiar with all aspects of their culture. They do expect and should receive the clinician's acceptance of their value system and a basic understanding of the intent of verbal and nonverbal behaviors. Many types of ethnic differences can have an impact upon clinical interactions. For many Asian cultures the outward display of certain emotions with non-family members would be unthinkable (Cheng, 1987), whereas the same emotions might be freely displayed by African Americans (Taylor, 1992) or Hispanics (Ramirez & Castaneda, 1974). Although the feelings may be identical for each client, their culture dictates how they will be displayed.

One area of major concern to speech-language pathologists is the general use of normative test instruments whose reference group is white, middle class Americans. With increased sensitivity to ethnic differences, standardized, age-related tests for language and articulation have now become available for African Americans, Hispanics, and Asians (Cheng, 1987; Cole & Deal, in press). Culturally sensitive test instruments have also been developed in the area of fluency (Culatta & Goldberg, in press).

A second area of concern is referral patterns for children needing speech and language services. Some studies show that an important determinant of whether or not a child is referred for special services is the ethnicity of the individual responsible for making referrals (Lambert et al., 1989). Cultural differences in speech and language may be incorrectly identified as disorders. For example, children who are learning a second language have normal disfluencies that are often identified as stuttering (Montes & Erickson, 1990). Conversely, a child with a genuine disorder may not be referred since the individual responsible for making the referral believes that "that's just the kind of problem *those people* have; it doesn't really bother them."

Religion. During an average week in the United States, approximately 42% of all adults attend a church or synagogue, and nearly 143 million individuals claim an affiliation with a religious group (Gollnick & Chinn, 1990). For many people, religion is a formal institution that has little influence on the development of their values and behaviors. For other people, it can serve as the culture having the greatest impact upon their lives. Awareness of a client's religious values can be important in avoiding embarrassing situations. Knowing that a client has strong Mormon values would prevent the clinician from offering a cup of coffee, since this beverage is forbidden by Mormon doctrine. Even having a Halloween party during the time designated for therapy might offend some fundamentalists who view the holiday as a form of Satanic worship. Similarly, scheduling an important clinical event on Yom Kippur would be viewed as insensitive by even mildly religious Jews.

Gender/Sex. The gender history of the United States has been one of clearly defined behavioral expectations (Frazier & Sadker, 1973). Little boys were expected to be dominating, strong, good in the sciences, and love baseball. Little girls were expected to be sweet, nice, loveable, great spellers, and collectors of cute dolls. The behaviors taught to children were considered to be the method of indoctrinating values that would carry over to adulthood (Stockard & Johnson, 1980). As the social values of America changed, the expectations of children's behavior also changed. The values that were once considered to be "male" and "female" now have less rigidly defined boundaries for both children and adults. Although some psychologists believe that many gender specific traits are "hard wired" into our genetics (Barfield, 1976), others see the blending of masculine and feminine traits as the logical extension of progressive societies (Sadker, Sadker, & Steindam, 1989). In treating children, one should be aware that what may have been considered to be "tom-boyish" or "sissy" behavior 20 years ago is now viewed as acceptable and appropriate. Activities should be designed for the gender values of the children and their family, not the clinician.

The gradual acceptance of homosexuality has allowed many men and women to openly express their sexual preferences. Many years ago the American Psychological Association removed homosexuality from its list of personality disorders; yet for many people the sexual preference of gays and lesbians becomes the one behavior that overrides an individual's values and beliefs. Just as stutterers are not their behavior, homosexuals are not their sexual preference. The values found in heterosexual parents and clients are the same as those found in homosexual parents and clients. In rare occurrences the sexual preference of a client may be a factor in clinical intervention, such as individuals wishing to change their vocal range. It is much more likely that it may be a factor affecting the clinician's responsiveness and understanding of the client or parents of a client. The concern that a gay father feels for his language-delayed child is no different than the concern felt by a heterosexual father.

Age. Certain cultural values are associated with age groups. As a society, we tend to identify individuals as belonging to one of eight different age categories (Kalunger & Kalunger, 1986): infancy (birth–2 years), early childhood (3–5 years), middle childhood (6–8 years), late childhood (9–12 years), adolescence (13–19 years), early adulthood (20–39 years), middle age (40–65 years), and elderly (beyond 65 years). Age-related values are primarily determined by experiences. For example, the 4-year-old child's view of the importance of money is very different from that of the 70-year-old retiree who must sustain herself on $450 a month.

The clinician must be aware of age-related values not only in interactions but also in the selection of appropriate clinical material. Choosing stimulus material for an adult aphasic from a child-oriented language kit may be effective in terms of the linguistic concepts to be taught, but it may inadvertently convey to the client a disrespect and condescension that can interfere with therapy. Some test instruments are designed only for a general age range, such as children (Shine, 1980), adolescents (Hammill, Brown, Larsen, & Wiederholt, 1980) or adults (Woolf, 1967). A few modify the instrument to be appropriate for more than one age range. One example of sensitivity to age factors is found in the Behavioral Cognitive Stuttering Therapy program (Goldberg, 1981). Goldberg designed three different sets of interview questions for children, adolescents, and adults. Although the information desired by the interviewer is identical for all ages, each set of questions uses age-appropriate terminology, phrasing, and concepts.

Exceptionality. Clients with communicative disorders confront their problem as soon as they attempt to understand another individual, respond, or ask for something. In the presence of people, it cannot remain a hidden disorder. When faced with a problem, an individual can accept it, compensate for it, or attempt to eradicate it. Regardless of the solution chosen, the choice results in the development of values that may be infused throughout the individual's behaviors. These values, associated with the limitations on communication and attempts to accommodate and change the behavior, constitute many of the cultural values of exceptionality.

For many individuals, exceptionality constitutes an insignificant microculture with limited importance. These individuals view their disorder as constituting only one aspect of their behavior and are determined not to have their problem define their personality. Unfortunately, for others exceptionality can become the predominant microculture, overshadowing all other cultural values. The adult stutterer who has been unable to control his speech may see life as a series of events on which he has little effect. The aphasic who was an articulate professor before his stroke may now view all interactions as painful vignettes, all designed to humiliate him. The most debilitating form of exceptionality occurs when the values associated with it constitute the macroculture. The young child whose language disability prevents her from telling her parents she is in physical pain may come to believe that physical pain is a normal part of life, to be accepted and endured. Continual communicative failures can lead to emotional scarring. Often these scars are masked by inappropriate behaviors, such as a child who acts out when asked to respond verbally in a way she knows she cannot.

The cultural values of exceptionality also develop from the reactions of society to the individual with the disorder. All too often the individual is viewed as his handicap, someone to be pitied or avoided, to bear the brunt of jokes. As a society, we have progressed significantly over the past 25 years. Yet, as Gollnick and Chinn indicate, the road to sensitivity is still largely untrodden. They point out that

> the general public may be required by law to provide educational and other services for the handicapped. The general public is prohibited by law against certain aspects of discrimination against the handicapped. No one, however, can require the person on the street to like the handicapped and to accept them as social equals. Many do not accept the handicapped. Just as racism leads to discrimination or prejudice against other races because of the belief in one's racial superiority, *handicappism* leads to stereotyping of and discrimination against the handicapped because of attitudes of superiority of some nonhandicapped individuals. (Gollnick & Chinn, 1990, p. 157)

Regional. Gollnick and Chinn view "geographic region" and "urban-suburban-rural" as two distinct cultural parameters. As a practical consideration, they have been condensed in this text into a single category called "regional." Often the importance of regional differences is ignored within clinical contexts. In the past, when we were a fairly immobile population, people generally trained and practiced within the region they would live. At one university in California the student enrollment in the graduate program in speech-language pathology over a 10-year period went from 95% enrollment from within the state of California to 50% enrollment of California residents. Most of the students graduating from the program continue to begin their practice in California. For many, coming from the Midwest and the South, some of the values they were accustomed to in interactions were either absent or modified by people living on the West Coast. Understanding the nature of these regional differences helped these new clinicians avoid misinterpreting their clients' behaviors.

Class. The socioeconomic class that one identifies with can have a significant influence on the development of values, forms of interaction, and language usage. The sociologist Max Weber (Parsons, 1947) believed that the values of individuals were primarily shaped by the socioeconomic class to which they belonged. For Weber, to understand why a person acted as he did, you must first understand his socioeconomic position in society. The effect of socioeconomic class values on the individual's behaviors has been documented in many studies ranging from the occurrence of neurosis and psychoses (Hollingshead, 1958) to the prevalence of stuttering in children (Morgenstern, 1956).

Insensitivity to socioeconomic values has lead to problems not only in therapy but also in diagnosis. A misdiagnosis can occur when an evaluation instrument is normed on one socioeconomic culture and then applied to another that is very different. There have been many examples cited in the literature where the instrument has been shown to be biased against one or more cultures. One example is the Northwestern Syntax Screening Test (Lee, 1971). Larson and Summers (1976) administered the NSST to 216 normal children in northern Texas, some from lower socioeconomic groups. The mean scores reported by these researchers were significantly below those reported by Lee, whose test population consisted primarily of normal children from white middle-class families from northern Illinois. The researchers concluded that the linguistic abilities of both groups of children were similar, but because the testing materials were culturally biased, the group from northern Texas appeared to be functioning at a lower linguistic level.

The effect of occupation on the development of values and behaviors is a phenomenon recognized by sociologists for many years. It can shape values as well as preferred styles of interaction. Take, for example, an elementary school teacher who spends six hours a day, five days a week, for nine months every year, instructing 6-year-olds on what they can and cannot do. As a client, she may present the impression of someone who is more interested in talking than listening. Similarly, the individual who is never afforded the opportunity to act independently in his job may appear confused when asked to choose between tasks. Although it is important to understand how clients' occupations shape their interactions, it is equally important not to stereotype clients based on what they do for a living. In his book *Working*, Studs Terkel has over 100 people describe their jobs and how they feel about them (1972). Two very revealing stories are told by a waitress and a telephone operator:

> Everyone says all waitresses have broken homes. What they don't realize is when people have broken homes they need to make money fast, and do this work. They don't have broken homes because they're waitresses. . . . People imagine a waitress couldn't possibly think or have any kind of aspiration other than to serve food. When somebody says to me, "You're great, how come you're *just* a waitress?" *Just* a waitress. I'd say, "Why, don't you think you deserve to be served by me?" (pp. 390–391).
>
> It's a strange atmosphere, You're in a room about the size of a gymnasium, talking to people thousands of miles away. . . . A lot of the girls are painfully shy in real life. You get some girls who are outgoing in their work, but when they have to talk to someone and look them in the face, they can't think of what to say. They feel self-conscious when they know someone can see them. At the switchboard, it's a feeling of anonymousness. (pp. 65–66).

Just as clients are not their disorders, they or their parents are not their occupations. It is important for the clinician to understand the relationship that occupation has to values and behaviors.

Combining Macro and Microcultures

Each person is the product of both macroculture and microcultures. Often values are so intertwined that they cannot be explained by referring to only one cultural category. For instance, the behaviors of a Vietnamese businessman who lives in and has embraced the life style of central Texas, votes Republican, and has remained a devout Buddhist, cannot be understood within any one cultural category. His beliefs regarding his daughter's disfluencies and how she should be treated may be both religious and socioeconomic. The way in which cultural values are combined should be of particular interest to speech-language pathologists in the areas of (a) child development, (b) rules for social interaction, (c) societal reactions, and (d) learning styles.

Child Development. There is no evidence that differences in motoric, cognitive, and linguistic development are related to racial genetic differences. Rather, environmental factors can enhance or impede the development of these abilities. The effects of the environment can occur very early in the child's life. A comparative study of Greek and Australian infants showed that by 9 months of age significant differences in temperament were evident (Kyrios et al., 1989). In older children, some of the differences can be more pronounced and affect areas more closely related to communication. For example, a study comparing Brazilian and British children at 4 years of age found that the British children performed better on fine motor and practical reasoning tasks, whereas the Brazilian children were more advanced on gross motor and speech tasks. If age was used as a primary criterion for differentiating between normal developmental disfluencies and stuttering, a misdiagnosis could occur within both populations of children.

There is much evidence to suggest that specific parental behaviors are conducive to the development of normal communication, while others reinforce the potential for communicative disorders (Cooper, 1979; Costello & Ingham, 1984a; Egolf, et al., 1972). The culturally sensitive clinician needs to determine which behaviors are expressions of traditional values and which are reflections of individual parental needs and beliefs. Counseling parents to change individual childrearing styles is easier and far less threatening than asking them to change a behavior that is an integral part of their heritage. If counseling is to be beneficial, it must be compatible with the parents' culture (Saleh, 1986). For example, a young child whose family recently immigrated from Cambodia was referred to the school speech-language pathologist. The pathologist recommended that the family engage in certain stimulation activities that the family viewed as an affront to their traditional childrearing activities. After apologizing for her ignorance, the pathologist asked them to suggest ways that the goals could be accomplished within the framework of their traditional childrearing practices.

Childrearing practices are not only an expression of an ethnic culture's values but also the primary method for its perpetuation. The father who teaches his son how to treat his elders may be conveying both ancient and personal beliefs. The child, to a large extent, is the product of his parents' behaviors and values. Critical comments directed toward the child's behaviors may unintentionally convey to the child a negative assessment not just of him, but more cruelly, of his parents. By understanding that the cultural components of parents' childrearing practices are expressed through their child's behaviors and values, the focus of counseling and suggestions for change can be more effective. Before the American Speech-Language-Hearing Association took a stand against labeling African American dialects as deviant, many children came to believe that the speech and language of their family, relatives, and community were something to be ashamed of, lacking the approval of authority figures such as school speech-language pathologists.

Even the early identification of communicative disorders as something requiring professional intervention may have cultural concomitants. Studies of parental reactions to children's behaviors indicate that parents from various cultures will react differently to the same behavior (Zeskind, 1983). Where the stuttering behavior of a child in one culture may be viewed merely as a different form of speaking requiring little attention, the same speech pattern in another culture may result in shame to the family and an intensive effort by the parents to find help. A classic error occurred when researchers maintained that North American Indians did not stutter (Snidecor, 1947). Their conclusions were based on interviews they had with the residents of one village. They were assured that not only did they not have a name for stuttering, but they had never heard any of the villagers speaking in the way stuttering was described by the interviewers. Only after many years did it become known that not only did the Indians have a word for stuttering, but they also had stutterers in the village. When outsiders came, the stutterers were routinely hidden because of the shame the entire village felt.

Interaction Rules and Behaviors. Interaction rules are analogous to the syntax of a language. The rules give form and structure to the interaction. The specific behaviors of the interaction are analogous to the words of a language. Understanding the interaction rules and behaviors of a culture can eliminate an enormous amount of communication problems. Individuals bring into the clinic their own cultural rules of interaction. Although specific differences can be found between various microcultures, the greatest differences exist between Eastern and Western cultures (Farver & Howes, 1988). Compare for example the Indian and American methods of introduction. In India the hands are clasped together and the head is bowed, signifying a reverence for the divine in the person who is being met (Campbell, 1988). Contrast this with the Western custom of extending an open hand and looking directly at the person, behaviors thought to symbolize to the person being greeted that the greeter has no weapons. The hand clasping in India and the extended open hand of Western cultures both signify a greeting. Yet, each contains within it a vastly different history and communicative intent.

Societal Reactions. The feelings individuals have about their problem may, to a large extent, be related to their culture and societal reactions. In the following three case examples, each society viewed communicative disorders very differently.

An individual immigrated to the United States from Japan primarily because of his stuttering. During the diagnostic interview he painfully explained that his speaking problem had brought shame to himself and to his family. Since he felt that services for stutterers in Japan were inadequate, he had no alternative other than to come to the United States. After becoming fluent, he intended to return to Japan and restore his and his family's honor.

During a trip to Egypt, the author had a lengthy conversation with a highly educated devout Muslim regarding a number of topics. When asked about the occurrence of stuttering in his country, the Egyptian said that there were many stutterers but no treatment facilities. When asked why, he responded that stuttering was a malady given to the individual by Allah and therefore was not something to be treated.

In 1991 only one trained speech-language pathologist practiced in Costa Rica. In fact, she was the only speech-language pathologist in all of Central America. She explained that the historical poverty of the region necessitated giving speech-language pathology a low priority. Speech and language disorders were accepted, not because of any religious belief but because everyone knew that no one was able to help.

In these three cases, societal reactions toward the communicative disorders determined how communicatively impaired individuals viewed their problem and the courses of action that it required.

Learning Styles. The development of new speaking patterns usually requires learning new strategies and behaviors. It may necessitate decisions to engage in activities, monitoring of feeling states, or the initiation of specific behaviors. The assumption has always been that these strategies and behaviors could be uniformly taught to clients. Whether one chose an operant approach (Shames & Egolf, 1976), a cognitive approach (Rubin & Culatta, 1971), a symptomatic approach (Van Riper, 1971), or any of the more eclectic approaches found throughout the history of speech-language pathology, an equality of client learning styles was assumed. Recent experiments on children's learning styles reveals a very different picture. Research in cross-cultural learning styles should not be confused with ill-conceived attempts to support arguments of genetic inferiority or superiority. On the contrary, the research offers explanations for why children with similar cognitive abilities from different cultures can have widely disparate scores on standardized tests even when they are culturally balanced. For many years, two explanations for the differences were offered. One referred to differences in genetics, and the other addressed the inappropriate referents used in some of the tests. It became disturbing for those who supported the inappropriate referent model to find that even when test referents were normed for different ethnic cultures, significant differences existed. It became apparent to researchers in the area of instructional technology (Cronbach & Snow, 1977) that many of the ethnically normed tests did not account for different learning styles. Large-scale cross-cultural studies revealed that children use culturally dependent learning styles (Dunn, 1990). If children were asked to respond to a standardized test or engage in a learning situation that was not compatible with their learning style, the results were negatively affected.

When teaching new speech or language behaviors to clients, clinicians need to be cognizant of the most appropriate method of instruction. For example, whereas learning through repetition may be compatible for children who were educated in Japanese schools, this learning style might be less effective with children from Mexico or other Latin American countries where repetition is not a cornerstone of education (Resendiz & Fox, 1985).

Language as the Expression of Culture

Whorfian Hypothesis. Language and culture have a symbiotic relationship, each deriving its vitality from the other. According to the linguist Benjamin Whorf (1956), language is shaped by the culture from which it came and in turn shapes that culture. In other words, the values and beliefs of a culture are codified in the culture's language. The words and grammatical forms are not just objective descriptions of a detached reality but rather represent the relationship that reality has to the culture. For example, Eskimos had many names for snow, since their ability to survive depended on correctly determining the condition of snow if their sleds were going to safely navigate an area covering crevasses and ice flows. Contrast this with someone who lives in Central America whose only contact with snow may be a picture in a grade school text of a snow-covered field in Pennsylvania. For the Central American, the lack of importance his culture places on snow relegates the word to an unimportant position, with no additional defining terms such as *slush, kernally,* or *crusty.*

An interesting regional language difference and its effect on clinical evaluation occurred in an early version of the Peabody Picture Vocabulary Test (Dunn, 1965). The purpose of the test is to estimate the subject's verbal development by measuring receptive ability. A page containing four drawings is shown to the subject. The examiner then says "Show me . . ." The subject points to one of the four drawings and the next page is shown. On one of the pages is a drawing of a hot dog. Although *hot dog* is the most common name for this type of sausage, in certain parts of the country it is also known as a *wiener, frank, frankfurter* or *red hot.* Conceivably, a child who used one of these alternative names might not be able to point correctly to *hot dog* if the words were not used in his culture. Although he understands the concept to which the words *hot dog* refer, he is scored as "incorrect" since the words used to identify the concept are not known to him. This problem was recognized by the author and addressed in the revised edition of the test (Dunn & Dunn, 1981).

Clearly, one's culture determines the language that one uses, and as Whorf maintains, the language one uses in turn shapes one's culture. We cannot escape the language we use in understanding and evaluating our world. This cyclical relationship is known as the *Whorfian hypothesis.* The Whorfian hypothesis has a direct relationship on how we understand our clients. There are various cultures within our country. Although there may be a homogeneity of certain ideas and values in the United States, the heterogeneity of our nation requires that one be sensitive to cultural differences, not only in social discourse but also in clinical interventions. Language differences resulting from cultural diversity need not be as great as that of the preceding example concerning snow. Often differences are more subtle.

Differences and Disorders. Cultural insensitivity has often resulted in identifying a child as having a language disorder, when in fact the problem is one of English as a second language (ESL). The two must be distinguished because the methods of correcting a language disorder are different from those of teaching a second language. A more complex problem arises when a child with limited English proficiency (LEP) also has a linguistic disorder in his native language. With so few speech pathologists fluent in languages other than English, these children are often misdiagnosed or do not receive adequate services.

Children who are using a cultural dialect have also been misdiagnosed as having a language disorder. A *dialect* is a variant of a language that has a structure and rules as logical and well-formed as those of the language. In the past, African American and Latino dialects were often labeled as deviant or disordered. Within the public schools, children having these dialects were identified as requiring remediation to correct their "disorder." Labeling a dialect as a "language disorder" has consequences far beyond that of language. Dialects spoken by children tend to reflect the language of their family and community. It is a primary cultural and familial marker. If children believe that their dialect is "deviant," then by association their family and culture are devalued, if not by them, then at least by authoritative individuals within their school system.

We are a nation of minorities, with a multitude of dialects and primary languages. According to Orlando Taylor (1989):

> Clearly, communication disorders specialists will increasingly work with culturally and linguistically diverse populations who will bring to the clinical situation a variety of cultural and linguistical behaviors that differ from the Eurocentric and English-speaking norms that predominate in our field. (p. 73)

If we are to meet the needs of our multicultural population, it is incumbent on speech-language pathologists to become familiar with the language, values, and culture of the populations they will serve. The importance of understanding the richness of language variants was emphasized by Bernard Spolsky (1972):

> Whatever language goals a society may set for its schools can be achieved only if they take into account the language competence that the pupils bring to school. There is no justification for the myth that children of lower socioeconomic class speak no language, or an inferior one, or a debased and inaccurate form of the standard language. Such children have learned the variety of language to which they have been exposed, a variety with as much semantic richness, structural complexity, and potential for communication as any other. If society believes they must also acquire some other language or variety, then the schools must develop sound and effective methods of language instruction. (p. 9)

Language variants should be treated as structurally intact, legitimate forms of communication that do not require remediation. If it is deemed important and correct to teach the standard language, it should be done as instruction in an additional language. The emphasis on treating dialects as different, and not disordered, is a position the American Speech-Language Hearing Association has included in its code of ethics.

Cognition

When one chooses words for communicating, it is with the assumption that the listener will understand the thoughts and objects that the words represent. In most cases, the assumption is correct. In a clinical situation, however, the assumption may be inappropriate. The meaning of a word depends on both cognitive functioning and past experiences. For example, the word *car* for a 40-year-old mechanical engineer probably means something very different than for a 4-year-old child. For the engineer, his concept of *car* may involve the intricate functioning of a vast amount of gears, nuts, and bolts, all being moved by the physical laws of thermodynamics. For the child, the word *car* means that red plastic thing he rides on in his room. Various theories of cognitive development and its relationship to semantics can help the clinician design therapy to be congruent with the client's intellectual abilities. By matching the therapy to the client's level of understanding, new behaviors are more easily learned.

Piaget. Jean Piaget (1954) maintained that the intellectual activity of a child is a form of *adaptive behavior* whereby the child adjusts and organizes thought and behavior as a result of environmental demands. The child is constantly assimilating and accommodating information. The *assimilation* of information involves putting new information into existing categories. *Accommodation* is the creation of new categories to account for new information. According to Piaget, the child's cognitive development goes through three stages: (a) sensorimotor activity; (b) concrete operations; and (c) formal or conceptual operations. During the *sensorimotor period,* the child's world view is shaped by his immediate sensorimotor experiences. During this developmental stage, the world begins to be divided into basic components, such as "food-provider," "warmth," and "twirling, flashing figure." When children begin *concrete operations,* their relationship with the world changes from passivity to active involvement. Children can now see a relationship between their behavior and the world. The toy which in the past was visually neutral can now become exciting when struck with a hand. During *formal* or *conceptual operations,* more complex relationships are understood by the child. All things with wheels now may be classified as objects that can transport people. Although much of Piaget's work is disputed by current neurological theory and cognitive psychology, his emphasis on examining the child as a logically evolving organism who is attempting to understand his world still has relevance today. Children are constantly redefining the labels they use and changing their understanding of the world. Young clients are constantly changing and continually assimilating and accommodating new information. Within a clinical setting, children should be viewed as dynamic entities, constantly changing, continually reformulating their perception of reality.

Semantics. Many people believe that an understanding of how children change their world view can best be derived by examining how children attach meaning to words. Eve Clark's (1973) semantic feature acquisition theory does this by relating cognitive development to semantics. Clark maintained that when a young child begins acquiring the meaning of words used by adults, initially only a few of the salient semantic features are identified. For example, the word *car* for a child may involve only the identification of anything with wheels. The child's early meanings therefore, are different from those of the adult. For the adult, the definition of *car* would involve enough salient features to eliminate things like *truck, bicycle, motorcycle, bus,* and *wagon*. As the child develops perceptive and cognitive skills, additional semantic features are added, eventually resulting in a semantic interpretation that is identical to the adult meaning. Constancy in semantics, therefore, is not something to be expected in young children.

Levels of Learning. But how does this developmental process occur? What is occurring cognitively that allows children to become more sophisticated in their perceptive and intellectual abilities? In other words, how do children learn? This question was addressed by Robert Gagné (1970). Gagné was interested in determining what sets of circumstances must be present for learning to occur. Learning, of course, can involve very simple or very complex processes. According to Gagné, there are eight different types of learning:

1. Signal learning
2. Stimulus-response learning
3. Chaining
4. Verbal association
5. Discrimination learning
6. Concept learning
7. Rule learning
8. Problem solving

Gagné maintained that each level depends on all levels that precede it. Therefore, a child who is experiencing difficulties in concept learning will most likely have difficulties in rule learning and problem solving. Gagné's learning model can be used for adapting intervention protocols to clients' cognitive capabilities. In Chapter 6 the eight levels of learning will be examined in depth.

Experience

The study of culture and cognition is not sufficient for understanding an individual's explicit and implicit communication. Together, they can provide reference points on which all can agree on the meaning of specific words or grammatical structures. However, initial semantic agreement does not necessarily result in uniform meanings. Group semantics are modified by individual experiences. The following example will illustrate this point.

A 4-year-old child sees an old car coming down the street and says, "Look, daddy, an old car!" In the culture of this child, the word *car* means a type of enclosed vehicle that has four tires and can move people from one place to another. Both the child and his father would agree on this conception. But this is only the base definition of the word *car*. For this child, the car may look like some of his favorite toy cars that he has played with for hours. The experience he is now having is related to past experiences. The relationship is close enough that it is appropriate to use the same words to describe it. *Old car* is a label the child is using to describe a current event that is related to his past, and it is also an expression of values. The father experiencing the same event also says, "Yeah, an old car," remembering the fun he and his high school sweetheart had in a similar car 25 years ago. Although both father and son used the words *old car,* the label clearly reflects significantly different past and present experiences. Therefore, the words one uses have not only a dictionary, or denotative meaning, but also a private or personal meaning. This highly individualized meaning becomes a part of the person's concept of *old car.*

Private Meanings. For centuries, philosophers have been struggling with problems associated with "private" meanings. In the 17th century, René Descartes (Lafleur, 1960) examined the dualism that existed between mind and body. For Descartes, knowledge was independent of experience. "Private" meanings, therefore, could be semantically correct, independent of the experienced world. *Old car* could have completely different and correct meanings for both father and son.

A reaction against this highly individualized concept of meaning occurred in the later half of the 17th and the early 18th centuries. British philosophers such as Locke, Berkeley, Hume, Reid, and Mill (Ayer & Winch, 1963) developed a conception of knowledge and meaning that was known as *radical empiricism.* They maintained that meaning was independent of thought and an integral property of the object itself. For them, *old car* would have a scientific and objective meaning, independent of either the father's or the son's past and present experiences. The concepts espoused by the radical empiricists were important for the development of much of current scientific thought in both the natural and social sciences. The notion that things can have a scientific and objective meaning was important not only for discerning the laws of nature but also for developing accountability in the helping professions. No longer did improvement depend solely on the intuitiveness or skill of individual therapists. If intervention protocols were scientific and objective, results could be replicated.

In the 1940s, a new philosophical approach to the study of knowledge and meaning was developed. Known as *phenomenology,* this approach was a synthesis of Descartes dualism and British empiricism (Kwant, 1963). Its major proponent, Maurice Merleau-Ponty (1962) maintained that meaning is derived through one's perception of reality. Perception is not something independent with its own separate existence, but rather it depends on the individual who is giving it meaning. When people observe an event or object, they are constantly relating it to experiences they have had with the same or similar events or objects. Their current perception incorporates past memories and also the field of sensation they are currently experiencing. Therefore, the meaning one gives to *old car* will depend on three elements: past experiences with a similar object, current physical sensations of the actual object, and current physical sensations of the field in which the object is observed. The philosophy of phenomenology was embraced by many psychologists who believed that the objectivity of the empiricists was having an adverse effect on how clients were being viewed. For them, clients were more than the sum of a collection of objective laws of human nature. They viewed their clients as unique individuals whose interaction with the world defined their characteristics, needs, and values.

Perception. The interplay between the physical world and an individual's mind is of crucial importance in understanding the role that experience has in the development of meaning. If the meaning of words partially depends on experiences, then semantics must be viewed as a dynamic process, changing with time and the individual's encounters with reality. With experience, the child's concept of *old car* will probably change, especially if the type of interactions he has with old cars changes. The importance of experience on the development of language should not be underestimated. When teaching concepts to clients, attention needs to be given to how and in what contexts the concept is presented. The manner in which the stimuli are presented to clients will determine the meanings they associate with it. Similar concerns are relevant in the language retraining of head-injured and aphasic clients. This area will be expanded in Chapter 6.

SUMMARY

In our attempts to be scientific and objective, we may forget that our clients have very diverse needs. For one client, receiving a smile of approval from a clinician may be very reinforcing, while another client may respond only if a tangible reinforcer, such as a piece of fruit, is offered. By understanding the needs of clients, clinicians can design clinical intervention programs that are sufficiently rewarding to elicit the type of responses desired. An understanding of personal needs may help the clinician determine when the importance of completing a planned activity must give way to allowing a client to discuss a problem of importance. No memory-enhancing task should be more important than an aphasic client's explaining how it feels to lose her ability to communicate. Nor should a lesson plan be forcefully implemented when it is obvious that what the child needs most is to be held by a caring adult. Clinicians must balance the cognitive and emotional needs of their clients. This concept is the central idea of a philosophy known as *Taoism,* which emphasizes the importance of balance and the avoidance of extremes. According to Suzuki (1955), the middle path should be taken. Clinicians who are determined to provide their clients with the best possible opportunity to gain communicative normalcy are obligated to take the middle path and to attend to both the emotional and cognitive needs of their clients.

SUGGESTED READINGS

Cheng, L. R. I. (1987). Cross-cultural and linguistic considerations in working with Asian populations. *ASHA, 29,* 33–37.
Cole, L. (1989). E pluribus pluribus: Multicultural imperatives for the 1990s and beyond. *ASHA, 31,* 65–70.
Cronbach, L. J., & Snow, R. E. (1977). *Aptitudes and instructional methods.* New York: Irvington Publishers, Inc.
Gagné, R. M. (1970). *The conditions of learning.* New York: Holt, Rinehart & Winston.
Gollnick, D., & Chinn, P. (1990). *Multicultural education in a pluralistic society* (3rd ed.). New York: Merrill/Macmillan.
Hall, E. T. (1966). *The hidden dimension.* Garden City, NY: Doubleday.
Korzybski, A. (1958). *Science and sanity.* Lakeville, CN: The International Non-Aristotelian Library.
Miller, E. S. (1979). *Introduction to cultural anthropology.* Englewood Cliffs, NJ: Prentice-Hall.
Perkins, W. H. (1986). Functions and malfunctions of theories in therapies. *ASHA, 28*(2), 31–33.
Taylor, O. L. (1992). in L. Cole & V. R. Deal (Eds.), *Communication disorders in multicultural populations.* Rockville, MD: American Speech-Language-Hearing Association.
Terkel, S. (1972). *Working.* New York: Avon Books.

Activity 1.1
Microcultural Values

Observe a client with a communicative disorder and identify the factors listed below. If the client is an adult, you may also wish to interview him or her. If the client is a child, an interview with the parent will be helpful. Identify as many microcultures of the client as you are able to and then hypothesize how the microcultures blend together to form a set of values. Interview him or her after receiving permission from the clinic supervisor.

Ethnic or National Identity:

Religion:

Gender/Sex:

Age:

Exceptionality:

Urban-Suburban:

Geographic Region:

Socioeconomic Class:

Summary of How the Microcultures Combine to Form a Value System:

Chapter 2
The Clinician as a Caring Scientist

STUDY GUIDE

- Describe the relationship between logic and knowledge.
- How is knowledge acquired by deductive reasoning?
- How is knowledge acquired by inductive reasoning?
- How does the knowledge gained through an academic context differ from the knowledge gained in a clinical context?
- How can intuition be used rigorously and scientifically within a clinical context?
- Describe the major components of the scientific method.
- Specifically, in what ways do a clinician's personality traits affect clinical interactions?
- Power can be used in clinical situations to advance the growth of the client or to reinforce the inadequacies of the clinician. Contrast each use.
- How are values related to clinical practice?
- New clinical students will have failures. How can these be transformed into positive experiences?
- How can a synthesis be formed between science and compassion?

The synthesis of being both caring and scientific may be one of the highest ideals for a clinician to achieve. Usually possessing only one of these qualities results in less than adequate therapy. The caring but unscientific clinician may falsely believe that compassion is sufficient to effect meaningful behavioral changes. Compassion is important for developing a therapeutic relationship, but without a careful analysis of the client's progress, compassion alone may result in little more than the client's acceptance of himself and his disorder. The reverse problem exists with the unfeeling scientific clinician. Although such clinicians may possess substantial knowledge of how to effect behavioral change, the client's perception of the clinicians as uncaring may result in rejection of their guidance. When the clinician is both scientific and caring, clinical procedures can be developed that are efficient, effective, and facilitative of the client's growth.

❑ ❑ ❑ THE SCIENTIFIC APPROACH

Science is based on the acquisition of knowledge. *Knowledge,* according to Bosanquet (1895) is the medium in which our world, as an interrelated whole, exists for us. It is a mental construction of reality that can be visualized as existing on two continua, one involving the method of acquisition and the other the context in which it is acquired (Table 2.1). At various times in the training of a clinician, each type of knowledge is required.

Types of Scientific Knowledge

We are constantly acquiring knowledge, sometimes through a concerted effort, often as a result of just being conscious. There are two methods by which information can be acquired: deductive and inductive reasoning. Each is important in developing clinical skills. Each involves different types of thinking.

Deductive Knowledge. *Deductive knowledge* involves the gradual, orderly acquisition of bits of information that, when formed into descriptive statements, allow one to identify a specific incidence of a model or theory. Take, for example, the following statement. "Stuttering is reduced when the client prolongs speech." To understand the statement, one first needs to have learned what types of behaviors are identified as "stuttering" and how speech is altered when it is "prolonged." The statement can now be viewed as a simple model of how something in the real world operates. That is, if someone who stutters reduces his rate of speech to below 30 syllables a minute, the number of disfluencies in his speech will be reduced. Armed with a model, incidence of the behavior can be identified. This would be an example of deductive knowledge. Most knowledge acquired through course work is deductive. The student learns the information through reasoning and a certain amount of memorization.

The amount of information to be learned is enormous, because the interdisciplinary requirements of the helping professions extend far beyond the parochialism associated with certain disciplines. Speech-language pathologists need to be familiar with the current state of deductive knowledge in many areas. Murphy (1982) lists 22 distinct professions or specialties related to the disorders

Table 2.1
Acquisition of knowledge

Setting	Logic	
	Deductive	**Inductive**
Academic	Learning basic definitions, concepts, rule behaviors of specific disorders	Formulating new relationships from existing information and positing the occurrence of specific events
Clinical	Directly applying specific procedures presented and discussed within an academic setting	Testing the relationship posited between specific variables that have not been previously known

of speech, language, and hearing (Figure 2.1). At first glance the list may appear intimidating. No one would expect the speech-language pathologist to be an expert in each of these areas. However, it is reasonable to expect the clinician to have deductive knowledge in each of the areas as it pertains to the practice of speech-language pathology.

Inductive Knowledge. *Inductive knowledge* is associated with the discovery of some regularity in nature that was unknown to the person experiencing it. It is the "Eureka" experience, when a person grasps something new that had been unknown. It might involve original insights never before thought of by anyone, or it could involve the child's first realization of how a doll wets itself after being given a bottle filled with water. In both examples, there is a willingness to posit relationships. In therapy, we may not know the effects of a certain procedure on a particular type of client. Possibly, the information gained through course work did not cover this type of problem. Our deductive knowledge provides us with a base for assessing the problem, but may not be adequate to predict the outcome of a procedure. We formulate an "if-then" statement where we posit, or hypothesize, that if certain things are done, specific types of outcomes are possible. For example, when taking a course on phonological disorders, a student learned that repetition was important for a child's acquisition of new phonemes. She also learned that new phonemes should be generalized as soon as they are established within words. When faced with her first client, she wondered if the amount of time required for therapy could be reduced if she taught the target phoneme in generalized settings. She developed a rigorous program to test her hypothesis, and both she and her supervisor were astounded by the results. Reichenbach (1961) emphasized the importance of using inductive knowledge in a world where certainty is a transitory feature:

> The man who makes inductive inferences may be compared to a fisherman who casts a net into an unknown part of the ocean—he does not know whether he will catch fish, but he knows that if he wants to catch fish he has to cast his net. Every inductive prediction is like casting a net into the ocean of the happenings of nature;

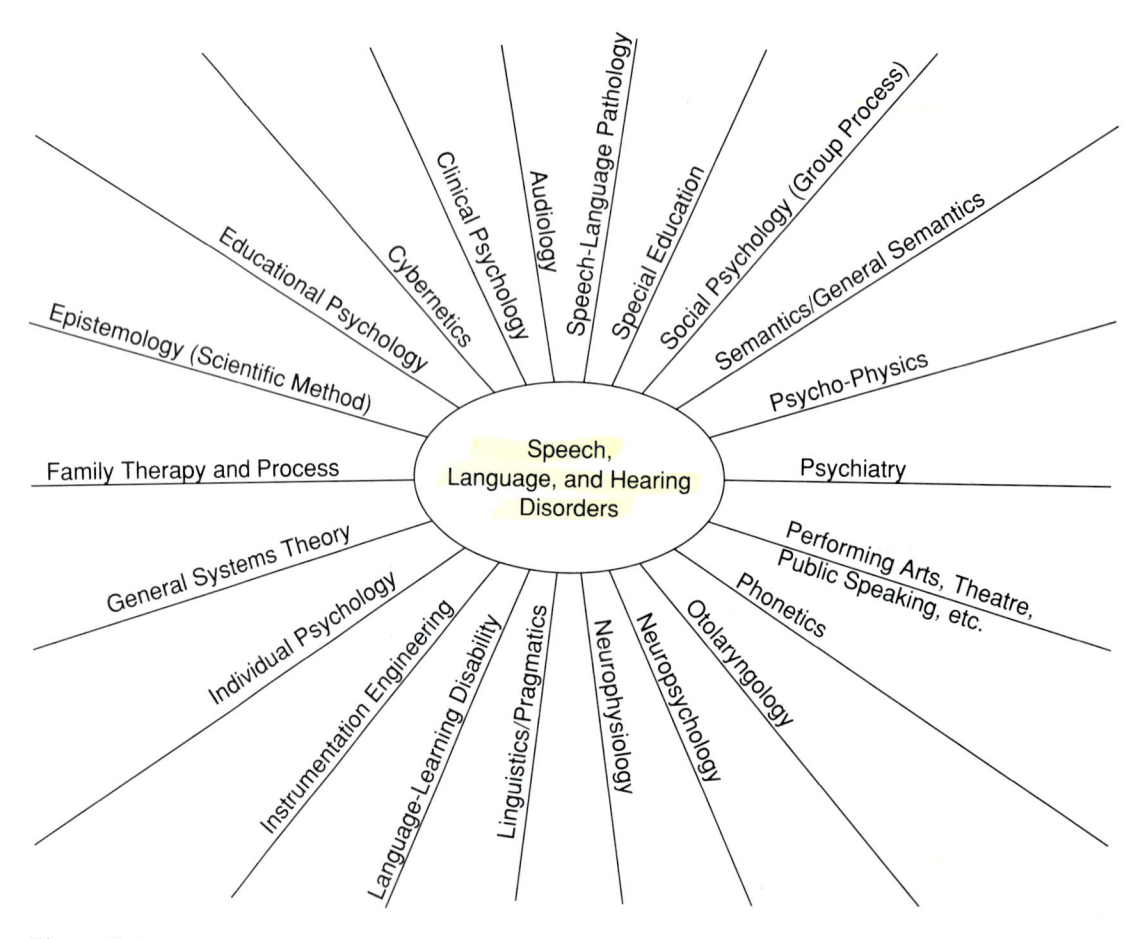

Figure 2.1
Professions related to human communication disorders
Source: Adapted from Murphy, 1982.

Spokes around "Speech, Language, and Hearing Disorders": Epistemology (Scientific Method), Educational Psychology, Cybernetics, Clinical Psychology, Audiology, Speech-Language Pathology, Special Education, Social Psychology (Group Process), Semantics/General Semantics, Psycho-Physics, Psychiatry, Performing Arts, Theatre, Public Speaking, etc., Phonetics, Otolaryngology, Neuropsychology, Neurophysiology, Linguistics/Pragmatics, Language-Learning Disability, Instrumentation Engineering, Individual Psychology, General Systems Theory, Family Therapy and Process.

we do not know whether we shall have a good catch, but we try, at least, and try by the help of the best means available.

We try because we want to act—and he who wants to act cannot wait until the future has become observational knowledge. To control the future—to shape future happenings according to a plan—presupposes predictive knowledge of what will happen if certain conditions are realized; and if we do not know the truth about what will happen, we shall employ our best posits in the place of truth. Posits are the instruments of action where truth is not available; the justification of induction is that it is the best instrument of action known to us. (p. 245)

Inductive reasoning involves a creative process that presupposes the individual already possesses deductive knowledge. It would be difficult to predict how the child's articulation would improve without knowing something about phonemic acquisition and generalization. With training and clinical experiences, the student will rely increasingly on inductive knowledge.

Contexts of Knowledge Acquisition

Academic. The primary method of acquiring deductive knowledge is through academic courses. Gagné (1970) wrote that problem solving does not occur in a vacuum, devoid of any prior knowledge. "The major condition for encouraging the learner to think is to be sure he already has something to think about" (p. 62). Academic knowledge reduces anxiety and allows clinicians to focus their attention on the clinical interaction. In specific disorder courses, definitions are learned, discriminations are made, concepts are learned, and theoretical models are understood. The models may be *descriptive* or *prescriptive*. That is, they may describe the conditions of a disorder or specify how the disorder should be treated. These are all necessary steps in skill acquisition. Academic knowledge is described by Dreyfus and Dreyfus (1986) as "knowing that" knowledge. Factual knowledge, usually acquired in the classroom, can be learned without actually experiencing or observing a person or event. The following would be an example of "knowing that" knowledge in the area of voice:

> The majority of phonation disorders are related to faulty use of the larynx, known as functional voice disorders. A common problem is vocal abuse, which involves using the laryngeal mechanisms excessively for such behaviors as continual throat clearing, yelling, or crying. (Boone, 1988, p. 2)

A student could amass a vast amount of knowledge about voice disorders and methods of remediation and still be unable to do voice therapy effectively. The actual knowledge of how to do voice therapy would be acquired within a clinical context.

Clinical Context. The clinic becomes the laboratory where knowledge acquired within academic settings is tested and applied. For Dreyfus and Dreyfus (1986), this is the setting where "knowing how" knowledge is developed.

> The know-how of cashiers, drivers, carpenters, teachers, managers, chess masters, and all mature, skillful individuals is not innate, like a bird's skill at building a nest. We have to learn. Small children, and sometimes adults, learn through trial and error, often guided by imitation of those more proficient. (p. 19)

Knowing how to do something depends primarily on experience. New clinicians must rely heavily on "knowing that" deductive knowledge during their initial clinical interactions. This form of knowledge should be applied almost as if the clinician were following a script. The script should be more than a lesson plan that merely specifies procedures and goals; it should be a scenario that hypothesizes both the various reactions clients can make and possible clinician responses. Reliance on the script is reduced with each application. "Knowing that" knowledge is gradually transformed into "knowing how" knowledge. With experience and more difficult clients, clinicians find that their reliance on deductive knowledge becomes inadequate. It is not possible to "script" interactions to account for the many variables that are present in an interaction. Inductive knowledge is required.

The use of inductive logic is often in the form of what is referred to as *clinical intuition*. Unfortunately, clinical intuition is viewed by many to be an innate characteristic that allows the practitioner to mystically have an insight into the correct clinical procedure or interaction that facilitates client growth. The mythology of intuition has been perpetuated throughout the history of our culture. The epitome of this concept is found in Frank Herbert's classic science fiction novel *Dune* (1965). In the novel, the leader of the planet Dune was able to develop pre-science, or the ability to see into the future, by ingesting a substance taken from the great sandworms. He was able to know what was going to happen before it occurred, thus allowing him to take the most appropriate actions.

Reliance on intuition can add a fascinating component to a novel, but it has limited value as an initial building block in the development of "knowing how" clinical skills. In the early days of aviation when pilots had little reliable information about the weather, condition of landing fields, or the aeronautical features of their plane, they referred to what they did as "seat-of-the-pants" flying. Early reliance on intuition in making clinical decisions can be called "seat-of-the-pants" therapy. It may have been appropriate in the 1930s when many of the helping professions were just developing, but it is an anachronism today because of the vast amount of "knowing that" knowledge available.

Intuition can have an important function within the development of "knowing how" knowledge. However, it should be relied on only after an extensive amount of academic and practical knowledge has been gained. Clinical intuition is a developed skill resulting from accumulated academic and practical knowledge. It involves the use of inductive reasoning to formulate a hypothesis instantaneously and apply the procedures for testing it. This concept of intuition has been a cornerstone of Eastern philosophical thought. In many Eastern philosophies, intuitive knowledge was used only after the application of rational thought (Watts, 1957). For example, in the training of Buddhist priests, many years are spent in studying the teachings of past masters. Only after the priest has successfully completed numerous stages in his formal education will his own Master help him develop intuitive knowledge. There is a Buddhist saying that a finger is needed to point to the moon, but one should not trouble with the finger once the moon is recognized. In speech-language pathology, the years of formal training involving careful analyses, data collection, experimentation, clinical practice, and continuous instruction from master clinicians can be seen as the finger that points the way to knowledge.

After the student has assimilated the massive amount of information and has applied it practically, then and only then can intuitive knowledge become an important tool of clinical practice. The use of intuitive knowledge becomes apparent in contingency planning. This involves the clinician's ability to plan for any eventuality of the therapy process, to predict client responses and the effect the clinician's counterresponses will have on the client; to change the course of therapy in midstream when things are not going well; and to choose immediately the most appropriate comment to a client's statement with what may be little or no time to compose a response. A master clinician can provide critical insight after the brilliant encounter. But it is obvious that the intricate, logical thought process gives way to the immediacy of intuitive knowledge during the encounter. Goldberg (1990) studied this skill in four clinicians who were identified as "outstanding" by a number of their peers. What he found was that after the session, each clinician was able to intricately trace the steps involved in specific clinical decisions but readily admitted that during the interaction the decision was instantaneous, with little conscious thought being given to it.

Clearly, knowledge gained through academic settings is different from knowledge derived within a clinical context. Although different, each is necessary for the development of the master clinician. In both contexts, deductive and inductive logic can be used. The developmental direction is from academic to clinical, deductive to inductive.

Clinical Experimentation

In the clinic, deductive and inductive knowledge are acquired through experimentation. Experimentation is not limited to objective studies of minute aspects of human behavior; it also includes diagnostic therapy. The term *diagnostic therapy* is used to describe the testing of various treatment protocols with a client to find the best method of teaching new communicative behaviors. The procedure to be used for both basic research in the social sciences and diagnostic therapy is called the *scientific method*. Although philosophers of science have devoted entire books to the subject (Nagel, 1961; Pap, 1962), a clinically useful condensation is provided by McReynolds and Kearns (1983). According to them, the steps in the scientific method that are most critical for the speech-language pathologist to follow are (a) specifying operational definitions; (b) differentiating between dependent and independent variables; (c) establishing control, and (d) applying reliable procedures.

Operational Definitions. The beginning of any study involves defining what is to be investigated. Many controversies in speech-language pathology involve differences in definitions. Stuttering is a prime example. Numerous articles have been written to attempt to define stuttering unambiguously only to be rebuked by authors in subsequent articles (Ingham, 1990; Perkins, 1990). The use of operational definitions is a way of avoiding semantic conflicts that may not be germane to what is being studied. An *operational definition* specifies the observable behavioral components of the subject being investigated. According to McReynolds and Kearns (1983), "No concept is described uniquely by a single operational definition. Instead, many definitions are possible; and the choice depends on which aspects the investigator wishes to study" (p. 2).

Although some individuals would reject the idea that more than one definition of a behavior is possible, it is an accepted scientific practice. By operationally defining the behavior or topic, discussions of whether or not the definition is "correct" are avoided. For example, Van Riper (1978) operationally defined stuttering as the speech occurring when "the forward flow of speech is interrupted abnormally by repetitions of sound, syllable, or articulatory posture or by avoidance and struggle behaviors" (p. 257). His definition is not necessarily correct or incorrect. Rather, as McReynolds and Kearns would maintain, the definition reflects either the theoretical or experimental interests of the author. Contrast

Van Riper's definition to that of Ham (1990), "Stuttering is a syndrome characterized by involuntary disruptions in the ongoing flow of speech, tending to occur on syllables or sounds in the form of clonic and/or tonic productions. Disruptions often are accompanied by stereotyped utterances, physical struggle, and distortions in parts of the speech mechanism and/or body areas." Ham's definition, just as Van Riper's, reflects the author's preferences and biases. An operational definition is crucial for clinical experimentation because it specifies what aspects of a behavior will be studied and tested.

Dependent and Independent Variables. Clinicians encounter two types of variables: dependent and independent. The *dependent variable* is the behavior that one wishes to change. An example would be a child's misarticulation of the /t/ phoneme. The *independent variable* is the procedure that the clinician will use to change the dependent variable (misarticulation of the /t/ phoneme). In this example, the clinician may wish to see if the production of a vowel sound (independent variable) immediately preceding the misarticulated /t/ phoneme (dependent variable) will change its production.

Control. When assessing the effects of a clinical procedure, control must be exerted over the independent variable. Without adequate controls, the clinician will not be able to determine if the selected independent variable resulted in the change, or whether other independent variables caused the change. If the clinician wished to test the belief that /i/ produced immediately prior to the production of /t/ will facilitate its correct production, a simple protocol could be constructed involving control over other independent variables. The clinician would first have the client say a list of words with /t/ in the initial position. This would be the baseline information for eventually determining if the clinical protocol worked. This is also known as the "A" condition in single-subject research designs. It refers to the behaviors of a client prior to the application of therapeutic procedures. In the second step, or "B" condition of the procedure, the client could be asked to engage in a number of speech activities, each requiring the production of /i/ followed by /t/. This might go on for a certain number of minutes, or for a specific number of productions. If the clinician was correct in believing that /i/ would facilitate the production of /t/, the client should show a marked improvement when compared with the productions made in the pre-therapy condition A. In the final stage of the experiment, the client is asked to again say the list of words produced in the pre-therapy condition, but this time without the preceding /i/ phoneme. If, with the removal of the independent variable (/i/) the client reverts back to the post-therapy condition, the clinician has strong evidence that the clinical procedure is an effective one. This important ABA single-subject research design could not have been conducted without controlling the effects of the independent variable.

Reliability. *Reliability* occurs when, over a number of trials, a procedure can be consistently applied. Without reliable procedures, it would be difficult to determine when a client has actually mastered a new behavior. For example, when teaching a child to use adjectives a clinician might rely on the following written description of a specific procedure:

> First identify four objects that the child can name consistently. Then select one color attribute you wish to teach. Assemble three examples of each of the four objects, all having the same color. Begin the treatment.

Regardless how many times the procedure is used, the rigor with which it was written should facilitate its consistent application, even if one clinician is substituted for another. Such a process would be an example of a reliable procedure. Contrast this with the following example:

> Identify some objects that the child has named in the past. Then select a few colors you wish to teach. Assemble some examples of the colored objects and begin the treatment.

In this example, it is very unlikely that any two clinicians independently working with the same client would use this procedure in a similar manner. Each time the protocol is used, it must be applied identically. To do this, the procedures must be objectively described. By objectively describing the procedures and consistently using them with each application, the clinician will introduce reliable procedures into the therapeutic process.

THE CARING APPROACH

Speech-language pathologists place great importance on the replicability of clinical procedures. A basic assumption is that if a specific technique or procedure is applied identically by a variety of clinicians, the results should be roughly similar. Although this "scientific" approach is necessary in the helping professions, it tends to minimize the effect that personality and values have on clinical interactions. Yet the importance of these factors becomes apparent to anyone who has witnessed the competent application of the same technique by two clinicians having radically different personalities. For example, a number of years ago a clinic supervisor was observing a student administer an intervention program he had developed. Although each step in the program was being competently administered, the warmth and humor that he thought typified his approach was transformed into a biting sarcastic assault upon the client. The interactive role of the clinician should not be ignored but rather be utilized and developed.

Personality Traits of the Clinician

The role of personality is evident to anyone who has ever witnessed the "laying on of hands" at a religious revival meeting or the way eloquent orators can move an audience to tears or action by the charisma they exude. The same type of phenomenon also exists in the area of communicative disorders. A number of years ago, a well-known professor was presenting his approach to stuttering therapy to an audience that included speech-language pathologists and their stuttering clients. He asked for a volunteer to come on stage so he could demonstrate his approach. A very disfluent young woman agreed. The professor was very clear that he would be demonstrating all of the steps in his program during the next 20 to 30 minutes. He cautioned both the woman and the audience that these steps would normally be applied over a period of several months and that this would be a demonstration, not therapy. After the 30-minute session was completed, the woman was completely fluent and she, as most people in the audience, held the professor in awe. To anyone witnessing the demonstration, it was similar to the "laying on of hands" seen at faith-healing meetings. Although the therapeutic program was very good, it was the style and personality of the professor that was critical. For whatever reason, he was able to convince the woman that she could be fluent by using the methodology he suggested. For those 30 minutes, the force of his personality was primarily responsible for her fluency. Unfortunately, her speech deteriorated to its previous disfluency level within a few days after the demonstration ended. This does not minimize the quality of the therapy program but rather emphasizes the importance of the clinician's personality.

Traits That Facilitate Positive Changes. If a clinician's personality is critical for effective therapy to occur, should training programs reshape or remold the student's personality? Probably not. However, specific personality traits have been shown to facilitate positive clinical interactions. New clinicians may wish to examine their own personalities in light of what more experienced clinicians in the helping professions have found to be effective.

Satir (1967) gave eight characteristics that she believed were important for those in helping professions to possess:

1. Reveal yourself clearly to others.
2. Be in touch with your own feelings.
3. Be realistic about yourself and your capabilities.
4. Regard each person as unique.
5. Differences should be viewed as learning experiences, not as a threat or signal for conflict.
6. Understand clients for what they are, not how you wish them to be.
7. Understand that clients are responsible for their own behaviors.
8. Be able to clarify the meaning of a client's utterances.

These are all laudable qualities for a clinician to have, but not necessarily inclusive or acceptable to everyone. Contrast Satir's personality characteristics with Murphy's classification of "closed-system" and "open-system" clinicians in Table 2.2 (Murphy, 1982). Murphy contrasts desirable and undesirable clinical skills. Although the terminology and specific traits differ from those listed by Satir, each author seems to be specifying the characteristics of a nondefensive, confident, and accepting individual.

Rogers (1965) was concerned how the clinician's personality affected the client. He maintained that a clinician's personality traits have tremendous consequences in the development of trust within a clinical situation. He believed that the client needs to feel that the clinician is competent and self-assured. Competency can be gained by knowledge and experience. But self-assurance is derived

Table 2.2
Characteristics of closed and open clinicians

Closed System	Open System
Need to reduce uncertainty	Admits and accepts uncertainty
Cautionary communicative style	Spontaneous communicative mode
Predictable	Unpredictable
Resistant to new information	Open to new information
Stereotyped behavior	Adaptable behavior
Solutions assumed known	Solutions assumed improvable
Steady goals	Variable, evolving goals
Resistance to change	Changeable
Rigid, static	Pliable, dynamic

Source: Adapted from "The Clinical Process and the Speech-Language Pathologist" by A. T. Murphy, 1982. In G. H. Shames and E. H. Wiig (Eds.), *Human Communication Disorders* (pp. 453–474). Columbus, OH: Merrill/Macmillan.

from the clinician's willingness to be "transparent," to allow the client to view him or her honestly without any false pretenses.

Traits That Impede Positive Behavioral Changes. One problem that can impede client growth is clinician ego glorification. *Ego glorification* involves an inflated judgment of a person's importance. Glorification results from two independent factors: the clinician's realization that she possesses an enormous amount of power and influence and the client's belief that the clinician is responsible for all changes. The client or client's parents come to the clinical setting willing to rely totally on the professional for help and advice. The relationship has dynamics similar to those described in Bertrand Russell's treatise on priestly power (1961). Russell was concerned about the amount of influence people had solely because of their position within society. His example was the priest or religious leader who was able to issue edicts that were respected and adhered to, regardless of what the followers thought of them. The fact that the instructions and pronouncements emanated from a glorified leader was sufficient for them to be followed. Speech-language pathologists share some of the same role characteristics of Russell's priests. As professionals, they generate respect and power often only because of their position within a societal structure. The ability to influence people and direct their lives may have little to do with their competence, intelligence, or compassion.

Russell's priestly power is not an "all or nothing" phenomenon in speech-language therapy. It is applied in varying degrees. Rollin (1987) examined the use of it in clinical relationships within a Jungian psychoanalytical framework. According to Jung, we all possess a "shadow side," a part of our personalities that we do not like and try to hide. Because of the nature of clinical interactions, this shadow side often emerges, resulting in specific styles of therapy, each utilizing various degrees of power. Rollin specified five different roles clinicians could assume, depending on their shadow side. Although one may question the relevance of a Jungian perspective, the following clinical roles are easily identifiable to anyone who has supervised clinicians.

The "benign dictator" is one who specifies all action and behaviors for the client. These clinicians assume that they know what is best for the client, and they use their position to intimidate the client into submission. The "benign super-therapist" is one who not only specifies the behaviors that are necessary for the remediation of a communicative disorder but also intrudes into other areas that are not necessarily related to speech and language. The "sophisticated therapist" is one who may examine very interesting aspects of the client's relationships at the expense of treating the actual communicative disorder. The "benevolent therapist" is one who allows a client to deviate from a prescribed remediation program, often at the expense of the program. Finally, there is the "powerless therapist," a clinician who gives up all power to the client.

Rarely does a clinician assume only one of these roles in therapy. Clinicians may assume one role for a specific purpose and then abandon it and substitute another because of other goals. It could be argued that each of these roles has its appropriate and inappropriate uses. It is important that the clinician recognize that each role will probably result in different interaction patterns.

The second factor that can result in ego glorification is the client's acknowledgment that the clinician has been responsible for tremendous positive changes in his or her life. It may prove difficult to assume the mantle of humility when client after client tells you how important you have been for their success in therapy and, more important, in life. Speech-language pathologists assume a central position in the rehabilitation of clients and the emotional well-being of their families. Often regaining the ability to communicate or understand communication is the most important thing in our clients' lives. The following passage by a woman who recovered from aphasia illustrates this point (Wulf, 1973):

> The door opened quietly and then I knew. No words told me that this was the one I needed so badly—a radiant smile did that, and the weights of uncertainty that seemed to be sitting all over me flowed, like mercury, into one great big ball, rolled off and vanished never to return again.
>
> And this was the first miracle speech therapy wrought for me. No word was needed—it was in the magic of a look—an instantaneous rapport partly because my innermost messenger had told me it would be that way. Speech therapy's rare talent is this: being able to hop on anybody's wave length and stay there until the aphasic has learned how to climb the unending tortuous crag facing him.
>
> This therapy develops a facility for relating to seriously ill patients who are trying to remember how to say anything, only by the time they think they may have found out they no longer remember what it was they had set out to discover. And then a therapist comes, a person who knows! And those dreadful empty spaces are of very little moment.
>
> The awful feeling of being a prisoner within myself! How could there be a rote, dispassionate, scientific discussion of what speech therapy can do for an aphasic, for aphasia is not a plain vanilla kind of disorder to which rules 1, 2, and 3 apply and that's it!
>
> A successful therapist has to be intuitively perceptive, attuned to using every clue, things nobody else would suspect were clues; a mind imaginatively sensitive to

our needs, wants, desires, frustrations, weariness, hopes, abilities and our obvious disabilities. There must be finesse with words to secure necessary information and patients never need to feel insecure with a therapist. How could they, bolstered as they are by lovely smiles, sweet talk when needed (which is nearly all the time), and genuine encouragement.

Two years post-stroke and I can still feel the indescribable relief when a rescuing therapist opened the door. There seemed to be a golden thread linking us, mind to mind, and I knew that this bit of gossamer gold was my means of getting thinking reorganized; of finding, in my bashed brain, new pathways to trot over or old ones to plod through. This was my life-line to sanity.[1]

Speech-language pathologists are often key figures in our clients' development as functional communicators. As Helen Wulf so beautifully wrote, we are viewed as a "bit of gossamer gold" that links the patient with the world they knew or the world they would like to know. We are given a tremendous amount of power by our clients because of what we are capable of doing. Along with this power comes a tremendous amount of responsibility.

The assumption of power by position (priestly power) or power by success can result in ego gratification at the expense of the client. When clinicians begin to rely routinely on the status they have as professionals to convince clients to take certain actions, they lose the ability to rationally justify procedures and actions. Assertions made on the basis of status may cloud the clinician's ability to critically self-analyze their own behaviors. When clinicians allow clients to assert that they have been responsible for the clients' successes, a kernel of clinical symbiosis develops, whereby clients become dependent on the clinician for all behavioral changes. If clients truly believe that the clinician is responsible for their progress, they may deny their own responsibility for change. Clients begin to feel that, without the clinician, already acquired changes may cease or new changes will not be possible. This becomes evident when clients say things like, "I was speaking real good after the session, but after four days I started to stutter a lot. Boy, I'm glad I'm here now for my fluency shot!" As clinicians, we need to reduce our importance to our clients if they are to assume responsibility for changing their own behavior.

A more complex problem can develop with success. A false sense of confidence may develop if the clinician's embryonic skills result in rapid success. Therapy appears to be an easy endeavor, requiring only a limited number of skills to achieve success. The clinician may assume that all cases will possess the same dynamics as the present one. The successful clinician may begin to place his or her development ahead of the client's. Success is a very positive stroke to receive. It can result in the clinician developing a sense of self-importance that adversely affects the clinical relationship. Clients may now be blamed for failures. By absolving oneself of responsibility for failure, the clinician may cause the client's already low esteem as a communicator to descend to even lower depths. When this occurs, therapy for the client constantly mirrors his or her inadequa-

---

[1] From *Aphasia, My World Alone* (pp. 50–51) by H. H. Wulf, 1973, Detroit, MI: Wayne State University Press. Copyright 1973 by H. H. Wulf. Reprinted by permission.

cies. With each new failure, the client's self-image as an inadequate individual is reinforced. It is little wonder that clients who experience minimal clinical success and are chastised for lack of progress drop out of therapy. Nobody likes to be punished, especially if they are told that their communicative problems are self-inflicted. An excellent example of this problem appears in a study conducted by Goldberg and Culatta (1991). A questionnaire was sent to members of a national self-help group. Over 80% of its members felt they were currently moderate or severe stutterers. Of these individuals over 90% had been involved in stuttering therapy. Of these individuals over 70% no longer continued with therapy, even though they acknowledged that they still had a communicative disorder that was extremely disruptive to their lives. For these individuals, the pain associated with clinical failures far outweighed its benefits.

Values

It is an exercise in self-deception to believe that clinical interactions in speech-language pathology are neutral and therefore outside of a specific value system. When we deceive ourselves about what is real, we tend to either ignore or misinterpret the consequences of our actions. One cannot help but make a statement of one's values during clinical interactions. As we decide on a clinical approach, offer advice, direct the outcome of therapy, or suggest alternative approaches to parents regarding childrearing practices, we are continually infusing our own values in our utterances and actions. The danger of misinterpreting the client's needs by superimposing our own values and beliefs has been emphasized by many nondirective psychologists. Carl Rogers (1965) implored counselors and therapists to use the client's frame of reference when evaluating goals and methods. He believed that by bringing into the clinical relationship the theoretical constructs and possibly false notions of causal relationships, the therapist reconfirms his own biases rather than helping the client solve his own problems.

Other psychologists are equally adamant in maintaining that their own specific approach, with its inherent values, is the most effective way of having the client achieve success. The father of psychoanalysis, Sigmund Freud (1933) maintained that most neurotic behavior resulted from early sexual thoughts or actions. Albert Ellis (1962) believes that most emotional disturbances result from irrational statements that people use to indoctrinate themselves. Frederick Perls (1969), the founder of Gestalt therapy, maintained that the individual was in constant search of balance. Neurotic behaviors were a result of the person's attempt to reach it through inappropriate means. These therapists, and many other notable ones, based a clinical approach on specific values.

What are values? The study of values and morals has taxed great minds since the time of the ancient Greek philosophers. In the *Nicomachean Ethics,* Aristotle (Ostwald, 1962) examined the relationship of values to everyday actions. For Aristotle, "good" values were universal. That is, they were, or should be, identical for all people. Throughout the history of philosophy, this belief was affirmed by other great minds such as Rousseau (Cole, 1950) and Kant (Infield, 1963) in the 18th century, and in the 19th century by Mill (Schneewind, 1965) and Nietzsche

(Golffing, 1956). Although each believed in a universal set of values, each differed as to what they were. A reaction to this approach to the study of values occurred in the 20th century in the form of the logical positivism movement. The logical positivists believed that the study of values is neither scientific nor objective. Values, therefore, are nothing more than preferences, and as such, should not be part of philosophic inquiry. A.J. Ayer (1936) wrote, "We shall set ourselves to show that in so far as statements of value are significant, they are ordinary 'scientific' statements; and that in so far as they are not scientific, they are not in the literal sense significant, but are simply expressions of emotion which can be neither true nor false" (p. 21).

Regardless whether one believes that values are universal or are merely expressions of belief and preference limited only to the person espousing them, values take the imperative form of "should" or "ought to." If one believes that values should be universally applied, then all clinicians should be expected to have similar values. If one is less egocentric, then one's values become guidelines for personal action. Let us begin with the less ambitious task of outlining the fundamentals of a personal value system and explaining how it is related to clinical behavior. The examination entails a three part process: (a) personal values; (b) clinical values; and (c) clinical behaviors.

Personal Values. Some philosophers have maintained that by their very nature, values are relativistic (Kockelmans, 1965). That is to say, they vary among cultures and change depending on the circumstances in which they are applied. This principle served as a foundation for existentialism, an approach to understanding human interactions that is still important in the helping professions. Rollo May (1961) said, "There is no such thing as truth or reality for a living human being except as he participates in it, is conscious of it, has some relationship to it." Even if one examines the ten commandments, the highest of all moral doctrines in the Judaic-Christian tradition, one might have difficulty rigidly adhering to its strict universal application without adding the phrase, "except when. . . ." For example, if one believes that under no circumstances should one kill, then were the only moral and ethical people in World War II those who did not fight against the Nazis? Were the Allied soldiers immoral in their struggle against Hitler's army? Or is it possible to find "special" occurrences where one value can be subordinated to another more compelling one? In his examination of religion and mythology, Joseph Campbell points out a biblical contradiction rarely discussed in religious circles (1988). On the one hand, in Deuteronomy, God gives the commandments to the Hebrews, "Thou shall not kill," and "Thou shall not covet your neighbor's wife," but later qualifies them as guides to behavior only within the Hebrew nation. Outside of the nation, Deuteronomy instructs the Hebrews to put all males to the sword and take women as their booty. If Campbell is correct in this analysis, it appears that the relativity of values was acknowledged even in the basic teaching of Judeo-Christian doctrine. Bertrand Russell (1961), one of the greatest of the 20th century philosophers, not only examined the hierarchical nature of values, but also how most were culturally based.

> In all ages and nations positive morality has consisted almost wholly of prohibitions of various classes of actions, with the addition of a small number of commands to perform certain other actions. The Jews, for example, prohibited murder and theft, adultery and incest, the eating of pork and seething the kid in its mother's milk. To us the last two precepts may seem less important than the others, but religious Jews have observed them far more scrupulously than what seem to us fundamental principles of morality.
>
> South Sea Islanders could imagine nothing more utterly wicked than eating out of a vessel reserved for the use of the chief.
>
> My friend Dr. Barogan made a statistical investigation into the ethical valuations of undergraduates in certain American colleges. Most considered Sabbath-breaking more wicked than lying, and extraconjugal sexual relations more wicked than murder.
>
> The Japanese consider disobedience to parents the most atrocious of crimes. I was once at a charming spot on the outskirts of Kyoto with several Japanese socialists, men who were among the most advanced thinkers in the country. They told me that a certain well beside which we were standing was a favorite spot for suicides, which were very frequent. When I asked why so many occurred they replied that most were those of young people in love whose parents had forbidden them to marry. To my suggestion that perhaps it would be better if parents had less power they all returned an emphatic negative.
>
> To Dr. Barogan's undergraduates this power of Japanese parents to forbid love would seem monstrous, but the similar power of husbands over wives would seem a matter of course. Neither they nor the Japanese would examine the question rationally; both would decide unthinkingly on the basis of moral precepts learned in youth.[2]

Personal values, therefore, are culturally related and may be linear or hierarchical. *Linear values* are all equal and are to be adhered to regardless of circumstances. In Russell's example, the ancient Jews and modern orthodox Jews would maintain that all kosher laws are linear. There is no difference between not eating pork and not eating shellfish. Because of the rigidity attached to linear values, they are most often associated with religious doctrine, although some may be nonreligious. In examining personal value systems, linear values tend to be fewer in number than hierarchical values.

Hierarchical values are those that are arranged in an ascending order, with the higher values having precedence over lower ones. Hierarchical values are those that end with the phrase "except when . . . ." An example would be, "Do not kill, except when there is no other way to defend yourself or your loved ones." In this example, "Defend yourself and your loved ones" would have a higher hierarchical order than "do not kill."

Personal value systems usually consist of both linear and hierarchical values. These values become the guidelines for behavior. They are abstract models that allow the user to make decisions regarding real behaviors. Until the values are applied, they are merely intellectual constructs, having only a theoretical rela-

---

[2] From *The Basic Writings of Bertrand Russell* (p. 345) by Bertrand Russell, 1961 (R. E. Egner and L. E. Denonn, Eds.). New York: Simon & Schuster. Copyright 1961 by Simon & Schuster. Reprinted by permission.

tionship to one's ethical behavior. Although personal values are intricately related to one's everyday behaviors, few people can explain their value system when asked to do so. Values tend to be regarded as amorphous edicts, identifiable only when they are put into action.

The first step in determining how one's values are related to clinical behavior is to identify those values that are important in guiding personal behavior. Once a list has been made, one can then determine which values are linear, which are hierarchical, and under what circumstances the relativistic values can be modified, or subverted. The task is formidable, as evidenced by the fact that ethics has been debated since human beings were able to think.

Clinical Values. The American Speech-Language Hearing Association has from its inception in 1926, when it was known as the American Academy of Speech Correction, been concerned about a clinical code of ethics (Paden, 1970). The latest revision to the code of ethics was completed in 1989 (ASHA, 1992) and is a good starting point in our examination of clinical values. An abridged form appears in Table 2.3. The entire Code of Ethics is reproduced in Appendix A.

The ASHA Code of Ethics provides a basic ethical and moral framework for practicing speech-language pathologists and audiologists. It serves as the foundation for ethical and professional practice. Matthews (1982) maintained that the code of ethics is more than a statement of "Thou shalt nots." For him, it is the basis on which clinical choices are to be made.

Table 2.3
ASHA code of ethics (abridged version)

PRINCIPLES OF ETHICS

Four principles serve as a basis for the ethical evaluation of professional conduct and form the underlying moral basis for the Code of Ethics. Individuals subscribing to this Code shall observe these principles as affirmative obligations under all conditions of professional activity.

Principle of ethics I

Individuals shall hold paramount the welfare of persons served professionally.

Principle of ethics II

Individuals shall maintain high standards of professional competence.

Principle of ethics III

Individuals shall promote public understanding, support development of services designed to fulfill unmet needs and provide accurate information.

Principle of ethics IV

Individuals shall honor their responsibilities to the public, their profession, and their relationships with colleagues and members of allied professions, uphold the dignity of the profession and accept the profession's self-imposed standards.

Source: From American Speech-Language-Hearing Association, 1992.

> The real basis of a code of ethics is giving highest priority to the welfare of the clients a profession is to serve. What is ethical or not ethical in your behavior as a professional boils down to the kinds of choices you make. You will very frequently be confronted with making choices which could be based on your answers to three questions:
> 1. What is the appropriate decision as far as the best interest of my client?
> 2. What is the best decision in terms of the organization I work for? and
> 3. What is the best decision for me personally? (p. 18)

Is the code of ethics authoritative enough to affect the transference of personal values into clinical values? It is not. It is merely a guideline that can set a course of travel but it is not explicit enough to indicate the appropriate turning points. Clinical values are a subset of personal values. In some cases there may be a direct correspondence between the two, such as "respect the worth of each individual." This value may be applied equally in the contexts of both nonclinical and clinical settings. But other values pose ethical dilemmas. For example, within a personal value system it may be abhorrent to manipulate the behaviors of others. If this value is transposed into a clinical setting, the therapist would be ineffectual in changing a client's communicative behavior, since change involves some forms of manipulation. A similar case may exist with the value of "truthfulness." Honesty and truthfulness may be very important values in a personal value system. To be truthful and forthright are laudable values. However, within certain clinical settings, the clinician might wish to withhold some information or change the character of it to benefit the client. The timing of when to present information and how it should be presented are areas of concern to all counselors. A clinician may believe that the freedom of an individual is a sacred value but find that physical restraint is the only way of maintaining eye contact with an autistic child. Or the clinician may believe that children should be free to explore without limitations but find that a hyperactive child must be given few choices in learning situations.

Rollin (1987) addressed the relationship between the client's problem and the clinician's role.

> As therapists, we not only vary our roles according to the clients with whom we work but also our clinical behavior for any one client. . . . Ideally, what we hope to learn, however, is that the therapist who guides and yet is flexible to the client's needs will provide a therapeutic environment where the client can grow and change within his or her greatest potential. (p. 309)

It is the importance of clinical growth, therefore, that is central to how we as clinicians should act. The centrality of the client's welfare may be the key to resolving what appeared above to be "ethical dilemmas" between personal values and clinical realities.

Can a clinical value be stated that incorporates the notion of client welfare? Is one clinical value possibly so powerful that all others are subsumed under it? Frederick Perls believed there was. For him, as well as other Gestalt therapists (Perls, Hefferline, & Goodman, 1951), "maturation" was the most important clinical value. He defined *maturation* as the development of the individual from environmental support to self-support. This is a process whereby you may initially offer support, strength, and guidance to your clients. Gradually, as clients begin to understand their problems and learn how to solve them, your support is reduced and eventually withdrawn, thus requiring clients to become responsible for their own behavioral and attitudinal changes. Within clinical contexts, you continually strive for your client's self-support. This may or may not be a value in your nonclinical relationships. If maturation is the most important clinical value, all others become secondary. When a conflict develops between maturation and another value, such as freedom to explore, maturation must be given the prime consideration. This concept of clinical growth is not unique to Gestalt therapy. Elements of this idea are found not only in psychology but also in Eastern and Western philosophy. It is identified as "nirvana" in Zen Buddhism (Watts, 1957), "self-actualization" in the writings of Maslow (1968), "personhood" for Buscaglia (1982), "order" for Krishnamurti (1970), and the "potential self" for Carl Rogers (1970). Virtually every eminent person in the helping professions has a similar value, regardless of the name it goes by. This concept of growth is the clinical value under which all personal values should be subsumed. It is the one value that justifies the subordination of personal values without compromising ethics.

Training Program Orientation. Clinical training programs are inherently biased as to the etiology and treatment of specific disorders and general clinical approaches. There is nothing wrong with this. On the contrary, a clinical training program that has no orientation would be suspect. We have legitimate preferences. Unfortunately, new students are rarely knowledgeable enough to question them. As a result, one's theoretical beliefs and clinical behaviors usually are a by-product of professional training. Goldberg's Behavioral-Cognitive Stuttering Therapy Program (1981) is the result of the influence of three of his former instructors. Matthews (1986) in an insightful introduction to a book that examined the history of stuttering therapy, traces his own development and how each of the great contributors in the field of speech pathology relied on their mentors.

The orientation of mentors and the training program philosophy will exert a tremendous influence on the development of a student's clinical approach. A problem develops only if the philosophy is never examined. Theories and approaches proliferate and develop. Each is acceptable only as long as it can explain phenomena and allow for effective and efficient positive change of the client's behaviors.

COMBINING SCIENCE AND COMPASSION

Speech-language pathologists are not merely professionals who modify or change one's ability to use speech and language. They are helping professionals who can and usually do have a fundamental impact on the lives of their clients and their clients' families. They remediate one of the most fundamental of human characteristics: the ability to communicate and be meaningfully involved in the communication process. Often, even the most seemingly insignificant change in a person's speaking pattern can result in lifelong changes. Speech-language pathologists obviously do more than merely change tongue positions and teach new linguistic forms. They possess immense power that can be used for either the benefit or detriment of their clients.

Clinicians find themselves in unique situations. During a session they might initially be empathetic and compassionate, but then become critical and confrontational. This vacillation may be necessary for the growth of the client. However, it requires an integrated personality to perform it. Giffen and Patton (1971) emphasized the importance of clinicians knowing and understanding their values, capabilities, and limitations. Clinicians do not have to be all-knowing or continually correct to be effective. They must, however, be realistic in assessing both their strengths and weaknesses.

Self-Image. The self-image of a new clinician is a fragile entity. New clinicians are expected to perform at least adequately, yet they generally possess minimal clinical competencies. The dilemma can be anxiety-producing unless it is viewed as a growth experience. New clinicians should expect to have failures and often use inefficient therapeutic techniques. If each new client is viewed as an educational experience, clinicians may avoid depicting themselves as failures. It can be very demoralizing for the new clinician to spend countless hours attempting to teach a client a new behavior and still be unable to make any headway. For example, one clinician questioned her clinical skills because she had been unable to teach a young client the correct tongue placement for a specific phoneme. After five frustrating sessions, she asked her supervisor for help. He listened to the child for one minute and then asked him to place his tongue slightly forward of where it usually was and produce the sound. The child instantly produced the target sound. The new clinician was distraught. After the session she said to her supervisor, "I spent five hours in therapy with this kid and failed. You spent less than two minutes and he's hitting the target sound consistently." The supervisor responded, "No, it didn't take me two minutes; it took me ten years." The knowledge gained with each new clinical experience cannot be underestimated.

Failure can be either growth enhancing or devastating to the development of clinical skills. When clients are blamed for failure, the clinician's skills may stagnate. When one does not accept responsibility for failure, one can avoid critical self-examination. When responsibility for failure is consistently shifted to the client, clinicians avoid confronting their own inadequacies. The ability to confront one's inadequacies and learn from failures is a distinguishing characteristic of "master clinicians," even those who have practiced for many years. To develop clinical skills, clinicians must constantly reassess their selection of procedures and their implementation.

Although critical self-examination is important, the new clinician should not assume the role of a Hindu holy man who takes on all the evils of the world as his salvation. If clinicians accept the entire responsibility for failure, an unhealthy humility can develop. Often, clients do not accept responsibility for behavioral change. An important clinical maxim is to accept the responsibility for clinical failure initially. Assume that the program or approach is not appropriate for this client. Give the client the benefit of doubt. Modify the approach or program to meet the client's real or perceived needs. If modifications are made and the client is still unable to achieve success, then it is appropriate to question the client's commitment to behavioral changes. Usually a combination of humility and confidence in one's clinical skills is a healthy mixture for both new and experienced clinicians.

SUMMARY

The personalities of clinicians, their needs, and insecurities affect clinical interactions. Clinicians need to be aware of their personality traits and critically examine them, not in terms of whether or not they are "good" or "bad," but whether they have a positive or negative effect on clinical interactions.

To be able to develop and implement an intervention plan that not only "corrects" a speech, language, or hearing problem but also has a positive effect on a client's life is exciting and fulfilling both for the client and the clinician. The experience of being creative and helpful is a powerful incentive for continuing in a profession. The clinician is compassionately translating intelligent thought into effective and ethical actions. In *The Teachings of Don Juan* (1968), Carlos Castenada has Don Juan asking, "Does this path have a heart? If it does, the path is good; if it doesn't, it is of no use." The lesson from this novel can be directly applied to speech-language pathology. The path to the development of functional communication involves the scientific application of human interaction principles. The foundation of the profession is the desire to help people achieve their full potential as normal communicators. The soul of speech pathology is an intertwined mixture of knowledge, compassion, and clinical ethics.

SUGGESTED READINGS

Dreyfus, H. L., & Dreyfus, S. E. (1986). *Mind over machine.* New York: The Free Press.
Matthews, J. (1990). The professions of speech-language pathology and audiology. In G. H. Shames and E. H. Wiig (Eds.), *Human communication disorders: An introduction* (3rd ed., pp. 2–27). New York: Merrill/Macmillan.
McReynolds, L. V., & Kearns, K. P. (1983). *Single-subject experimental designs in communicative disorders.* Baltimore: University Park Press.
Reichenbach, H. (1961). *The rise of scientific philosophy.* Berkeley, CA: University of California Press.
Rogers, C. R. (1965). *Client-centered therapy.* New York: Houghton Mifflin.
Rollin, W. J. (1987). *The psychology of communication disorders in individuals and their families.* Englewood Cliffs, NJ: Prentice-Hall.
Russell, B. (1961). *The basic writings of Bertrand Russell.* R. E. Egner and L. E. Denonn (Eds.). New York: Simon & Schuster, p. 345.
Satir, V. (1967). *Conjoint family therapy* (rev. ed.). Palo Alto, CA: Science and Behavior Books.
Wulf, H. H. (1973). *Aphasia, my world alone.* Detroit, MI: Wayne State University Press.

❑ Activity 2.1
A Clinical Experiment—ABA Design

Describe the ABA design you would use to determine if a clinical procedure you have selected to change a behavior is appropriate. The activity has four components. First, observe a client for at least 15 minutes. Second, select one very small behavior or a component of a more complex behavior. Third, briefly describe, as reliably as possible, the procedure you will be testing. Fourth, construct your ABA design.

Time the Client Was Observed: _____ minutes.

Behavior to Be Changed _____

Procedure Used to Change Behavior:
    Materials:

    Application:

Experimental Design:
    A Condition (Pre-therapy)

    B Condition (Application of therapy protocol)

    A Condition (Post-therapy)

❑ **Activity 2.2**
A Self-Evaluation of Values and Ethics

This exercise in self-analysis is intended to help you focus your attention on issues that will be critical in the development of clinical skills.

1. What would be the worst type of clinical failure you could imagine happening?

2. How could this become a learning experience?

3. What was the most successful interpersonal experience you have ever had?

4. What did you learn from it?

5. In your nonclinical interactions, to what extent and how do you exert power?

6. Based on your nonclinical interactions, how would you see yourself using power in a clinical setting?

7. What is the most important thing you have ever done for another person?

8. What was their perception of you after the important event occurred?

continues

Activity 2.2 continued

9. How did this make you feel?

10. List five personality traits of yours that you believe will be positive clinical traits. Why?
    a.

    b.

    c.

    d.

    e.

11. List five personality traits of yours that you believe will be negative clinical traits. Why?
    a.

    b.

    c.

    d.

    e.

12. List your five most important personal values in descending order.
    a.
    b.
    c.
    d.
    e.

Activity 2.2 continued

13. How could you translate each of the personal values you listed in question #12 into clinical values?

   a.

   b.

   c.

   d.

   e.

14. Are there any ethical standards of ASHA that you disagree with? If so, please list them and state why.

15. What do you believe is the orientation of your training program? Do you agree or disagree with it? Why?

16. People may feel that most things in their life are going well and form an integrated whole. Conversely, they may feel a tremendous amount of conflict and uncertainty, causing them to feel fragmented. On a scale of 1 to 10, with 1 being "very fragmented" and 10 being "very integrated," how would you rate your personality?

17. What could you do for yourself to become more integrated?

PART II
Clinical Behaviors

We must use all available weapons of attack, face our problems realistically and not retreat to the land of fashionable sterility, learn to sweat over our data with an admixture of judgment and intuitive rumination, and accept the usefulness of particular data even when the level of analysis available for them is markedly below that available for other data in the empirical area.

Binder, 1964, p. 294

Clinicians are inundated with sensory data at the same time they are attempting to apply strategies or implement therapeutic protocols. Without training and practice, these tasks can be formidable. However, they can be simplified by using the scientific technique called *reductionism*, a procedure whereby a complex situation or physical entity is reduced into its smallest meaningful components (Nagel, 1961). Each component is individually examined and then reassembled and analyzed as a whole. By reducing a phenomenon into smaller units, one is better able to understand its operation. In this part, the clinical situation will be reduced into its major component units: (a) speech and language behaviors; (b) metalinguistic behaviors; and (c) nonverbal behaviors. Chapter 3 serves as the foundation for the reduction by presenting basic principles of clinical observation and methods of recording and analyzing behaviors.

Chapter 3
Observation and Measurement

STUDY GUIDE

- Data can be collected for many reasons. What are they?
- What are the various methods of collecting data? What are the advantages and disadvantages of each?
- Describe how you would calculate the percentage of correct responses.
- How is the percentage of correct responses used in graphing a learning curve?
- Why would one wish to determine the learning curve of a client's progress?
- What is a type-token ratio and why would one wish to determine it?
- What can the latency of response tell you about your client?
- When would one wish to use a rating scale? What are the advantages and disadvantages of rating scales?

"Why collect data when all I want to do is help my client?" This is an often heard lament of many new, well-meaning, but unscientifically oriented students. They tend to contrast the research scientist with the clinical practitioner. The dichotomy is false and results in the creation of two stereotypes that represent the worst any helping profession has to offer. On one hand is the rigorous researcher who is so concerned with investigating the basic scientific elements of speech and language that she fails to see the pain that communicatively disordered clients are experiencing. On the other hand is the dedicated, caring, humanistic clinician who views data collection with as much anathema as one would a self-imposed lisp. The effective clinician is the one who understands the tragedy of communicative failures and realizes that the path to normalcy or improved communicative ability requires the rigorous application of scientific methods in a concerned, compassionate manner. The first step in the process is the objective observation of clinical behaviors.

REASONS FOR DATA COLLECTION

One often hears the statement, "I don't mark down every little correct answer; that interferes with therapy." Pleading that objectification of therapy dehumanizes clinical interactions usually is an attempt to hide sloppy and inefficient methods. The collection of objective data is important for reasons of assessment, accountability, and client motivation.

Assessment

Assessment procedures enable the speech-language pathologist to distinguish one communication problem from other problems that it may resemble (Johnson et al., 1959). These procedures may involve normative assessments or the recording of speech and language samples. The data gathered not only will be used for diagnostic purposes but also can serve as baseline data for assessing the effectiveness of therapeutic programs. Assessment needs to be continual because therapy is a dynamic process that involves continual behavioral and attitudinal changes. When these changes occur, the clinician will need to adjust the clinical program. If one relies on inappropriate intuitive knowledge or periodic assessments, either time may be wasted or clients may be placed in a new phase of therapy for which they are not yet ready. By continually assessing progress, therapy can be efficient and effective.

Accountability

We live in an era of accountability. It is no longer sufficient to describe a client's progress or lack of progress by using terms such as *better, worse,* and *somewhat improved*. Clients and their parents have a right to know just how much improvement has occurred and how the clinician has made the determination. Additionally, school districts, insurance carriers, and university supervisors tend to be unimpressed with the use of ambiguous terms such as *better*. In a school district in Illinois, a Down syndrome child was seen twice a week by a speech-language pathologist for language therapy. For an entire semester only marginal progress notes were kept. At the scheduled IEP meeting, the mother asked to see the progress the child had made. When she was presented with short, general, descriptive paragraphs of her child's progress, she said, "This doesn't tell me anything. Show me how you know my daughter has progressed. Where's your data?" The embarrassed therapist had to indicate that she did not keep data records. Her descriptive paragraphs reflected her "feelings" about the child. The case raised some difficult ethical issues for the speech-language pathologist and legal ones for the school district.

Lawsuits in the area of speech-language pathology were unheard of 30 years ago. With increased interest in client rights and the possibility of large malpractice insurance awards, the speech-language pathologist's legal vulnerability has increased (Silverman, 1983). By keeping adequate and detailed records, speech-language pathologists can minimize their exposure to lawsuits.

Motivation

Clients often have difficulty detecting subtle changes in their own behavior. It is not enough for the clinician to assure them that progress is being made. It is more impressive and meaningful to refer to objective data. For example, a stutterer's speech may display little difference to the listener when comparing an 84% fluency rate to an 87% fluency rate. The stutterer himself may not even be able to detect the difference. However, in clinical terms, any movement towards fluency is significant. Unless the clinician can convince the client that progress has occurred, important attitudinal shifts may not occur. If the clinician can refer the client to baseline data showing an 84% fluency rate prior to therapy and an 87% fluency rate after three therapy sessions, the client may begin to realize that fluency is in fact an obtainable goal.

The importance of providing feedback on achievement has been recognized by cognitive psychologists (Deci, 1975). Knowing that you are succeeding at a task that in the past appeared unobtainable is very motivating. Various studies have shown that, although achievement is not necessarily reinforcing for all people, a significant portion of both children and adults studied were intrinsically reinforced by achievement (de Charms, 1968).

❑ ❑ ❑ *PRINCIPLES OF OBSERVATION*

Before a problem can be corrected it should be observed. It is important not only to diagnose the specific speech, language, or hearing disorder but also to observe and identify all factors that can have a bearing on therapy. If observation is to be useful, it must be precise. Precision requires objective measurement through data collection. Observations involve multidimensional analysis that should not be contaminated by value judgments. They can be conducted within various contexts and involve precise recordings by the clinician or an individual whose function is to observe the client's behaviors.

A Multidimensional Process

When observing and describing a clinical interaction, it is imperative to remember that the interaction is constantly changing as a result of each participant's production and reception of messages. If the clinician asks a threatening question, the feelings it engenders in the client change a pleasant interaction into one filled with hostility. A child with limited conversational skills, who has always been reticent to converse with adults, becomes an animated storyteller in the presence of a sensitive accepting clinician. In these situations and in hundreds of other real examples, the interaction is a continually changing event that can be better understood by examining the multidimensional communication processes that are simultaneously occurring. Take, for example, a clinical diad consisting of a very defensive parent and a nervous new clinician who is conducting her first interview. The clinician sits down, smiles, and says to the parent, "I'm very happy for the opportunity to meet you." While smiling and indicating verbally that she has been looking forward to the interaction, the clinician's hand trembles slightly, the muscles of her neck are tensed, and her legs are rigidly crossed. The parent also smiles and responds, "Yes, I also have been looking forward to our meeting." While saying this the parent leans far back in her chair away from the clinician, avoids direct eye contact, and displays a staccato vocal pattern. Without making an interpretation, one might question whether the clinician and parent have really been looking forward to this interaction. The interaction is very complex, and the verbal messages of both parent and clinician may not be truthful. An examination of each interactant's nonverbal behaviors might clarify the true feelings of each person. Although the tendency in observing interactions of this type is to make an immediate judgment regarding affect, it should be avoided until sufficient observational data are obtained.

A Nonjudgmental Process

It is difficult to observe something without including a judgment in the observation. Yet the importance of objective observation is critical within a clinical context. If an observation contains an evaluative judgment, the information that is being collected becomes inherently distorted. For example, a clinician used the following statement to describe a child in the clinic:

> This child entered the clinic wearing a dirty blouse and skirt, both of which were not ironed, nor matched in colors.

This seemingly nonjudgmental statement is value-loaded. The blouse was covered with peanut butter following a hurried lunch eaten in the car. The child's skirt was covered with finger paint that had spilled on it during a creative activity at the day-care center. Because the mother was told that the children would be finger painting, she purposely chose the oldest skirt she could find for her daughter. The impression one gets from reading the clinician's description of the child is very different from the reality of the situation. To label the blouse and skirt as "dirty" denotes a judgment about the child's cleanliness and possibly parental child care practices. Also saying that the blouse was "not ironed" reinforces the image of an unkempt, sloppy little girl. This would be a more objective and less judgmental description:

> She was wearing a blue blouse spotted with peanut butter. The blouse was wrinkled on both the front and back panels. Her brown skirt was covered with large areas of finger paint.

The observer should not only write the report in this manner but also begin thinking in this way. The child may have in fact been both dirty and sloppy. However, to make that assumption without further evidence could seriously bias the observer's assessment of the child and her parents.

Can we avoid making judgments about our clients while we are observing and interacting with them? According to the linguist Edward Sapir (1921) it is not possible to escape injecting judgment in our observations because our observations are in the form of language, and language involves concepts that are based on our cultural values. Does this mean that it is not possible to make objective observations? The question of whether it is possible to make "purely" objective observations is of less clinical importance than examining how we can minimize the effects of value judgments on observation.

In the early 20th century this problem was addressed by the philosopher Edmund Husserl (1964). To Husserl, questions of epistemology, or knowledge, were of critical importance. He was concerned with how one can observe the "essence" of an object or event without allowing other things to color the observation. His solution to the problems of knowledge has relevance for clinical observations. For Husserl, the solution involved a process called *bracketing*, whereby the sensations we are having are reduced to their elemental form, devoid of judgment and interpretation.

> Thus to each psychic lived process there corresponds through the device of phenomenological reduction a pure phenomenon, which exhibits its intrinsic (immanent) essence (taken individually) as an absolute datum. (p. 35)

He called this process "phenomenological reductionism." A complex event is observed and bracketed into its elemental parts. This reductionism allows the observer to "see" each of the elements individually, experiencing them prior to making a judgment. After the observation is complete, the observer can then reformulate the experience and have a clear understanding of what occurred. Clinically, this process allows us to understand complex interactions objectively. Events are reduced to their most elemental forms and then reassembled with maximum objectivity.

Contexts for Observing

The bracketing of events usually occurs in four settings in which observations take place: (a) home, (b) school, (c) clinic waiting area, and (d) clinic room. Within each setting, the client can be observed with various individuals, engaging in formal and informal activities. Each type of observation may provide information on different aspects of the client's behavior. By assembling all the bits, a more or less complete picture of the client may be developed. This collage, sometimes referred to as an "approximation of knowledge" (Webb et al., 1966), can provide important information to the clinician.

By observing the client in a variety of contexts, the resulting picture is likely to be more representative of the client's behaviors than if only one or a few contexts were used. Within each context, clients should be observed both in low-structured and elicited tasks. By combining both types of observations, the clinician will be best able to develop a representative sample of the client's speech and language behaviors (Lahey, 1988).

Number and Length of Observations

Regardless of where the behaviors are observed, it is important that the clinician specify the duration of the observation. Duration is the length of time behaviors are observed. The criteria for determining whether responses or time are specified usually depend on what is being observed. In many forms of language sampling, for instance, the number of utterances is the criterion used. Tyack and Gottsleben (1974) suggest that 100 utterances be used for a representative language sample, as does Brown (1973) for calculating the mean length of utterance. Lahey (1988) prefers that 200 or more utterances are recorded for a representative language sample. When analyzing articulation disorders, McDonald suggests that each sound is observed in various phonemic contexts (1964). Fisher and Logemann have a 31-item test that examines the production of phonemes in initial, medial, and final position (1971).

Time as the unit of measurement is also appropriate for recording language samples. Lahey (1988) suggests that if 200 utterances cannot be obtained because of time restrictions, then the observation should last for at least 30 minutes. Time is the preferred unit of measurement in the area of stuttering. Goldberg (1981) records 5-minute samples of stutterers' speech in three different contexts. Costello and Ingham (1984a) use a 1-minute ABAB probing design.

Unfortunately, there is little research indicating what is the "best" number of responses or duration for recording representative samples of different speech and language disorders. A useful rule of thumb is that the larger the sample in various contexts, the more likely it will be representative.

Observer Roles

The types of observations that are possible and the effect observers will have on the interaction may be determined by their roles. In general, three observer roles can be assumed within a clinical context.

Participant Observer. An important function of a clinician is to serve as an observer. Since speech-language pathologists are observing while engaging in the clinical interaction, they are participant observers. Although observation by the clinician is something that is always required, it is the most difficult kind of observation to perform for two reasons. First, clinicians are usually so intent on conducting instructional or manipulative activities, that they may not notice important pieces of client information. This problem can be overcome by recording each session after written permission has been received from the client or parent. In a study conducted by the author, even very experienced, highly competent clinicians were often unable to recount immediately after a session certain important events that occurred.

The second problem with assuming the role of a participant observer is one that has historically created problems for anthropologists. That is the loss of objectivity by becoming too immersed within a culture (Naroll & Naroll, 1963). The clinical equivalent would be losing sight of behaviors or problems because of the desire to see the client or program succeed. For example, the clinician who feels a personal commitment to a nonverbal psychotic child she has been working with may unconsciously avoid seeing the resurfacing of autistic behaviors that had been eliminated months ago by a brilliant program published by the clinician.

Visible Observer. The visible observer is usually the person who is sitting within the therapy room while a session is progressing. Although their presence may initially distort the behaviors of those being observed, their disruptive effects tend to be diminished after a relatively short amount of time (Bales, 1950; Deutsch, 1949). If the observer becomes a somewhat permanent fixture, the effects on the client's behaviors are continually reduced with each session. The author has found that usually after the first 10 minutes of a session, the behaviors exhibited by the client tend to be indicative of the behaviors present when observers are not present. The same general rule of thumb should be applied when observable audiotape or videotape recorders are introduced for the first time.

Nonvisible Observer. The nonvisible observer usually sits behind a one-way glass, concealed in an observation booth. Often the nonvisible status of the observer is illusionary. Even very young clients often know that people are observing them from behind the large mirrors that serve no apparent purpose in a room. When this occurs, or when in training programs, clinicians routinely explain to clients that they may be observed; the same admonitions given about visible observers apply.

DATA COLLECTION DEVICES

Data can be recorded through various methods ranging from the sophistication of electrical responses triggered by muscular movements to the simplicity of writing checks on a piece of paper. Data can be collected in speech pathology and audiology in four major ways: (a) videotapes, (b) audiotapes, (c) electronic or mechanical counting devices, and (d) written forms.

Videotapes

Videotape provides the clinician with a permanent, accurate record of an entire interaction. It records nonverbal behaviors, verbal behaviors, and the environment in which the interaction occurred. It is imperative that prior to video- or audio-recording a client, a written permission is obtained. Microphones and cameras placed within the therapy room usually lose their "interfering" qualities after the initial 10 or 15 minutes. The devices tend not to inhibit clients' behaviors in subsequent sessions. The sound quality of the newer VHS recorders is adequate for analysis, provided that the remote microphone is sufficiently sensitive or an omni-directional microphone is placed close to the client. A videotape may be technological "overkill" if one is merely interested in counting something as simple as the number of verbal interactions that occurred. Additionally, the use of a VHS system may not be available to the clinician. A reasonable alternative in many cases is a good quality audio recorder.

Audiotapes

The recording quality of audio recorders tends to be less a problem than their playback abilities. Mini-recorders with very small speakers are almost useless for doing phonetic transcriptions. The dynamic range of these speakers makes it difficult to distinguish between phonemes that differ from each other only in a few distinctive features, such as /p/ and /t/. Playback features are critical in selecting audio recorders. If the speaker is not adequate, a good set of earphones should be used. Two useful features available on some more expensive models are instantaneous pausing and modifiable speeds. With instantaneous pausing, when the tape is stopped and then restarted, very few or no gaps in playback occur. This can save time when transcribing a language sample, where the tape must be continually stopped and restarted. Some audiotape recorders allow for increasing and decreasing the speed by up to 20%. Although the speaker's pitch becomes distorted, the audiotape recorder can either allow the listener to reduce the amount of time necessary to hear the content of a recording, or reduce the rate of speech, allowing for easier transcribing of a language sample.

The advantage of both audio and video recorders is that they allow the observer or clinician to record behaviors that may be too fast or too complicated to observe "live." For example, a written transcription would be required if one wished to count the various types of linguistic units a child uttered during a session. It would be very difficult to write down all of the child's utterances as they are occurring. Audio- and videotapes allow us to repeat segments of the interaction so we can accurately record data. However, this also is its disadvantage. When one uses recording devices, the assumption is that the material will be reviewed after the session has occurred. Therefore, if the session lasted one hour, you will probably spend at least an additional hour in assessing your data. This is appropriate when the data are complicated or occur too rapidly to record. However, a significant amount of data collected by speech pathologists and audiologists can be recorded instantaneously through the use of counters or a checkmark system.

Counters

Often, the behaviors we wish to record are very simple and can be noted by a simple recording method. For example, if we wished to record merely the number of verbs a child used during a session, it would not be necessary to use an audio- or videotape. Each time a verb is used, the observer or clinician could press a lever on an electronic or mechanical counting device. Each new student should have in their possession two mechanical counters. The simplest and least expensive type is the "grocery" counter, priced at less than a few dollars. With a simple click, the observer records the occurrence of a behavior and continues the observation. A simple calculator may serve the same function if you press the "+" and "1" keys following each occurrence of a behavior.

Written Forms

When counters are unavailable or inappropriate, another simple way of recording data is to use a checkmark table, where a column of numbers is written and a checkmark is placed next to each number as a behavior occurs. Table 3.1 is one example of this method. For clinicians recording data while doing therapy, it is important that they list as much information as possible on the form prior to beginning the clinical interaction. The goal is to limit record keeping during therapy to a simple checkmark.

SAMPLING PROCEDURES

It is not always possible or necessary to observe a complete session to develop a representative picture of the client's behaviors. Certain types of behaviors are so constant that a fairly small sampling will result in an accurate description of the behavior. For example, a person with a motor speech problem will most likely display the problem throughout the session (Dworkin, 1991). The stutterer's rate of speech will probably remain constant during any 5-minute segment of the session (Peters & Guitar, 1991). An individual with pitch breaks will probably exhibit them during a controlled 15-minute segment of a 60-minute session (Aronson, 1990). Various procedures can be used to sample behaviors. Two of the most common are timed segments throughout the session and designated segments.

Timed Segments Throughout the Session

Recording certain types of responses for an entire session can be tedious. The speech rate of stutterers is a good example. Instead of counting all syllables spoken throughout the session, a sampling technique devised by Costello and Ingham (1984b) and modified by the author can be used. It involves initially recording 10 one-minute samples of the stutterer's speech, evenly spaced throughout the session. An analysis of the 1st, 5th, and 10th sample may provide a rough estimate of the client's speech rate. The remaining 7 samples should be analyzed to confirm the rates recorded on the first 3 samples. A similar procedure may be used when attempting to measure other behaviors that have a constancy of occurrence, such as pitch breaks or distortions caused by motor speech disorders.

Designated Segment

An alternative method of sampling involves designating a timed segment during the middle of the session which will function as the observation period. The

Table 3.1
Data collection form

Correct Behavior:_____

Criteria for Advancement to Next Task: 90%___

√ = correct response
X = incorrect response

Response Number for Each Trial	Trial 1	Trial 2	Trial 3
1			
2			
3			
4			
5			
6			
7			
8			
9			
10			
11			
12			
13			
14			
15			
16			
17			
18			
19			
20			
Correct Responses			
Percentage Correct			

advantage of this procedure is that it provides the observer with an opportunity to record variations in the behavior that might not be evident by recording more observations of shorter duration. For example, with individuals who have a cognitive disorder, the ability to concentrate on a task may deteriorate rapidly after 10 consecutive minutes have passed. By sampling only a series of one-minute segments, the collected data might not indicate the existence of the problem.

UNITS OF MEASUREMENT

Numerous types of data can be collected, ranging from the occurrence of a behavior to a measurement of its strength. The type of data collected depends on its purpose. One should not collect data just for the sake of appearing objective. The clinician should first identify the goals of therapy and then determine the most appropriate form of data that will facilitate its completion. Various authors have listed the general methods of behavior analysis that are commonly found in clinical situations (Emmert & Brooks, 1970; Mowrer, 1982). Eight very useful techniques for describing clinical behaviors will be explained in this section. They are (a) simple enumeration, (b) number of correct responses, (c) percentage of correct responses, (d) learning curve, (e) type token ratio, (f) latency of response, (g) amplitude of response, and (h) rating scales. In this section, these and other common forms of clinical analysis are discussed.

Simple Enumeration

Simple enumeration involves counting the number of responses in a given period of time or during a specific activity. For example, we could specify the number of words a client spoke during a 10-minute period of observation or the number of words spoken while a child was playing a specific game. Much important observational data can be gathered by simply counting responses. With little training this easy method of data collection can provide the clinician with critical information. Of prime importance is to collect data without being judgmental. To describe an event or interaction in non-judgmental terms requires the clinician to be as objective as possible. Value loaded terms such as *good, better, nice,* and *enjoyable,* for example, should be scrupulously avoided. In simple enumeration, only the number of occurrences are recorded. In Table 3.2, three examples of counting behaviors are given: the number of times a client left her seat, the number of times she said "I don't know," and the number of times she did not respond verbally. Every time one of the three behaviors occurs, a "√" is placed in the appropriate column. At the end of the session, the occurrences of the three behaviors are totaled and appear at the bottom of each column.

Number of Correct Responses

When counting correct responses one must first specify the contents of two categories, "correct" and all others. Only responses that meet specific criteria are designated as correct. All others are incorrect. Criteria are the standards by which we determine the presence of correct responses. This may seem self-evident and simplistic. However, the clinician should begin the practice of behaviorally specifying the criteria for a correct response. For example, if the clinician is going to record the number of times that the client correctly identifies specific objects, the criterion for a correct response might be "A correct response occurs only when the *first* pointing gesture of the client is to the target object." Criteria for "correctness" should be as objective as possible.

Percentage of Correct Responses

Often, we wish to know more than the number of correct responses a client is producing. A percentage of correct responses may be a critical indicator of when

Table 3.2
Counting behaviors: Three examples

Instructions: Place a "√" when a behavior occurs under each appropriate category.

Length of Time for the Observation: 30 minutes

	Number of Times Client Left Seat	Number of Times Client Said "I Don't Know"	Number of Times Client Did Not Respond Verbally
1	√		
2	√	√	√
3	√	√	√
4	√	√	√
5		√	√
6		√	√
7		√	√
8		√	
9		√√	
10			
11			
12			
13			
14			
15			
16			
17			
18			
19			
20			
Total Behaviors	4	8	6

to advance the client to a more complicated task. This is known as the *criteria for advancement.* The criteria for advancement tell the clinician when the client has mastered a specific task. Various research studies have been done to determine when mastery occurs. Dietrich & Bangert (1980) maintain that a criterion of 75 to 80% is sufficient to advance to the next task. Costello (1982) uses a 85 to 90% criterion. Hedge and Davis (1992) believe that a minimum criterion should be 90% and that some disorders, such as stuttering, require a 97 or 98% criterion. Obviously, the closer clients get to 100% the more we can be assured that they have learned whatever it is we are teaching them. However, to use 100% would be too severe, since it would not allow for errors of inattention or errors not related to learning. A figure of 80% may be marginal, since research indicates that it is approximately the lowest criterion for learning. A good compromise, then, would be 90%, because it assures us that the client has mastered the task.

To compute the percentage of correct responses, divide the number of correct responses by the total number of responses:

$$\text{Percentage of Correct Responses} = \frac{\text{Number of Correct Responses}}{\text{Total Number of Responses}}$$

An example of how one would compute the percentage of accurate responses appears in Table 3.3.

Table 3.3
Computing percentage of correct responses

Correct Behavior: Client points to specified object on first attempt.

Criteria for Advancement to Next Task: 90% of 20 responses correct

√ = correct response
x = incorrect response

Number of Responses for Each Trial	Trial 1	Trial 2	Trial 3
1	√	√	√
2	√	√	√
3	√	√	√
4	x	√	√
5	x	√	√
6	√	√	√
7	√	√	√
8	√	√	√
9	√	√	√
10	x	√	√
11	√	√	√
12	√	√	√
13	x	x	x
14	x	x	√
15	x	√	√
16	x	x	√
17	x	√	x
18	x	√	√
19	x	x	√
20	x	x	√
Correct Responses	9	15	18
Percentage Correct	(9/20) = 45% (Repeat activity)	(15/20) = 75% (Repeat activity)	(18/20) = 90% (Go to next activity)

Learning Curve

In Table 3.3, we can see that our client seemed to improve with each new trial. Initially, only 45% of his responses were correct. This was followed by 75% accuracy and finally 90% accuracy. If we looked only at these three percentages, we could conclude that he seems to be learning more on each additional trial. However, our assessment of the client or our program would be different if the percentage of accuracy figures were respectively, 45%, 47%, and 45%. Learning curves are also useful for comparing the abilities of different clients. Let us assume that we are working with two clients who have a similar problem. For example, in a school setting you may be seeing two 7-year-old children together who both have w/r misarticulations. Since both children have the same type of error, are the same age, and are in the same class, you may decide to use the same intervention program for both. After three attempts to reach a criterion of 90%, you notice a significant difference in their abilities to perform the task. The first child's percentages of correct responses were respectively 45, 75, and 90. The second child's were 45, 47, and 45. If the results from our two hypothetical children were plotted on a graph, the comparison of their abilities becomes more dramatic (Figure 3.1). This graph indicates to us that our second child may require a significantly greater number of trials to achieve success than is expected

Figure 3.1
Learning curves of two different clients

PERCENTAGE CORRECT

	Trial 1	Trial 2	Trial 3
Client 1	45	75	90
Client 2*	45	47	45

Criterion for advancement = 90%

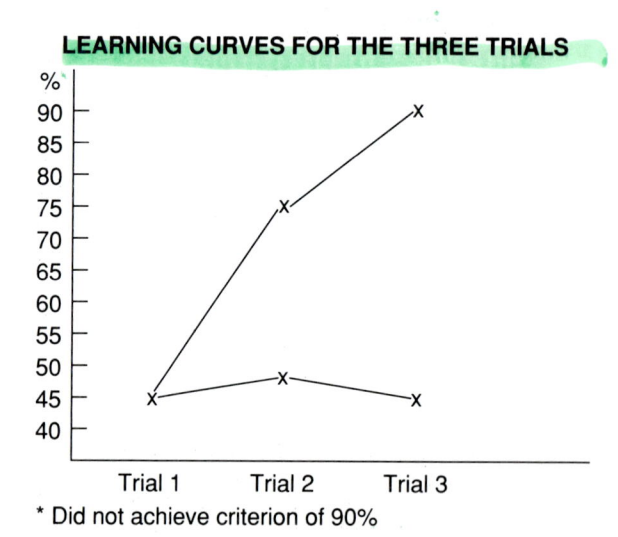

LEARNING CURVES FOR THE THREE TRIALS

* Did not achieve criterion of 90%

with other clients, or the program is too difficult. With this information, we might adjust our expectations of the client, or redesign our program so that it better fits the needs of the client. It is also possible to examine various learning curves of a single client. This would be done to see if the mastery of one task had any effect on other related tasks. For example, let us assume that we want to teach a client to identify four different objects when we say, "Point to the (object)." The tasks are similar since they involve the identification of objects, yet dissimilar because the objects—a ball, car, block, and doll—are used in varying ways by the client. In each learning activity various sizes and shapes of the target object are juxtaposed to other types of objects. There may be, for example, three different balls, each a different size and color. Since we are teaching the concept of ball, we want our client to identify all three objects as "ball" when we ask him to respond. In this example, we use this same procedure in the identification of the other three objects. On task 1 (ball) and on task 2 (car), it took the client 4 trials to achieve our 90% criterion (Figure 3.2a and b). On task 3 (block), the 90% criterion was reached in 3 trials (Figure 3.2c). On task 4 (doll), criterion was achieved in only 2 trials (Figure 3.2d). If we superimpose all four graphs, it becomes apparent that our client has been able to apply what he has learned in one task to other similar but different tasks (Figure 3.2e).

Type Token Ratio

Often when we count behaviors, we may wish to note the ratio of one type of behavior to all other behaviors. This is known as a *type token ratio.* It is most often used in language analysis when we wish to determine the ratio of different words children use to all of the words. To obtain this measure, a language sample is taken of either a specified number of utterances or the utterances spoken during a given number of minutes. A transcription is made, and each individual word and the number of times it occurs is noted. The number of different words are then divided by the total number of words to determine the type token ratio.

$$\text{Type Token Ratio} = \frac{\text{Number of Different Words}}{\text{Total Number of Words}}$$

Type token ratios can indicate a lack of richness or sophistication in children's language, since it can show that a child who is very verbal may in fact be using a small repertoire of different words. Type token ratios can also be determined for other aspects of language. For example, one may wish to determine a ratio of questions to all types of utterances a client uses. Type token ratios may also be determined for nonverbal behaviors. When working with a psychotic child, the clinician may wish to determine the ratio of communicative nonverbal behaviors to all nonverbal behaviors. An example of how to perform a type token ratio for individual words appears in Table 3.4.

Latency of Response

The *latency of a response* is the period of time that occurs between the presentation of a stimulus and the occurrence of a response. This measurement may be

Figure 3.2
Advancing learning curves of a single client across tasks

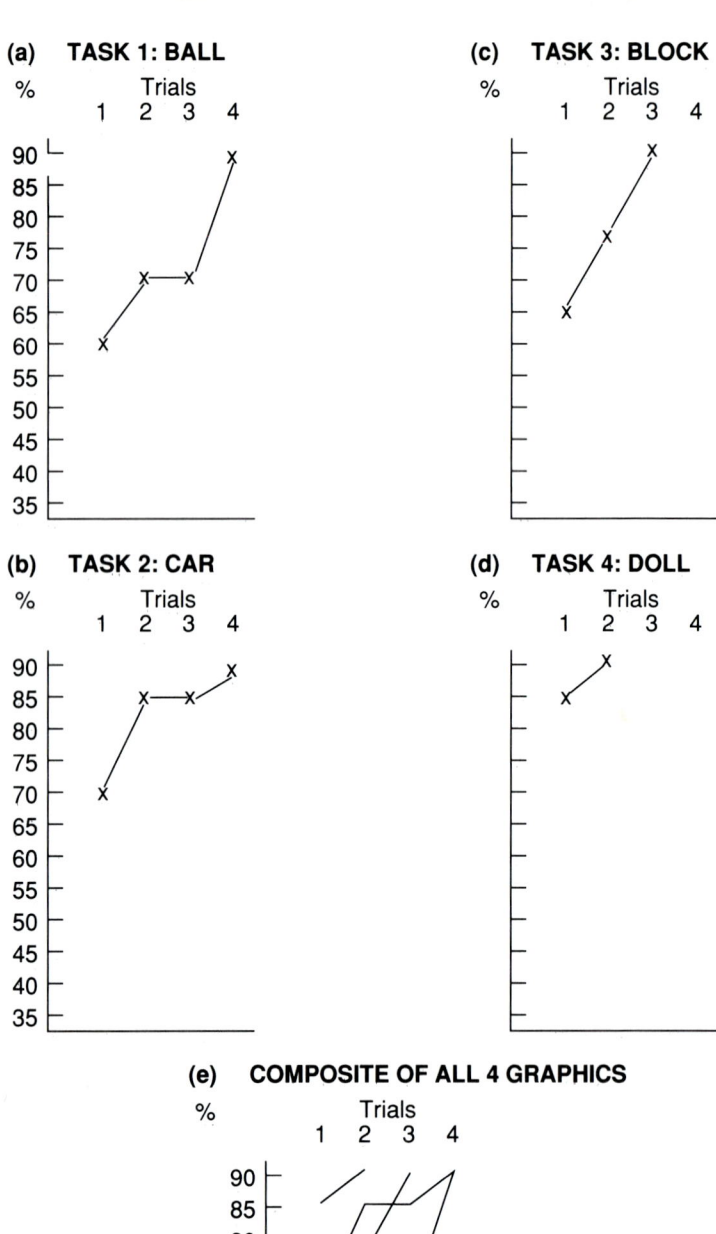

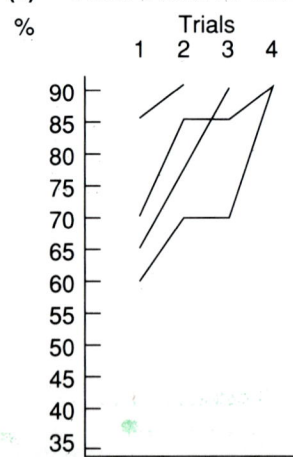

Table 3.4
Type token ratio example

Sample Size: 5 utterances

1. I want to go home.
2. My mommy is at home.
3. Do you have a mommy and a home?
4. My daddy and my mommy go home.
5. My home is over there, with mommy and daddy.

Analysis:

Number of Different Words	Word	Occurrences	Percentage of Total Sample
1	I	1	2.6
2	want	1	2.6
3	to	1	2.6
4	go	2	5.1
5	home	5	16.1
6	my	4	10.3
7	mommy	4	10.3
8	is	2	5.1
9	at	1	2.6
10	do	1	2.6
11	you	1	2.6
12	have	1	2.6
13	a	2	5.1
14	and	3	7.7
15	daddy	2	5.1
16	over	1	2.6
17	there	1	2.6
18	with	1	2.6

Total Number of Words = 39
Number of Different Words = 18

TTR = 18/39
    = .41

---

important in assessing either the client's motivation or ability to process the information contained in the stimulus. The following example will clarify the distinction. A clinician has been presenting a language disordered child with a simple classification task. When shown a picture of a form, the child has to identify it as either a circle, square, triangle, or rectangle. In a trial of 20 items containing equal numbers of each form, the child identifies 95% of them correctly. Although a 95% correct figure may be high enough for the clinician to proceed to the next task, she is concerned about the amount of time the child required before responding. The latency of response ranged between 5 and 30 seconds. At the most superficial level, the child may just be bored. If that is the case, the clinician may decide to increase the child's motivation by either presenting more interesting stimuli or introducing some form of reinforcement for correct responses. A new, more interesting stimulus could take the form of blocks having the four shapes. Reinforcers, such as tokens, for correct responses could be used at the end of the session to purchase a desirable item. If after trying both modifications of her program the child's latency of response does not significantly improve, the clinician may conclude that for this child, the processing of incoming information requires a longer amount of time than would be necessary for most children. To accommodate the child's processing problems, the clinician would provide the client an ample amount of time to respond before assuming that the child did not know the answer.

Amplitude of Response

In certain situations a clinician may wish to measure the strength of a response. The lowest strength at which a stimulus can elicit a response is known as the *response threshold*. In audiometry, a *threshold* is defined as the point at which a stimulus is recognized 50% of the time. The meaning of response threshold in speech-language pathology is somewhat different.

Measures of amplitude can be subjective or objective. One way of subjectively measuring a response is through the use of rating scales or evaluative terms. The problems associated with either approach will be discussed in the next section. The objective assessment of response amplitude depends on careful instrumentation. For example, the loudness of a client's voice can be measured by noting the excursion of the needle on a VU meter when voicing occurs. Other examples are the galvanic skin response (GSR) readings a stutterer would record while speaking or the strength of alpha waves a client may generate while using a biofeedback device.

Rating Scales

It is not always possible to be as objective as one would like. Although clinical impressions may be important, they tend to lack the objectivity necessary for accurately assessing the status of a communicative disorder. Take for example a clinician who refers to a client as a "moderate" stutterer. Unless one clearly understands what "moderate" means to the clinician, the term will be confusing to the listener or reader of a report. Various researchers have attempted to minimize the problem by anchoring judgments to numbered rating scales and uniformly training observers. For example, in describing a stutterer's speech the following scale may be used:

Very Severe	Severe	Moderate	Mild	Very Mild
1	2	3	4	5

By arranging value judgments on a 5-point rating scale, a certain degree of objectivity is introduced. Rating scales can contain a smaller or larger point spread.

Although the introduction of a rating scale does help in objectifying value judgments, it still leaves much to be desired. When possible, category names should be related to specific behavioral measurements. For example, if someone is to be labeled "severe," two of the following hypothetical criteria must be met:

1. 30% of their speech during a 10-minute sample must be disfluent.
2. Blocks must be at least 10 seconds in duration.

When both criteria are met, the person can then be called a "severe" stutterer. Disagreement, however, is still present, since one might reasonably question whether a 30% disfluency rate is too high or the 10-second block criterion is too short. Rating scales, therefore, although not as precise as other methods of describing behaviors, may be the only reasonable alternative a clinician has to saying or writing nothing that could be interpreted as "subjective." Rating scales provide "soft," but often important information.

SUMMARY

In this chapter the principles of observation and measurement were discussed along with methods of recording data. It was emphasized that the observer should have minimal impact on the clinical interaction. To observe objectively and accurately requires that the observer forgo evaluations until the observation process is completed.

Throughout the therapy process clinicians function both as observers and interventionists. At times, the requirements of one role result in inadequate functioning in the other. Unfortunately, clinicians usually must do both, simultaneously observing and intervening. By developing observational skills prior to engaging in therapy, the new clinician will be better able to deal with the complexities of the clinical situation.

SUGGESTED READINGS

de Charms, R. (1968). *Personal causation: The internal affective determinants of behavior.* New York: Academic Press.

Deci, E. L. (1975). *Intrinsic motivation.* New York: Plenum Press.

Mowrer, D. E. (1982). *Methods of modifying speech behaviors.* (2nd ed.). Columbus, OH: Merrill.

Silverman, F. H. (1983). *Legal aspects of speech-language pathology and audiology.* Englewood Cliffs, NJ: Prentice-Hall.

Webb, E. J.; Campbell, D. T.; Schwartz, R. D.; & Sechrest, L. (1966). *Unobtrusive measures.* Chicago: Rand McNally & Co.

❏ **Activity 3.1**
Simple Enumeration

Ask a clinician to identify a specific behavior that she or he will be attempting to teach the client and the number of times it will be attempted during each trial. For example, a clinician may attempt to have a child correctly use target verb phrases. A list of 10 pictures will be shown to the child. The target behavior is the correct use of a verb phrase with each picture. There would be 10 possible responses for each trial. First, record the correct and incorrect responses for three different trials, and then graph the child's learning curve. Share this analysis with the clinician.

Correct Behavior:_____

Criteria for Advancement to Next Task: 90%

√ = correct response   X = incorrect response

Response Number for Each Trial	Trial 1	Trial 2	Trial 3
1			
2			
3			
4			
5			
6			
7			
8			
9			
10			
11			
12			
13			
14			
15			
16			
17			
18			
19			
20			
Correct Responses			
Percentage Correct			

Activity 3.1, continued

Learning Curve for Three Trials

%	Trial 1	Trial 2	Trial 3
90	-	-	-
85	-	-	-
80	-	-	-
75	-	-	-
70	-	-	-
65	-	-	-
60	-	-	-
55	-	-	-
50	-	-	-
45	-	-	-
40	-	-	-
35	-	-	-
30	-	-	-
25	-	-	-
20	-	-	-
15	-	-	-
10	-	-	-
5	-	-	-
0	-	-	-

❑ **Activity 3.2**
Type Token Ratio

It will be your task to perform a type token ratio of a client's language. Inform the clinician that you will be doing this and share your analysis with him or her. Begin by completing a transcription of the child's first 50 utterances. Write one utterance on each line. The sample you will be transcribing will be used in Chapter 5 when you perform a mean length of utterance (MLU) analysis.

After completing the transcription, list each word and indicate the number of times it was used. Then compute the percentage of occurrences for each word.

Sample Size: _____ minutes
Transcription (Only the child's language)

1. _____
2. _____
3. _____
4. _____
5. _____
6. _____
7. _____
8. _____
9. _____
10. _____
11. _____
12. _____
13. _____
14. _____
15. _____
16. _____
17. _____
18. _____
19. _____
20. _____
21. _____
22. _____

Activity 3.2, continued

23. _____
24. _____
25. _____
26. _____
27. _____
28. _____
29. _____
30. _____
31. _____
32. _____
33. _____
34. _____
35. _____
36. _____
37. _____
38. _____
39. _____
40. _____
41. _____
42. _____
43. _____
44. _____
45. _____
46. _____
47. _____
48. _____
49. _____
50. _____

Notes:

continues

Activity 3.2, continued

Analysis

	Word	Occurrences	Percentage of Total Sample
1.			
2.			
3.			
4.			
5.			
6.			
7.			
8.			
9.			
10.			
11.			
12.			
13.			
14.			
15.			
16.			
17.			
18.			
19.			
20.			
21.			
22.			
23.			
24.			
25.			
26.			
27.			

Activity 3.2, continued

Word	Occurrences	Percentage of Total Sample
28.		
29.		
30.		
31.		
32.		
33.		
34.		
35.		
36.		
37.		
38.		
39.		
40.		
41.		
42.		
43.		
44.		
45.		
46.		
47.		
48.		
49.		
50.		

Total Number of Words = _____

❑ *Activity 3.3*
Rating Scales

This activity should be done with at least three people. While observing the same sample, each person should individually rate the severity of the disorder. Then compare your ratings. Rate each sample from 1 (mild) to 5 (severe) and indicate the variables you used to arrive at your ratings.

Stuttering   Circle Appropriate Number

	Mild		Moderate		Severe
Subject 1	1	2	3	4	5

Explanation for Ratings:

Aphasia   Circle Appropriate Number

	Mild		Moderate		Severe
Subject 2	1	2	3	4	5

Explanation for Ratings:

Chapter 4
Speech Behaviors

STUDY GUIDE

- Describe three types of phonological disorders.
- What is a distinctive feature analysis and how is it applied to vowels and consonants?
- Describe the ways overt and covert stuttering behaviors can be measured.
- What are the various types of rate measurements that can be used in analyzing stuttering behaviors?
- List the major disorders of phonation.
- Describe the major disorders of resonance.
- What are the distinguishing features of cleft palate speech?

In this chapter the behaviors associated with four major types of speech disorders will be described: phonology, stuttering, voice, and cleft palate speech. Cleft palate speech is identified as a separate category because it involves disorders of both articulation and voice. The information in this chapter should be used as guidelines for the identification of behaviors, not as diagnostic tools. A comprehensive list of speech diagnostic tools appears in Appendixes C through G. Courses in each of these disorders and seminars in diagnostic procedures will provide the student with the appropriate knowledge of assessment instruments.

PHONOLOGY AND ARTICULATION

Phonological and articulatory disorders constitute a significant portion of most clinicians' caseload. Although most are developmentally related, some are physiologically based. In this section the behaviors that are considered disordered will be described. No distinction will be made between developmentally related and physiologically based disorders. Regardless of the etiology, the behaviors can be described using the same methods.

Phonemes

When describing a client's normal and disordered phonology, we are interested in describing as objectively as possible the manner in which sounds are produced. A list of sounds, or phonemes, in the English language appears in Table 4.1. Students unfamiliar with phonetics should continually refer to this table until they acquire a knowledge of phonetic transcription. Students who know phonetic transcription can ignore Table 4.1. These phonetic symbols are used to describe both normal articulation and misarticulations. A *misarticulation* is the absence, addition, or production of a sound that is different from the one that should occur within a word. Not all misarticulations are considered to be disorders, since the ability to correctly produce all phonemes is gradually acquired over a period of six or seven years. For example, a 2-year-old child who is substituting /w/ for /r/ in the word *rabbit* is misarticulating the /r/ phoneme, but does not have a phonological disorder since the ability to produce the /r/ phoneme does not develop for another two years. Guidelines for distinguishing between a misarticulation and a phonological disorder have been derived from three major, classic studies on the acquisition of English phonemes by children. A comparison of them appears in Table 4.2 (Templin, 1957).

Types of Disorders

Four different types of phonological disorders can be identified: (a) additions, (b) distortions, (c) omissions, and (d) substitutions. Each of these phonological disorders can occur at the beginning, middle, or end of words and may involve vowels, diphthongs, or consonants.

Table 4.1
English phonemes

Vowels

[i] meat	[a] ask	[u] tool	[ɚ] onward
[ɪ] hit	[ɑ] calm	[ʊ] pull	[ʌ] but
[e] rate	[ɔ] tall	[ə] about	[ɛ] bet
[æ] hat	[o] moat	[ɝ] word	

Consonants

[b] big	[l] laugh	[s] some	[ŋ] sung	[h] happy
[k] cake	[m] many	[t] tie	[θ] thigh	
[d] dog	[n] nice	[v] vacuum	[ð] thy	
[f] fan	[p] pig	[w] watt	[ʃ] shame	
[g] game	[r] run	[z] zoo	[ʒ] azure	

Diphthongs

[eɪ] pail
[aɪ] mile
[ɔɪ] foil
[oʊ] foal
[aʊ] fowl

Combinations

[tʃ] chum
[dʒ] jam
[hw] when
[ju] youth

Additions. *Additions* involve the placement of an extraneous phoneme in the beginning, middle, or the end of a word. This type of articulation error is rarely encountered. When it does occur, it has little effect on the intelligibility of the speaker. Errors of this type are usually heard when a child is learning a new word. In attempting to match his production with that of a speaker, a certain amount of experimentation occurs. Often the misarticulation is in the form of an additional sound. With instruction from the speaker or increased opportunities to practice the word, the addition will often disappear without any need for direct intervention by the clinician. The occurrence of additions is so rare and so rarely requires remediation that many speech-language pathologists do not even consider it to be an articulation error (Bernthal & Bankson, 1981). An example of an addition would be "Mommy, please give me some more milky (milk)."

Distortions. A *distortion* that has been occurring within a child's phonetic repertoire consistently and over a long period of time would constitute an articulation disorder requiring remediation. These stable distortions need to be distinguished from distortions that are intermediary steps in the child's progress

Table 4.2
Comparison of the ages at which subjects correctly produced specific consonant sounds in the Templin, the Wellman, and the Poole studies

	Age Correctly Produced		
Sound	Templin (1957)	Wellman et al. (1931)	Poole (1934)
m	3	3	3.5
n	3	3	4.5
ŋ	3	—[a]	4.5
p	3	4	3.5
f	3	3	3.5
h	3	3	3.5
w	3	3	3.5
j	3.5	4	4.5
k	4	4	4.5
b	4	3	3.5
d	4	5	4.5
g	4	4	4.5
r	4	5	7.5
s	4.5	5	7.5[b]
ʃ	4.5	—[c]	6.5
tʃ	4.5	5	—[c]
t	6	5	4.5
θ	6	—[a]	7.5[b]
v	6	5	6.5[b]
l	6	4	6.5
ð	7	—[c]	6.5
z	7	5	7.5[b]
ʒ	7	—[c]	6.5
ʤ	7	6	—[c]
hw	—[a]	—[a]	7.5

Source: From "Certain language skills in children, their development and interrelationships" by M. C. Templin, 1957, *Institute of Child Welfare, Monograph Series,* No. 26, p. 54. Minneapolis: University of Minnesota Press. Reprinted by permission.

* In the Wellman et al. (1931) and Templin (1957) studies a sound was considered to be mastered if it was articulated correctly by 75% of the subjects. The criterion of correct production was 100% in the Poole (1934) study.

[a] Sound was tested but was not produced correctly by 75% of the subjects at the oldest age tested. In the Wellman data the "hw" reached the percentage criterion at 5 but not at 6 years, the medial "ŋ" reached it at 3, and the initial and medial "θ" and "ð" at 5 years.

[b] Poole (Davis, 1938), in a study of 20,000 preschool and school-age children reports the following shifts: s and z appear at 5.5 years and then disappear and return later at 7.5 years or above; θ appears at 6.5 years and v at 5.5 years.

[c] Sound not tested or not reported.

from producing an incorrect to a correct production of a phoneme. A both are considered to be distortions, the first requires remediation, whe second is the result of self- or other-directed remediation. For example, compare two 8-year-old children who are distorting /r/. The first has always distorted /r/ as a result of a too forward tongue placement. The second child's placement of her tongue is also too forward, but her distortion has resulted from efforts to eliminate her /w/ for /r/ substitution.

Vowel distortions are often identified as substitutions. For example, the difference between producing the phoneme /i/ as b*eat* and /I/ in b*i*t involves a difference of a fraction of an inch in tongue placement. A vowel distortion will more likely be perceived as a substitution rather than a distortion because a slightly missed target position of the tongue often results in the correct target position for an adjacent vowel. Distortions of consonants are more likely to be perceived as distortions.

Although each sound can be uniquely distorted, the majority of distortions that are heard can be classified as sounds associated with frontal and lateral lisps. A *frontal lisp* occurs when there is an excessive amount of air emission through the front of the mouth. Children who have a condition called "tongue thrust" frequently have frontal lisps. *Tongue thrust* involves the movement of the tongue toward the front of the mouth during the production of most sounds. A *lateral lisp* occurs when there is an excessive amount of air emission through the side of the mouth.

Omissions. *Omissions* can have the greatest effect on intelligibility because they significantly reduce the important cues a listener depends on for deriving meaning from an utterance. Children with auditory memory problems or cognitive deficits often omit the final sounds of multisyllabic words. The listener is more likely to understand utterances with final phoneme omissions than omissions that occur at the beginning or middle of a word. Contrast the following omission types with the same sentence, "Daddy, give me some more milk."

Initial Omission	: addy ive me ome ore ilk
Medial Omission	: Day, ge me so moe mk
Final Omission	: Dad, gi me some mo mil

Substitutions. The most common form of misarticulations in children are *substitutions* involving consonants. The substitution pattern is rarely random. The substituted phoneme usually involves features similar to those of the target phoneme. Intelligibility is minimally affected when there is only one or a few errors. However, when multiple substitution errors are present, a significant loss of intelligibility is likely.

Vowels

A vowel sound is formed as sound energy from the vibrating vocal folds escapes through an open vocal tract. There are two different ways of describing how vowels are produced: traditional and distinctive feature analysis. Each provides unique information on vowel production.

Traditional. Although various parts of the oral musculature are involved in the production of vowels, of critical importance to the speech-language pathologist are the position of the tongue and lips and the amount of tension used to produce the vowel. In Figure 4.1 the vowels are graphed on two placement continua and marked as having lip rounding and tension.

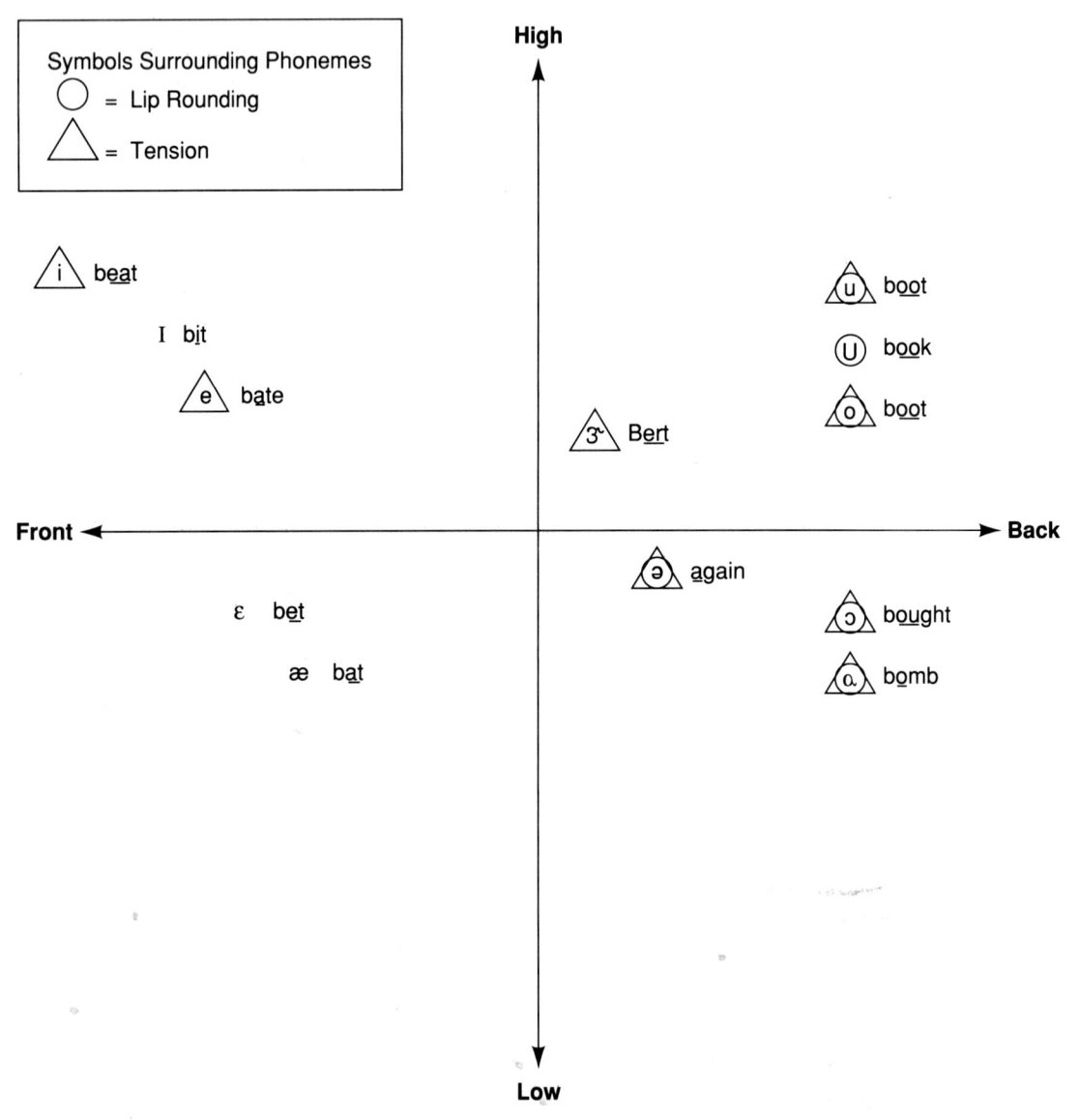

Symbols Surrounding Phonemes
○ = Lip Rounding
△ = Tension

High / Low

Front ← → Back

△i beat
I bit
△e bate
△ɜ˞ Bert
△ə again
ɛ bet
æ bat

△⊙u boot
⊙ʊ book
△⊙o boot
△⊙ɔ bought
△⊙ɑ bomb

Figure 4.1
Vowel productions

The tongue moves on two continua, *front* and *back*, and *high* and *low*. In Figure 4.1 the oral cavity is viewed from a side or midsagittal position. The tongue placement for each vowel is shown. For example, if one wished to describe the tongue placement of /i/, it would be high front. The vowel /ɜ/ would be described as midcenter on both continua. To produce the target sound correctly, placement of the tongue must be relatively precise. A slight incorrect placement can change b<u>e</u>t to b<u>a</u>t or b<u>a</u>te to b<u>i</u>t.

The production of vowels is also affected by the extent of lip rounding. In Figure 4.1 vowels that have lip rounding are indicated by a circle around the phonetic symbol. Vowels without lip rounding are not circled. Vowels can have only a bimodal classification in terms of lip rounding. In other words, sounds are produced with either rounded lips or unrounded lips.

A third clinically important feature of vowels is *tension*. Vowels can be classified as either *tense* (long) or *lax* (short). The tenseness or laxity of vowels refers to the amount of muscular tension necessary to produce them. In Figure 4.1 a triangle appears around each vowel that is identified as tense. Vowels with no triangles are lax.

Distinctive Feature Analysis. The uniqueness of vowels can be attributed to their distinctive features. The nine features Chomsky and Halle (1968) identified appear in Table 4.3. For any sound, the presence or absence of each feature is noted. A system such as this can provide the speech-language pathologist with a method for determining not only which sound substitution or distortion has occurred but also the specific feature error. Table 4.4 is a matrix of the 9 vowel features and 10 vowel sounds. The presence of a feature is indicated by a + and the absence of the feature by a −. The use of this table can aid the clinician in determining why an incorrect vowel was produced. For example, if a client was producing /I/ for /i/, a distinctive feature analysis would determine that the problem involved an error in the manner of production. The client was attempting to produce the sound with an insufficient amount of tension. Most vowel misarticulations usually result from only a few distinctive feature errors.

Diphthongs

A second group of sounds in the English language are called *diphthongs*. These are actually combinations of two vowels, such as the phoneme /aɪ/, in the words <u>I</u>, b<u>uy</u>, and n<u>i</u>ght. Since each is a combination of two sounds, diphthongs can be divided into *on glides* and *off glides*, corresponding to the first and the second phoneme portion of the diphthong. The four diphthongs in English are:

/aɪ/	<u>I</u>, b<u>uy</u>, wh<u>y</u>, <u>i</u>ce, n<u>i</u>ght
/oʊ/	tr<u>ou</u>t, d<u>ow</u>n, <u>ow</u>l
/ɔɪ/	b<u>oy</u>, <u>oi</u>l, h<u>oi</u>st
/aʊ/	b<u>ow</u>, n<u>o</u>, l<u>oa</u>d

Table 4.3
Distinctive features

Class Features

Sonorant sounds have a vocal configuration that permits spontaneous voicing, which means that the airstream can pass virtually unimpeded through the oral or nasal cavity. This feature distinguishes the vowels, glides, nasal consonants, and lateral and rhotacized consonants from the stops, fricatives, and affricates (the class of obstruents).

Vocalic sounds do not have a radical or marked constriction of the vocal tract and are associated with spontaneous voicing. The voiced vowels and liquids are vocalic; the voiceless vowels and liquids, glides, nasal consonants, and obstruents (stops, fricatives, and affricates) are nonvocalic (that is, -vocalic).

Consonantal sounds have a radical or marked constriction in the midsagittal region of the vocal tract. This feature distinguishes the "true" consonants from vowels and glides.

Cavity Features

High sounds are made with the tongue elevated above its neutral (resting) position.

Low sounds are made with the tongue lowered below its neutral position.

Back sounds are made with the tongue retracted from its neutral position.

Rounded sounds have narrowed or protruded lip configuration.

Nasal sounds are produced with lowered velum so that sound energy escapes through the nose.

Manner of Articulation

Tense refers to the amount of muscular tension necessary for producing the sound.

Source: From *Articulation disorders* (pp. 34–35) by J. E. Bernthal and N. W. Bankson, 1981, Englewood Cliffs, NJ: Prentice-Hall, Inc. Copyright 1981 by Prentice-Hall. Adapted by permission.

Table 4.4
Vowel distinctive features

	i	ɪ	ɛ	æ	ə	ɝ	u	ʊ	ɔ	ɑ
Class Features										
Sonorant	+	+	+	+	+	+	+	+	+	+
Vocalic	+	+	+	+	+	+	+	+	+	+
Consonantal	−	−	−	−	−	−	−	−	−	−
Cavity Features										
High	+	+	−	−	−	−	+	+	−	−
Low	−	−	−	+	−	−	−	−	+	+
Back	−	−	−	−	−	+	+	+	+	+
Rounded	−	−	−	−	−	+	+	+	+	−
Nasal	−	−	−	−	−	−	−	−	−	−
Manner of Articulation										
Tense	+	−	−	+	−	+	+	−	+	+

Consonants

Consonants differ from vowels and diphthongs primarily in terms of vocal tract openness. Whereas vowels are produced with an open vocal tract, consonants require the vocal tract to be constricted. Consonants, like vowels, can be analyzed using a traditional or a distinctive feature analysis.

Traditional Analysis. A traditional method of describing consonants involves reference to place of articulation, manner of articulation, and the presence or absence of voicing. Table 4.5 provides definitions for each term used to describe the place, manner, and voicing of consonants. In Table 4.6 these terms are applied to each consonant. When describing misarticulated consonants using the traditional method of analysis, it becomes possible to determine not only what major component of the phoneme's production is in error (place, manner, or voicing) but also the specific behavior within the compo-

Table 4.5
Traditional consonant analysis terminology

Place of Production

Bilabial. (*b*oth) Two lips together.

Labial/velar. (*w*hen) Involves two lips together while forming a constriction between the back of the tongue and the velum.

Labiodental. (*v*ery) Upper teeth resting on lower lip.

Linguadental (interdental). (*th*at) Tip of tongue is placed against upper teeth.

Lingua-alveolar. (*n*ice) Tip of tongue is placed against the alveolar ridge.

Linguapalatal. (*sh*ame) The blade of the tongue is placed against the palatal area immediately behind the alveolar ridge.

Linguavelar. (for*k*) The back of the tongue is pressed against the roof of the mouth in the velar area.

Glottal. Refers to sounds emanating between the two vocal folds.

Manner of Production

Stop. (*d*addy) The articulators completely block the flow of air, then release it suddenly, causing the escape to create a sound.

Fricatives. (*z*en) A narrow opening is created causing the air escaping to make a noisy sound.

Affricatives. (*ch*ow) The sound has the feature of a stop followed by a fricative. First there is the complete blockage of air and then the air is released through a narrow opening.

Lateral. (*l*azy) Sounds that are produced when the air is released through the sides of the mouth.

Nasals. (*n*o) Sounds that are produced when the air passes through the nose rather than the mouth.

Rhotic. (*r*un) A complex sound created by the tongue moving toward the back of the mouth.

Voicing

Voiced (*y*es) A sound created by the vibrating of the vocal folds.

Unvoiced. (*sh*oe). A sound that is created without vibrating the vocal folds.

Table 4.6
Traditional consonant classification

Consonant Developmental Sequence		Place of Articulation	Manner of Articulation	Voicing
m	mother	Bilabial	Nasal	+
n	nice	Lingua-alveolar	Nasal	+
ŋ	bang	Linguavelar	Nasal	+
p	pen	Bilabial	Stop	−
f	fun	Labiodental	Fricative	−
h	hot	Glottal	Fricative	−
w	where	Labial-Velar	Glide	+
j	yes	Linguapalatal	Glide	+
k	cat	Linguavelar	Stop	−
b	boy	Bilabial	Stop	+
d	done	Linguadental	Stop	+
g	go	Linguavelar	Stop	+
r	run	Linguapalatal	Rhotic	+
s	sun	Linguadental	Fricative	−
ʃ	shoe	Linguapalatal	Fricative	−
tʃ	church	Linguapalatal	Affricate	−
t	tie	Linguadental	Stop	−
θ	thumb	Linguadental	Fricative	−
v	very	Labiodental	Fricative	+
l	laugh	Lingua-alveolar	Lateral	+
ð	this	Linguadental	Fricative	+
z	zoo	Lingua-alvelar	Fricative	+
ʒ	azure	Linguapalatal	Fricative	+
ʤ	jump	Linguapalatal	Affricate	+
hw	what	Bilabial	Fricative	+

nent. For example, compare the speech pattern of a young child who substitutes /d/ for /b/ (*doy*) for *boy*). An examination of Table 4.6 indicates that the source of the child's error is in his place of articulation. All other aspects of the phoneme were correctly produced. He is using a linguadental rather than a bilabial place of articulation.

Distinctive Features. Many clinicians prefer to use a more complex method for analyzing articulation disorders. Their methods involve identifying the distinctive features of each consonant. Chomsky and Halle (1968) identified 15 features of consonants. A definition of each feature is given in Table 4.7. The features have been grouped into the traditional categories of place, manner, and voicing. In this method of analysis, the presence of each feature is indicated by a + and the absence by a −. The classification chart for all consonants appears in Table 4.8. Clinically, one of the main purposes for doing a distinctive feature analysis

Table 4.7
Distinctive features of consonants

Manner of Production

Consonantal sounds have a radical or marked constriction in the midsagittal region of the vocal tract. This feature distinguishes the "true" consonants from vowels and glides.

Vocalic sounds do not have a radical or marked constriction of the vocal tract and are associated with spontaneous voicing. The voiced vowels and liquids are vocalic; the voiceless vowels and liquids, glides, nasal consonants, and obstruents (stops, fricatives, and affricates) are nonvocalic (that is, −vocalic).

Sonorant sounds have a vocal configuration that permits spontaneous voicing, which means that the airstream can pass virtually unimpeded through the oral or nasal cavity. This feature distinguishes the vowels, glides, nasal consonants, and lateral and rhotacized consonants from the stops, fricatives, and affricates (the class of obstruents).

Interrupted sounds have a complete blockage of the airstream during a part of their articulation.

Strident sounds are those fricatives and affricates produced with intense noise: /s/, /z/, /ʃ/, /ʒ/, /tʃ/, and /dʒ/. The amount of noise produced depends on characteristics of the constriction, including roughness of the articulatory surface, rate of air over it, and angle of incidence between the articulatory surfaces.

Nasality refers to the emission of air through the nasal cavity.

Place of Production

High sounds are made with the tongue elevated above its neutral (resting) position.

Low sounds are made with the tongue lowered below its neutral position.

Back sounds are made with the tongue retracted from its neutral position.

Anterior sounds have an obstruction that is farther forward than that for the palatal /ʃ/. Anterior sounds include the bilabials, labiodentals, linguadentals, and lingua-alveolars.

Coronal sounds have a tongue blade position above the neutral state. In general, consonants made with an elevated tongue tip or blade are + coronal.

Rounded sounds have narrowed or protruded lip configuration.

Distributed sounds have a constriction extending over a relatively long portion of the vocal tract (from back to front). For English, this feature is particularly important to distinguish the dental fricatives /θ/ and /ð/ from the alveolars /s/ and /z/.

Lateral sounds are coronal consonants made with midline closure and lateral opening.

Voicing

Voiced sounds are produced with vibrating vocal folds.

Source: From *Articulation disorders* by J. E. Bernthal and N. W. Bankson, 1981, Englewood Cliffs, NJ: Prentice-Hall, Inc. Copyright 1981 by Prentice-Hall. Adapted by permission.

Table 4.8
*Chomsky and Halle distinctive feature analysis**

Feature	m	n	ŋ	p	f	h	w	j	k	b	d	g	r	s	ʃ	tʃ	t	θ	v	l	ð	z	ʒ	dʒ	hw
Consonantal	+	+	+	+	+	−				+	+	+	+	+	+	+			+	+	+	+			
Vocalic	−	−	−	−	−	−				−	−	−	+	−	−	−			−	+	−	−			
Sonorant	+	+	+	−	−	−				−	−	−	+	−	−	−			−	+	−	−			
Interrupted	−	−	−	+	−					+	+	+	+	−	−	+			−	−	+	−			
Strident	−	−	−	−	+					−	−	−	−	+	+	+			+	−	+	+			
High	−	−	−	−						+	−	−		−	−	−			−	−	−	−			
Low	−	−	−	−						−	−	−		−	−	−			−	−	−	−			
Back	−	−	−	−						+	−	−		−	−	−			−	−	−	−			
Anterior	+	+	−	+						−	+	+	+	+	+	+			+	+	+	+			
Coronal	−	+	−	−						−	+	+	−	+	+	+			+	+	−	+			
Rounded	−	−	−	−						−	−	−	−	−	−	−			−	−	−	−			
Distributed	+	−	−	+	+					−	+	−		−	−	−			−	+	−	−			
Lateral	−	−	−	−	−					−	−	−	−	−	−	−			−	+	−	−			
Nasal	+	+	+	−	−					−	−	−	−	−	−	−			−	−	−	−			
Voiced	+	+	+	−	−					+	+	+	+	−	−	−			+	+	+	+			

* Partial list only

Chapter 4 ❑ Speech Behaviors

is to identify the type of error the client is making. For example, a client who is substituting /p/ for /t/ and /θ/ for /f/ has a problem with tongue placement. Although the method of analysis developed by Chomsky and Halle allows us to do this, it may be too complex for some clinical purposes, especially for new students. A more simplified method of analysis was developed by Miller and Nicely (1955). Their method for analyzing consonants contains only five distinctive features (Table 4.9). For the beginning student or one who has not yet completed a course on articulatory disorders, the Miller and Nicely method offers a simplified approach to doing distinctive feature analysis.

Table 4.9
Miller and Nicely distinctive feature analysis

Voicing	0 = unvoiced	1 = voiced	
Nasality	0 = nonnasal	1 = nasal	
Affrication	0 = nonaffricated	1 = affricated	
Duration	0 = short	1 = long	
Place	0 = front	1 = middle	2 = back

Consonant	Voicing	Nasality	Affrication	Duration	Place
p	0	0	0	0	0
t	0	0	0	0	1
k	0	0	0	0	2
f	0	0	1	0	0
θ	0	0	1	0	1
s	0	0	1	1	1
ʃ	0	0	1	1	2
b	1	0	0	0	0
d	1	0	0	0	1
g	1	0	0	0	2
v	1	0	1	0	0
ð	1	0	1	0	1
z	1	0	1	1	1
ʒ	1	0	1	1	2
m	1	1	0	0	0
n	1	0	0	1	1

Source: From "An analysis of perceptual confusions among some English consonants" by G. A. Miller & P. E. Nicely, 1955, *Journal of the Acoustical Society of America, 27,* p. 347. Copyright 1955 by the *Journal of the Acoustical Society of America.* Adapted by permission.

STUTTERING

Fluency relates to the flow of speech sounds in words, phrases, and sentences. One of the early researchers in the field of stuttering, Johnson (1959) maintained that there was a sharp demarcation between fluent and disfluent speech. Other researchers, such as Bloodstein (1961) and Shames and Sherrick (1963) believed that the distinctions between fluency and stuttering were not that clear. They believed that stuttering should be viewed as falling on a continuum of smoothness in speech production. During the ages of 3 and 5, children experience what is known as "normal developmental disfluencies" (Johnson, 1959; Rubin & Culatta, 1974), which are usually easy repetitions of syllables, words, or phrases. They tend to occur when children are beginning to use new and sometimes not quite mastered linguistic structures. When the repetitions become excessive or the child begins to "block" on the production of sounds or words, the child may be identified as a stutterer. Three categories of behaviors relate to a stutterer's speech: covert behaviors, overt behaviors, and listener reactions.

Covert Behaviors

Covert behaviors refer to behaviors that cannot be identified by observation. These involve beliefs the stutterer has about his speech. The usual method of obtaining information about covert behaviors is through questionnaires or interviews. The covert behaviors that are routinely examined in stuttering therapy are self-perception, estimates of anxiety, and expectations of fluency.

Self-Perception. Many authors believe that stuttering involves a self-perception that may be independent of the actual behavior (Bloodstein, 1960; Johnson, 1934). The stuttered speech of an individual who identifies himself as a stutterer may in fact be less disfluent than the speech of speakers who identify themselves as "normal." For these individuals, the fear of stuttering may be more debilitating than the actual behavior. To examine this aspect of stuttering, Shames and Florance (1980) used five categories of self-perception to assess the results of their therapy program. Clients were asked to select one of the following categories to describe how they viewed themselves at the end of therapy:

1. Still a stutterer
2. No longer a stutterer—does not monitor
3. No longer a stutterer with occasional monitoring
4. Perceived as a stutterer who speaks fluently
5. Perceived as a mild stutterer who exhibits mild stuttering
6. Perceived as a non-stutterer who exhibits mild stuttering

When assessing self-perceptions of stutterers, clinicians can use this classification system throughout therapy to determine if the stutterer's self-perception is changing as a result of therapy.

Estimates of Anxiety. Most stutterers are fearful of saying certain sounds and speaking in various situations. For example, an individual may believe that it is impossible to say words beginning with the phoneme /b/ and to speak fluently when speaking with a supervisor. Many forms of therapy concentrate on reducing the level of anxiety stutterers feel in various situations. To identify these situations and develop a hierarchy, the clinician asks the stutterer to describe each situation and the degree of anxiety he feels when placed in it. Many questionnaires have been developed to assess anxiety, often with significant overlaps. One of the first and most comprehensive was developed by Williams, Darley, and Spriestersbach (1978). Forty questions are answered on four domains: avoidance, reaction, stuttering, and frequency.

Expectations of Fluency. In some approaches to stuttering therapy, the emphasis is on improving fluency. In these approaches, clients are asked to focus on their fluent speech and situations in which they achieve the greatest amount of fluency. Goldberg (1981) developed a checklist that clients use to indicate how fluent they usually are in various situations. The assessment instrument contains 40 questions for adults and adolescents and 20 questions for children. The questionnaire for adolescents appears in Table 4.10.

Overt Behaviors

Overt behaviors are those behaviors that can be seen or heard and therefore empirically measured. Overt behaviors identified with stuttering can be grouped into two classifications: those directly related to the disfluency (primary) and those that are attempts by the person to avoid or terminate the disfluency (secondary). The terms *primary* and *secondary* have been used to describe these behaviors since the 1930s (Bluemel, 1932). Since these terms imply that stuttering develops in two stages, many researchers believe that the terms are inadequate for describing the development of stuttering and its specific behaviors (Bloodstein, 1975). For the current analysis, the terms *primary* and *secondary* will not be used to classify behaviors. Rather, four types of behaviors related to stuttering will be identified: (a) types of disfluencies, (b) associated behaviors, (c) speech rate, and (d) disfluent phonemes.

Types of Disfluencies Present. Williams et al. (1978) identified nine different types of disfluencies that stutterers exhibit. Table 4.11 provides a definition and an example of each behavior. Although this list is an excellent starting point, it can be strengthened with two revisions. The first involves expanding the repetitions category. Goldberg (1981) differentiates between two types of repetitions, single and multiple. A *single repetition* occurs when a sound, word, phrase, or sentence is repeated only once. An example of a single repetition is "I w-want to go home." A *multiple repetition* occurs when a sound, word, phrase, or sentence is repeated more than once. An example of a multiple repetition would be "I w-w-w-w-want to go home." These repetition measures are important for assessing probable length of therapy. Goldberg found that the greater the percentage

Table 4.10
Fluency checklist—Adolescent

Below you will find a list of situations with which you may be familiar. For each situation, circle either 1—*Always*, 2—*Most of the Time*, 3—*Sometimes*, 4—*Hardly Ever*, or 5—*Never*. Answer only those items that apply to you. We are interested in knowing how fluent you are in various situations.

	Fluent Speech				
	Always	Most of the Time	Sometimes	Hardly Ever	Never
1. Talking on the telephone	1	2	3	4	5
2. Talking to a stranger	1	2	3	4	5
3. Giving your name	1	2	3	4	5
4. Ordering food	1	2	3	4	5
5. Talking to an animal	1	2	3	4	5
6. Talking with a good friend	1	2	3	4	5
7. Talking in a rap session	1	2	3	4	5
8. Being criticized	1	2	3	4	5
9. Meeting someone for the first time	1	2	3	4	5
10. Saying hello	1	2	3	4	5
11. Reading aloud	1	2	3	4	5
12. Answering questions in class	1	2	3	4	5
13. Asking for information	1	2	3	4	5
14. Arguing with friends	1	2	3	4	5
15. Arguing with strangers	1	2	3	4	5
16. Giving directions	1	2	3	4	5
17. Talking when "high"	1	2	3	4	5
18. Talking when happy	1	2	3	4	5
19. Talking when sad	1	2	3	4	5
20. Speaking with 1 person	1	2	3	4	5
21. Speaking with 2–3 people	1	2	3	4	5
22. Speaking with 4–10 people	1	2	3	4	5
23. Speaking with more than 10 people	1	2	3	4	5
24. Apologizing	1	2	3	4	5
25. Speaking when angry	1	2	3	4	5
26. Speaking with someone of the same sex	1	2	3	4	5
27. Speaking with someone of the opposite sex	1	2	3	4	5
28. Speaking with someone your same age	1	2	3	4	5
29. Speaking with someone who is younger than you	1	2	3	4	5

	Fluent Speech				
	Always	Most of the Time	Sometimes	Hardly Ever	Never
30. Speaking with someone who is older than you	1	2	3	4	5
31. Speaking with someone who is angry	1	2	3	4	5
32. Speaking with someone who is very calm	1	2	3	4	5
33. Talking with teachers	1	2	3	4	5
34. When you talk to your mother	1	2	3	4	5
35. When you talk to your father	1	2	3	4	5
36. When you talk to your					
sister/brother	1	2	3	4	5
sister/brother	1	2	3	4	5
sister/brother	1	2	3	4	5
sister/brother	1	2	3	4	5
37. When you talk to your					
aunt/uncle	1	2	3	4	5
aunt/uncle	1	2	3	4	5
aunt/uncle	1	2	3	4	5
aunt/uncle	1	2	3	4	5
38. When you talk to your					
grandmother/grandfather	1	2	3	4	5
grandmother/grandfather	1	2	3	4	5
grandmother/grandfather	1	2	3	4	5
grandmother/grandfather	1	2	3	4	5
39. Buying something in a store	1	2	3	4	5
40. Talking when tired	1	2	3	4	5
Total Number (Add the number of circles in each category)	_____	_____	_____	_____	_____
Total Scores (Add the scores in each category)	_____	_____	_____	_____	_____
Grand Total (Add the *Total Scores*)	_____				
Mean (Divide *Grand Total* by sum of *Total Number* scores)	_____				
Mode Score (Category above that had the greatest *Total Number*)	_____				

Source: From *Behavioral Cognitive Stuttering Therapy* by S. A. Goldberg, 1981, Tigard, OR: C.C. Publications. Copyright 1981 by Quest Publishers, San Francisco. Reprinted by permission.

Table 4.11
Observable characteristics of stuttering

Behavior	Definition	Example
Hesitation	Any non-tense break in the forward flow of speech	I _____ am going home.
Broken Words	Partially uttered words with unacceptable within-word hesitations	I am going home.
Repetition	Repeated utterances of parts of words (PWR), words (WR) and phrases (PR)	I am g_ going. (PWR) I am am going. (WR) Iam Iam going. (PR)
Interjections	Use of sounds, syllables, and words that are independent of context of utterance	I er er am uh going.
Prolonged Sounds	Unacceptably prolonged sounds, usually at the start of a word	I am s-s-s-so late.
Dysrthymic Phonation	Distortion of the prosodic elements *within* a word with improper stress, timing, or accenting	I am going (rising inflection) home.
Tension	Audible manifestation of abnormal breathing or muscular tightening *between* words, parts of words, or interjections	I am (forced breathing) going home.
Revisions/modifications	Grammatical or content	I am, I was going.
Imcomplete Phrases	Failure to complete an initiated unit of speech	I am—but not today.

Source: Adapted from *Diagnostic Methods in Speech Pathology* by D. E. Williams, F. L. Darley, and D. C. Spriestersbach, 1978, New York: Harper & Row.

of multiple disfluencies present, the more sessions were required for developing normal fluency.

The second revision involves adding a category of behaviors known as blocks. A *block* occurs when the vocal folds are severely adducted, preventing or impeding the normal flow of air required for phonation. Because blocks are more visual than auditory, they are sometimes difficult to identify or measure on audiotapes. Aurally they are identified by either breaks in speech or a strident vocal quality. A block can be measured in absolute time or, more frequently, is evaluated subjectively as either *short* or *long*.

Single repetitions and blocks can be reported in two different ways. The first is to merely record the occurrence of each behavior and then report the percentage of all stuttered behaviors that it represents. An example of this method appears in Table 4.12. An analysis of this type may provide the clinician with an objective method of tracking the course of a client's disfluencies throughout

Table 4.12
Example of percentages of stuttering behaviors

Behavior	Number of Occurrences	Percentage of Total
Hesitation	5	6.09
Broken Words	10	12.20
Single Repetitions	25	30.50
Multiple Repetitions	20	24.39
Interjections	14	17.07
Prolonged Sounds	2	2.44
Dysrthymic Phonation	0	0.00
Tension	5	6.10
Revisions/modifications.	1	1.21
Incomplete Phrases	0	0.00
	82	100.00

Table 4.13
Percentage of stuttered syllables and words

Transcript (Stuttered syllables are underlined)

Yesterday when I went to the store I found a pair of gloves that were perfect. I would have bought them if I had the money. I'll get my paycheck on Thursday. If I have time, I'll go back to the store and get them. You should've seen them. They were terrific.

Minutes: 2

Syllable Analysis		Word Analysis	
Total Syllables Spoken	60	Total Words Spoken	52
Syllables Spoken per Minute	30	Words Spoken per Minute	25
Syllables Stuttered	12	Words Stuttered	12
Percent of Syllables Stuttered	20%	Percent of Words Stuttered	23%

therapy. The second way of reporting stuttering behaviors involves the percentage of syllables or words that the client stutters on in a given period. In this form of analysis, the clinician makes no reference to the type of disfluency that occurred. An example of how to perform this analysis of syllables and words appears in Table 4.13.

Associated Behaviors. *Associated behaviors* are attempts by the stutterer to prevent, reduce, or terminate a stuttering episode. The behavior most widely used to prevent a stuttering episode is circumlocution. *Circumlocution* involves the substitution of a word or series of words that have a similar meaning for a word containing a feared sound. Although this behavior can prevent stuttering, the resulting utterance may be either unclear or fragmented. Since no obvious stuttering behaviors are present, it is often difficult to identify. The following example of a circumlocution was given by a very severe stutterer. The underlined words are those on which he stuttered.

> You know, I live over in <u>Berkeley</u>. You see how hard it is for me to say <u>Berkeley</u> or other words that begin with <u>B</u>. So <u>what</u> I say <u>when</u> I'm <u>hitchhiking</u> and <u>someone</u> asks <u>where</u> I'm <u>going</u>, I say "over at the Ashby exit."

A second type of associated behavior present in stuttering includes those identified as superstitious. *Superstitious behaviors* were originally developed because of an erroneous causal relationship the stutterer assumed existed between the behavior and the reduction or termination of the stuttering episode. These behaviors may appear to be normal, such as a finger casually tapping a table; moderately disruptive, such as lip pursing; or very bizarre, as when a person's head will jerk violently backwards. Take, for example, the young stutterer who tried to push the words out by pursing his lips forward whenever a block occurred. Whether or not he pursed his lips, the block would most likely end. At the moment of the termination of the stuttering episode, the stutterer's lips were pursed. If lip pursing and block termination occur together with sufficient regularity, the stutterer may assume that the associated behavior can end the stuttering episode. The association results in the development of a conditioned learned behavior. A superstitious behavior is fallaciously assumed to have causal properties and will either coexist with the block or immediately precede it. Initially the behavior may help end the block, but eventually it loses its helping power. Although the usefulness of the behavior has vanished, the behavior itself remains. Many stutterers will then develop other equally superstitious behaviors. The result is often a layering effect, where the stutterer has multiple superstitious behaviors occurring immediately before and during a stuttering episode. These associated nonverbal behaviors can be grouped into various body areas: (a) eye movements; (b) facial contortions; (c) jaw movements; (d) hand/arm movements; (e) posturing; and (f) feet/leg movements.

A third type of associated behavior includes behaviors that the stutterer has developed or been taught to use as a way of reducing the severity of the stuttering episode. Over the past 40 years a variety of behaviors have been taught to stutterers (Van Riper, 1978). These include rate reduction, substituting a "bounced" sound rather than a hard block, easy repetition of a word or phrase, and the termination of speech that is stuttered. Often it is difficult to tell if these behaviors are used instead of more severe behaviors or are the stutterer's usual behaviors.

Speech Rate. Because many therapists focus on rate as one of the key variables in stuttering therapy, speech rate is an important measure. When recording a speech rate, a good rule of thumb is that the longer the sample, the more reliable the measurements. Therefore, a reliable sample should be at least 15 consecutive minutes or three 5-minute segments randomly selected from an hour session. Three different types of rate measurement can be obtained. The first is the syllable rate per minute that is favored by some therapists (Costello & Ingham,

1984). An example of this method appears in Table 4.14. To record the client's rate, each syllable is counted once and the total is then divided by the number of minutes contained in the sample. A second rate measure involves counting words rather than syllables (also shown in Table 4.14). Although less precise than a syllable count, it does offer the clinician an easier and less time-consuming method of analysis. A third rate measure involves an analysis of only the fluent portion of the sample. This measure provides a more realistic picture of the stutterer's rate of speech, because extensive and excessive blocks can reduce the stutterer's true rate of speech.

Disfluent Phonemes. Some forms of stuttering therapy involve modifying only those phonemes on which the client is disfluent. For these forms of therapy, the phonemes are identified by having the stutterer either read a standard passage, record conversational speech, or list difficult sounds and words. The production of disfluent phonemes will rarely be consistent, since stutterers are not disfluent in all situations. The list of disfluent phonemes may be "situationally bounded," that is, occur only in certain settings.

Listener Reactions

Societal reactions to the stutterer's speech can affect his self-perception and the development of fluent speech. In the past, assessment categories such as mild, moderate, and severe provided the clinician with a general indication of how the stutterer's speech was perceived. However, if stuttering is viewed as a behavior existing on a continuum of fluent and disfluent speech, a less disordered method of describing it may be more appropriate. Martinson, Haroldson, and Triden (1984) developed a 9-point naturalness scale that is used by listeners. On this scale a rating of 1 signifies highly natural speech and 9 signifies highly unnatural speech. They found that the scale was very reliable in assessing the naturalness of speech.

The naturalness scale is useful not only for assessing a stutterer's degree of disfluency but also for assessing the type of fluency being taught to the client. There are many forms of stuttering therapy, each with specific procedures that may result in the development of different forms of fluent speech. The naturalness scale becomes an excellent tool to assess the "treated" speech of stutterers.

VOICE

Vocal behaviors can be identified as being related to either phonation or resonance. *Phonation* is the production of sound through the movement of air over the vocal cords. Phonatory behaviors can be further divided into behaviors of pitch, loudness, duration, and quality. *Pitch* refers to the intonation pattern that allows the speaker to convey information beyond the meaning of each individual word. It is also referred to as *prosody*. *Loudness* and *duration* are self-explanatory. *Quality* is difficult to define. Although quality measures of voice can be instrumentally defined, it is usually clinically identified by subjective judgments. Terms such as *harsh* and *strident* are commonly used in the clinic. Disruptions in any of

Table 4.14
Disorders of phonation*

Aphonia. Complete loss of voice as a result of hysteria (conversion), growths, paralysis, disease, or overuse of the vocal folds which may develop suddenly or over a period of time; in a less severe form, often referred to as *dysphonia*.

Breathiness. Excessive amount of air loss accompanying vocal tone; an audible escape of air is usually observed as the approximating edges of the vocal folds fail to make optimum contact.

Diplophonia. Vibration of the ventricular folds concurrently with the vocal folds to produce a "two-toned voice"; the ventricular folds usually produce the lower pitch and the vocal fields the higher pitch.

Falsetto. High-pitched voice produced by the vibration of the anterior one-third of the vocal folds, the posterior cartilaginous portion being so tightly adducted that only minimal, if any, vibration is possible; falsetto range overlaps much of the normal range.

Glottal Catch. Extreme glottal closure prior to the initiation of the air flow which disturbs the normal synchrony of timing and results in the vocal folds being blown widely apart.

Glottal Fry. Syncopated vocal fold vibration that generally occurs over the lower part of the pitch range; usually described as a bubbling, cracking type of low-pitched phonation; gravel or pulsated voice; vocal fry.

Gutturophonia. Form of dysphonia characterized by a throaty or low-pitched voice.

Harshness. Usually perceived in a phonatory milieu of hard vocal attacks, pitch and intensity problems, and overadduction of the vocal folds.

Hoarseness. One of the more common dysphonias which can be produced by anything that interferes with optimum vocal fold adduction; pitch level is usually low and the range is restricted; pitch breaks and/or aphonic episodes may also be observed. Three types of hoarseness are (a) dry hoarseness, characterized by increased intensity and air loss; (b) rough hoarseness, a two-toned voice resulting from vocal fold vibration occurring in two different locations along the vocal folds; and (c) wet hoarseness, a voice consisting of air loss and lowering of pitch often accompanied by glottal fry.

Hyperfunction. Excessive forcing and straining, usually at the level of the vocal folds, but which may occur at various points along the vocal tract.

these areas can result in a voice disorder. A disorder of phonation may be functional or organic. The auditory features of a phonation disorder are determined by the various anatomical structures that are affected.

Resonance refers to a physical property known as the natural frequency of vibration. This is determined by two things, the mass of a body and its tension. The more mass, the lower its frequency of vibration. The greater the tension, the higher the frequency of vibration. Disorders of resonance usually involve nasality. It should be noted that some authors classify nasality as an articulation problem since it does not involve the vocal folds. The characteristics of both phonation and resonance disorders will be described in this section.

Hypofunction. Reduced vocal capacity resulting from prolonged overuse, muscle fatigue, tissue irritation, or general laryngeal or specific problems relating to the opening and closing of the glottis; characterized by air loss and sometimes hoarseness and pitch breaks.

Hypophonia. Form of dysphonia characterized by a whispered voice.

Macrophonia. Voice characterized by extensive intensity.

Monotone. Voice characterized by little or no variation of pitch or loudness; pitch range is usually restricted to one of four semitones.

Pitch Break. Sudden abnormal shift of pitch during speech, usually related to an individual's speaking at an inappropriate pitch level; the typical pitch break is one octave higher (ascending pitch break) or one octave lower (descending pitch break) than the normal voice.

Spastic Dysphonia. Momentary interruption of phonation that results from sudden overadduction of the vocal folds; speech lacks fluency.

Strident. Voice usually perceived as having high frequency resonance; produced by elevation of the larynx and hypertonicity of the pharyngeal constrictors, resulting in a decrease of both length and width of the pharynx.

Stridor. Voice quality that accompanies respiration and is characterized by the presence of a tense, non-musical laryngeal noise; typically appears in young children during sleep.

Syllabic Aphonia. Brief absence of sound during the effort to produce speech commonly known as "frog in the throat."

Tremulous Speech. Quavering speech, consisting of an irregular vibrato with amplitudes and frequencies approaching the tremolo.

Ventricular Dysphonia. Voice produced by the vibration of the ventricular folds which may occur as a substitute form of vocalization or concurrently with normal phonation; hoarseness, weak intensity, and low pitch with little inflection are characteristic.

Voice Fatigue. Deterioration of vocal quality due to prolonged use; may be the result of vocal abuse or indicate a pathological condition.

Source: From *Terminology of communication disorders: Speech, language, hearing* (pp. 221–222) by L. Nicolosi, E. Harryman, & J. Kresheck, 1978, Baltimore: Williams & Wilkins. Copyright 1978 by Williams & Wilkins. Reprinted by permission.

Disorders of Pitch

Three different types of pitch disorders are treated by speech-language pathologists. They are monotone, abnormally high pitch, and abnormally low pitch.

Monotone. A lack of pitch, or prosody, typifies the speech of individuals who have been severely hearing impaired or deaf from birth or early childhood. The inability to hear intonation patterns during language learning presents a formidable obstacle to learning normal prosody patterns. A monotone pattern is also present in the speech of some individuals with severe language problems. *Monotone speech* is characterized by the perception of flatness, or equal stress on all parts of words. In some cases it may sound like the speech produced by early forms of computerized synthesizers, where the syllables of all words had equal stress. Or it may be less severe, as in the case of some severe language-impaired individuals, who may be using some stress patterns only in certain parts of speech.

High Pitch. The most commonly occurring example of high pitch is a persistent falsetto in males. During puberty the vocal fold mass of males increases dramatically, resulting in a pitch drop of up to one octave. The change in pitch is not instantaneous but rather occurs gradually as the individual attempts to maintain the same pitch he is accustomed to, fails, and has a pitch break in his voice. The pitch breaks, which abruptly drop the voice up to an octave, signal the preparation of the larynx for engaging in a lower pitch. Most adolescent males gradually adapt to the new limitations of the larynx and automatically lower their pitch. In a small number of males, the change is resisted, resulting in a persistent falsetto. A persistent falsetto can also result from physiological problems such as *Froehlich's syndrome,* a condition resulting from a defect in the pituitary gland, which regulates hormone secretion, growth, and adolescent development.

Too high a pitch is not limited to persistent falsetto. Occasionally, women and men are seen in the clinic who, for social or psychological reasons, are using a pitch that is not appropriate for the mass of their larynx. An inappropriate pitch can result in various vocal problems such as vocal fatigue.

Low Pitch. Froehlich's syndrome has the reverse effect on women. It results in a pitch that is abnormally low. Most cases of low pitch are not organic. Many individuals attempt to present a particular social image through their voice. A television anchor person may wish to appear more authoritative by lowering his voice, or a rock singer who emulates blues musicians may lower her voice during singing to sound like her idol. Just as an inappropriate high pitch can lead to vocal problems, so can an inappropriate low pitch.

Disorders of Loudness

Inadequate Loudness. Most cases of inadequate loudness are functional. That is, the person does not have a physiological problem that is causing the soft voice. For a variety of reasons, the person is choosing to speak at a level that either cannot be heard or can be heard only with great effort. An example was a child being seen for speech-language therapy in a public school. He had recently arrived from Guatemala and was still uncomfortable speaking in English. Despite the best-planned therapy activities, the clinician was unable to convince the boy to increase the loudness of his speech. During a parent conference she learned that when he spoke in Spanish, he had no problem in the loudness of his speech. In fact, the parents had to continually tell him to speak softer. Clearly in this case, the inadequate loudness of the boy's speech was related to other issues.

Excessive Loudness. The use of excessive loudness by children may result in a condition known as *vocal nodules* or *screamers nodules*. The child may be using his voice to attempt to assert his position within his peer group. If the behavior continues, small callous-like growths, or nodules, develop on the edges of the vocal folds. With appropriate loudness and vocal rest, they may be reabsorbed by the tissue and not require any intervention. In resistant cases, they may require surgical or laser removal. The condition is also prevalent in singers who routinely sing at an abnormally high level.

Disorders of Duration

Function disorders of duration are not that common. They result from inadequate breath control. Most duration disorders result from physical problems, such as cerebral palsy or other organic problems that affect control of the diaphragm.

Disorders of Quality

Most disorders of quality result from organic laryngeal problems causing an abnormal vibration of the vocal cords. The etiology in some cases may have been functional, such as the inappropriate use of voice, but resulted in organic problems. For example, the singer who has an ulcerated laryngeal vocal fold may have developed it by continuous, excessive screaming. Table 4.14 shows the various terms used to describe vocal quality. Some of the terms are used to describe the speech of individuals with different etiologies. Most of the terms rely on subjective evaluations on the part of a listener. One way of organizing the terms is to use West and Ansberry's (1968) categories of organic problems. They divided all disorders of quality into three morphological areas: (a) defects on the edges of the vocal folds, (b) problems with the adduction of the cords, and (c) constriction or obstruction of the glottal opening.

Vocal Fold Edge Problems. Defects on the edges of the vocal folds can have both organic and functional etiologies. They can be caused by cancerous growths, tuberculosis, injury, or vocal abuse. The resulting sounds that are produced have a noisy quality and can be described by terms such as *breathiness* or *hoarseness.*

Adduction Problems. Difficulty with proper vocal fold adduction can result from a variety of reasons including paralysis or fatigue of the adductor muscles, immobilization of the arytenoid cartilages, or a decision on the part of the speaker to use breathy phonation. Terms that are used to describe adduction problems are *breathiness, hoarseness, hypofunction, hypophonia,* and *vocal fatigue.*

Constriction or Obstruction of the Glottal Opening. Constriction or obstruction of the glottal opening can result from excessively tense adduction of the vocal folds, growths, moist deposits resulting from postnasal drips, or inflammations of vocal folds. Terms associated with this type of disorder are *harshness, hyperfunction, macrophonia, spastic dysphonia,* and *strident.*

Disorders of Resonance

When we produce a sound such as *ah* with our mouth barely open, a certain quality is present. If the same sound is now uttered, but this time with the mouth wide open, a very different quality is heard. The vibratory features of all parts of our anatomy that are involved in producing sounds affect resonance. When these structures are changed in an abnormal way, disorders of resonance occur. Most disorders of resonance involve either too much or too little nasality, or in some cases a mixture of too little and too much nasality.

Hypernasality. *Hypernasality* results when the amount of air emission through the nose is excessive. It is most noticeable on vowels and vowel-like consonants such as /l/, /r/, /j/, and /w/. Although a cleft palate results in hypernasality on all phonemes, some authors do not consider it to be a true voice disorder (Bloodstein, 1979). Because cleft palate results in the inability to compress air in the oral cavity, it affects both voice and articulation. The term *hypernasality* in this section will refer to an excess of nasality due to functional reasons.

Hyponasality. *Hyponasality* refers to the change in resonance when the nasal cavities are partially or completely blocked. The most usual contributing factor to hyponasality is the closing of the nasal mucous membrane because of infection from the common cold. However, other conditions can have a similar result, such as allergies, enlarged tonsils or adenoids, or a deviated septum.

Cul-de-sac Nasality. *Cul-de-sac nasality* results when both hypernasality and hyponasality occur simultaneously. The hypernasality results from either too large a posterior aperture or too posterior a placement of the tongue. The hyponasality occurs because of an anterior nasal obstruction. The resulting vocal quality is often described as *hollow.*

CLEFT PALATE SPEECH

Cleft palate speech, which is characterized by hypernasality, is differentiated from voice disorders since the inability to have complete velopharyngeal closure results not only in extreme hypernasality but also in articulation disorders and nasal fricatives.

Hypernasality

The speech of individuals with unrepaired or partially repaired cleft palates is typified by its nasal quality. The extent of the nasal quality is determined by the lack of velophyrangeal closure that the individual is capable of executing. Anterior clefts that have not affected the pharyngeal walls or the velum are completely repairable and often result in speech that is quite normal. However, the more extensive the damage to the pharyngeal wall and the velum, the more difficulty the individual will have in producing velopharyngeal closure. The less closure, the more nasality. Hypernasality will have the greatest effect on the production of vowels and semivowels.

Articulation

The communication problems of an individual with cleft palate are attributable more to misarticulations than to the resonance problem of hypernasality. The inability to generate air pressure causes severe problems with two classes of consonants: stop-plosives and fricatives. In both cases, the consonants are substituted by a nasal distortion of the sound that often makes speech unintelligible. In the following example, each phoneme that is either a stop-plosive or a fricative is underlined.

To<u>d</u>ay I <u>p</u>layed soccer wi<u>th</u> my <u>fri</u>en<u>d</u>s.

To understand the extent of the problem, substitute an /n/ phoneme for each underlined phoneme. At best, the sentence is very difficult to understand.

Nasal Fricative

As the individual with a cleft palate is speaking, the listener can often hear a friction noise. This occurs for two reasons. First, with insufficient velopharyngeal closure there will be a continuous emission of air through the nose. Second, on sounds such as /p/, /t/, and /k/, requiring an extensive amount of intraoral pressure, the individual may attempt to compensate for lack of closure by exerting a greater amount of breath.

SUMMARY

The purpose of this chapter was to identify the components of commonly observed speech behaviors. Before behaviors can be changed they must be observed. When possible, the observation of behaviors should not include subjective evaluations. Unfortunately, certain characteristics of speech are inherently subjective since they involve listener evaluations. Observations of this type, although not precise, may be the best or only measurements available.

The identification of behaviors occurs within a complex context. The behaviors that have been precisely described in this chapter may appear vague in the speech of real clients or be distorted by the presence of other behaviors. For example, is the /r/ being substituted by a /w/, or is it a distorted /r/? Is the stutter a combination of two different behaviors? Is the vocal quality simultaneously harsh, hoarse, and tremulous? In previous chapters the importance of understanding the differences between models and reality was discussed. Just like theories of communication, behavioral descriptions are models that are intended to provide the clinician with a road map of the territory. Clinicians should not be concerned that the real, uncontrolled behaviors of clients do not fit neatly within a textbook category. Variability in behaviors is to be expected.

SUGGESTED READINGS

Bernthal, J. E., & Bankson, N. W. (1981). *Articulation disorders.* Englewood Cliffs, NJ: Prentice-Hall, Inc.
Bloodstein, O. (1979). *Speech pathology: An introduction.* Boston: Houghton Mifflin.
Boone, D. R. (1988). *Voice and voice therapy.* Englewood Cliffs, NJ: Prentice-Hall.
Case, J. L. (1991). *Clinical management of voice disorders.* Austin, TX: Pro-Ed.
Culatta, R., & Goldberg, S. A. (in press). *Stuttering therapy: An integration of theory and practice.* New York: Merrill/Macmillan.
Ingram, D. (1989). *Phonological disability in children.* San Diego, CA: Singular Press.
Nicolosi, L.; Harryman, E.; & Kresheck, J. (1978). *Terminology of communication disorders: Speech, language, hearing.* Baltimore: Williams & Wilkins.

Activity 4.1
Phonological and articulatory disorders

The behavioral checklist that follows will aid in the analysis. Use the following procedure.

1. Observe a client for 15 minutes without performing any analysis or forming a judgment. Just listen.
2. For the next 15 minutes record the child's articulation with the aid of a tape recorder. While the tape is recording, observe the client and record your data on the checklist.
3. Listen to the tape at least two times, each time recording the data on the checklist. Note differences on each of the listening sessions.
4. Summarize and correct your data on the following checklist.

Understand that this analysis should not take the place of a formal diagnostic test. This is an exercise in phonological and articulatory observation. The data collected can be used to supplement the results from a diagnostic evaluation.

1. Substitutions

Check the appropriate boxes.

No Problem	Substitutions Present				
[ ]	[ ]				
Substitute Sound	Target Sound	Distinctive Feature Error(s)	Distinctive Feature Target(s)	Consistent Error	Inconsistent Error
_____	_____	_____	_____	[ ]	[ ]
_____	_____	_____	_____	[ ]	[ ]
_____	_____	_____	_____	[ ]	[ ]
_____	_____	_____	_____	[ ]	[ ]
_____	_____	_____	_____	[ ]	[ ]
_____	_____	_____	_____	[ ]	[ ]
_____	_____	_____	_____	[ ]	[ ]
_____	_____	_____	_____	[ ]	[ ]

2. Omissions

Check the appropriate boxes.

No Problem   Omission Present
[ ]   [ ]

Omissions	Initial	Medial	Final	Consistent Error	Inconsistent Error
_____	[ ]	[ ]	[ ]	[ ]	[ ]
_____	[ ]	[ ]	[ ]	[ ]	[ ]
_____	[ ]	[ ]	[ ]	[ ]	[ ]
_____	[ ]	[ ]	[ ]	[ ]	[ ]
_____	[ ]	[ ]	[ ]	[ ]	[ ]
_____	[ ]	[ ]	[ ]	[ ]	[ ]
_____	[ ]	[ ]	[ ]	[ ]	[ ]
_____	[ ]	[ ]	[ ]	[ ]	[ ]

continues

Activity 4.1, continued

3. Additions

Check the appropriate boxes.

No Problem　　**Additions Present**

[ ]　　　　　　　　[ ]

Additions	Initial	Medial	Final	Consistent Error	Inconsistent Error
____	[ ]	[ ]	[ ]	[ ]	[ ]
____	[ ]	[ ]	[ ]	[ ]	[ ]
____	[ ]	[ ]	[ ]	[ ]	[ ]
____	[ ]	[ ]	[ ]	[ ]	[ ]
____	[ ]	[ ]	[ ]	[ ]	[ ]
____	[ ]	[ ]	[ ]	[ ]	[ ]
____	[ ]	[ ]	[ ]	[ ]	[ ]
____	[ ]	[ ]	[ ]	[ ]	[ ]

4. Distortions

Check the appropriate boxes.

No Problem　　**Distortions Present**

[ ]　　　　　　　　[ ]

Target Sound	Distortion	Initial	Medial	Final	Consistent Error	Inconsistent Error
____	____	[ ]	[ ]	[ ]	[ ]	[ ]
____	____	[ ]	[ ]	[ ]	[ ]	[ ]
____	____	[ ]	[ ]	[ ]	[ ]	[ ]
____	____	[ ]	[ ]	[ ]	[ ]	[ ]
____	____	[ ]	[ ]	[ ]	[ ]	[ ]
____	____	[ ]	[ ]	[ ]	[ ]	[ ]
____	____	[ ]	[ ]	[ ]	[ ]	[ ]
____	____	[ ]	[ ]	[ ]	[ ]	[ ]

◻ **Activity 4.2**
Fluency

Observe a person with disfluencies and analyze behaviors in terms of (1) type of repetitions; (2) blocks; (3) associated behaviors; (4) word rate per minute; (5) disfluent sounds, and (6) speech naturalness.

1. **Repetitions**

Check the appropriate boxes.	None	Single Repetitions	Multiple Repetitions
a. Initial sounds	[ ]	[ ]	[ ]
b. Medial sounds	[ ]	[ ]	[ ]
c. Final sounds	[ ]	[ ]	[ ]
d. Words	[ ]	[ ]	[ ]
e. Phrases	[ ]	[ ]	[ ]
f. Sentences	[ ]	[ ]	[ ]

2. **Blocks**

Check the appropriate boxes.	None	Short Less than 1 Second	Long More than 1 Second
	[ ]	[ ]	[ ].

   Description:

3. **Associated Behaviors**

Check the appropriate boxes.	None	Present
a. Single-sound interjections	[ ]	[ ]
b. Single-word interjections	[ ]	[ ]
c. Multiple-word interjections	[ ]	[ ]
d. Circumlocutions	[ ]	[ ]
e. Eye movements	[ ]	[ ]
f. Facial contortions	[ ]	[ ]
g. Jaw movements	[ ]	[ ]
h. Hand/arm movements	[ ]	[ ]
i. Posturing	[ ]	[ ]
j. Feet/leg movements	[ ]	[ ]

4. **Word Rate**

   a. *Continuous Speech*

   Number of words for 5-minute sample   =   _____
   Divided by 5   =   _____

   b. *Fluent Speech*

   Number of words for _____-minute sample   =   _____
   Divided by _____   =   _____

continues

Activity 4.2, continued

5. **Disfluent sounds**

   Circle each disfluent sound.

   a. *Vowels*

[i] beat	[a] ask	[u] fool	[ɚ] onward
[ɪ] bit	[ɑ] calm	[ʊ] full	
[e] bait	[ɔ] fall	[ə] above	
[æ] bat	[o] boat	[ɝ] word	

   b. *Consonants*

[b] bowl	[l] lot	[s] seal	[ŋ] sung	
[k] coal	[m] sum	[t] toll	[θ] thigh	
[d] dole	[n] sun	[v] vat	[ð] thy	
[f] fat	[p] pole	[w] watt	[ʃ] ash	
[g] goal	[r] rot	[z] zeal	[ʒ] azure	[h] happy

   c. *Diphthongs*

   [eɪ] fail
   [aɪ] file
   [ɔɪ] foil
   [oʊ] foal
   [aʊ] fowl

   d. *Combinations*

   [tʃ] choke
   [dʒ] joke
   [hw] what
   [ju] youth

❏ **Activity 4.3**
Voice

The following checklist should be used when listening to a person who may have a voice disorder. Assessing vocal quality involves a greater degree of subjectivity than most other disorders because you must rely on an auditory perception to make a clinical judgment. It is reasonable that there may be disagreements as to the type of phonatory or resonant disorder that may be present.

1. Listen to each person with a vocal disorder without performing any analysis or making a judgment. Just listen.
2. For the second observation note any phonation disorder on the checklist.
3. For the third observation identify resonation disorders.

Voice Disorders of Phonation

Check the appropriate boxes.	No Problem	Problem Present
Aphonia	[ ]	[ ]
Breathiness	[ ]	[ ]
Diplophonia	[ ]	[ ]
Eunuchoid Voice	[ ]	[ ]
Falsetto (High Voice)	[ ]	[ ]
Glottal Catch	[ ]	[ ]
Glottal Fry (Vocal Fry)	[ ]	[ ]
Gutturophonia	[ ]	[ ]
Harshness	[ ]	[ ]
Hoarseness, Dry	[ ]	[ ]
Hoarseness, Rough	[ ]	[ ]
Hoarseness, Wet	[ ]	[ ]
Hyperfunction	[ ]	[ ]
Hypofunction	[ ]	[ ]
Hypophonia (Dysphonia)	[ ]	[ ]
Macrophonia	[ ]	[ ]
Monotone	[ ]	[ ]
Pitch Break, Ascending	[ ]	[ ]
Pitch Break, Descending	[ ]	[ ]
Spastic Dysphonia (Laryngeal Stuttering)	[ ]	[ ]
Strident	[ ]	[ ]
Stridor	[ ]	[ ]
Syllabic Aphonia	[ ]	[ ]
Tremulous Speech	[ ]	[ ]
Ventricular Dysphonia (Ventricular Phonation)	[ ]	[ ]
Vocal Fatigue (Phonasthenia)		

Voice Disorders of Resonance

Assimilated Nasality	[ ]	[ ]
Cul De Sac	[ ]	[ ]
Hypernasality (Denasality)	[ ]	[ ]
Hyponasality	[ ]	[ ]
Mixed Nasality	[ ]	[ ]

Chapter 5
Verbal Behaviors

STUDY GUIDE

- What is a language disorder?
- Describe the elements of language.
- Describe the procedures for analyzing the mean length of a child's utterance.
- What advantages does transformational grammar have over phrase-structure grammar?
- What information can be derived from a case grammar analysis?
- Why do many people believe pragmatics is the most important element of language to consider?
- How does a metalinguistic analysis complement other forms of linguistic analysis?

The term *verbal behaviors* will be used here to refer to language units that involve semantics, syntax, morphology, pragmatics, and metalinguistics. Many formal diagnostic tests allow the clinician to assess functioning in each of these areas. A synopsis and review of 30 developed prior to 1978 appear in an excellent book edited by Frederic Darley (1979). An even more exhaustive list of diagnostic tests developed prior to 1978 with short summaries of their uses was compiled by Nicolosi, Harryman, and Kresheck (1978). Compton's review of 28 speech and language tests is more current (1990). Appendixes E and G contain lists of diagnostic tests appropriate for the assessment of language. An examination of these tests is better left to courses on diagnostic testing. For the purposes of observation, simplified behavioral recording instruments are presented in this chapter. The chapter is divided into three components: child and adolescent language disorders, adult language disorders, and metalinguistic analysis.

❏ ❏ ❏ **CHILD AND ADOLESCENT LANGUAGE DISORDERS**

Language Disorders

The purpose of an operational definition is to provide a focus of study. Since the purpose of this section is to provide the information necessary to identify linguistic disorders, a *language disorder* will be operationally defined as the absence or distortion of receptive or productive linguistic abilities in the areas of lexicon, syntax, morphology, or pragmatics.

Lexicon. A *lexicon* is simply the list of the words that a person understands or uses. These words are related to the person's culture, experience, cognitive functioning, and the situation in which the individual is speaking. Words are acquired in a systematic manner. Generally, a child will initially comprehend a word prior to using it, resulting in a delay of approximately 1 to 3 months between the child's comprehension and production of a word. Table 5.1 provides the approximate number of words that a child understands and uses at various age levels.

Morphology. *Morphology* refers to the smallest units of meaning within language. These include "markers" such as possessive *'s* and plurals indicated by *s*. These are also known as *inflections*, or alterations to the form of a word by the addition of a prefix or suffix. For example, the words *boy* and *airplane* each have only one unit of meaning. However, the words *boy's* and *airplanes* each have two morphemes: *boy* + possessive, and *airplane* + plural. *Boy*, the possessive marker (apostrophe), *s*, *airplane*, and the plural marker *s* are each considered to be a separate morpheme. Inflections that appear in English are listed in Table 5.2.

The number of morphemes used within an utterance can provide the clinician with a gross estimate of a young child's language development. This measure of utterance length is called the *mean length of utterance (MLU)* and is appropriate to use for children whose maximum linguistic age is 5. Beyond age 5, the MLU does

Table 5.1
Lexicon development

Chronological Age	Number of Words in Lexicon (Average)
0.8	0
0.10	1
1.0	3
1.3	19
1.6	22
1.9	118
2.0	272
2.6	446
3.0	896
3.1	1,000
3.8	1,300
4.0	1,540

Source: Data from Brown, 1973; Dale, 1976; Lahey, 1988.

Table 5.2
Inflections

Inflection	Example
Simple Present Progressive	is going
Simple Future Progressive	will be going
Simple Past Progressive	he went
Present Perfect Progressive	has been going
Future Perfect Progressive	will have been going
Past Perfect Progressive	had been going
Plural	cars
Past Irregular	went
Past Regular	kicked
Contractible Copula	she's (is) my friend
Uncontractible Copula	she was my friend
Articles	a, the, an
Third Person Singular Regular	he walks
Third Person Singular Irregular	he ate
Contractible Auxiliary	he'll (will) go home
Uncontractible Auxiliary	can

not provide an adequate or reliable measure of language development. Brown (1973) specified rules for determining the MLU. These appear in Table 5.3.

After the number of morphemes in each utterance has been determined using Brown's rules, the average MLU for all the utterances is determined by adding the number of morphemes and then dividing by the number of utterances. An example of how to determine the MLU for a small sample is provided in Table 5.4. Although an MLU can provide a gross measure of a child's language development, often a more precise method of examining language disorders is needed, such as measures of syntax.

Syntax. *Syntax* refers to the order in which words are placed according to agreed upon linguistic rules. There is more than one way to describe the syntax of a client's language. Two common ones are presented here: phrase-structure grammar and transformational grammar.

One of the simplest syntaxes used to describe a child's language is *phrase-structure grammar,* which divides an utterance into constituent units of language, such as a sentence, noun phrase, verb phrase, or article. Although this type of analysis can provide the clinician with an easy method of describing language, it

Table 5.3
Brown's procedures for determining MLU

1. Start with the second page of the transcription unless that page involves a recitation of some kind. In this latter case start with the first recitation-free stretch. Count the first 100 utterances satisfying the following rules.
2. Only fully transcribed utterances are used; none with blanks. Portions of utterances, entered in parentheses to indicate doubtful transcription, are used.
3. Include all exact utterance repetitions (marked with a plus sign in records). Stuttering is marked as repeated efforts at a single word; count the word once in the most complete form produced. In the few cases where a word is produced for emphasis or the like (no, no, no) count each occurrence.
4. Do not count such fillers as *mm* or *oh,* but do count *no, yeah,* and *hi.*
5. All compound words (two or more free morphemes), proper names, and ritualized reduplications count as single words. Examples: *birthday, rackety-boom, choo-choo, quack-quack, night-night, pocketbook,* and *see saw.* Justification is that there is no evidence that the constituent morphemes function as such for these children.
6. Count as one morpheme all irregular pasts of the verb (e.g., *got, did, went, saw*). Justification is that there is no evidence that the child relates these to present forms.
7. Count as one morpheme all diminutive words (e.g., *doggie, mommie*) because these children at least do not seem to use the suffix productively. Diminutives are the standard forms used by the child.
8. Count as separate morphemes all auxiliaries (e.g., *is, have, will, can, must,* and *would*), also all catenative *(gonna, wanna, hafta).* These latter are counted as single morphemes rather than as *going to* or *want to* because evidence is that they function so for the children. Count as separate morphemes all inflections, for example, possessive (s), plural (s), third person singular (s), regular past (d), progressive (ing).

Source: Reprinted by permission of the publishers from A FIRST LANGUAGE by Roger Brown, Cambridge, MA: Harvard University Press. Copyright © 1973 by The President and Fellows of Harvard College.

Table 5.4
Performing an MLU

Utterance	Number of Morphemes
1. Hi mommy	2
2. I want milk	3
3. He, ah, is gone	3
4. He, ah, has daddy's shoe	5
5. I wanted it	4
Total =	17
Divided by 5 (number of utterances) =	3.4 MLU

is usually inadequate for identifying the more complex aspects of a client's language competency.

A more sophisticated method of analysis can be achieved through the use of *transformational grammar* (Chomsky, 1972). Transformational grammar provides a list of linguistic rules that purports to show how speakers go from the intent of their communication to the actual production. Examples of commonly appearing normal transformations are shown in Table 5.5. A language disorder would occur if any of these rules are absent or altered. A list of transformation errors (restricted forms) appears in Table 5.6.

Semantics. *Semantics* refers to the meaning of individual words and word combinations. When the child's utterances consist primarily of two-word combinations, an appropriate method of describing them is Brown's semantic relationships (1970). These semantic relationships appear with examples in Table 5.7.

As the child begins to use three words in a single utterance, various semantic relations are combined, such as nomination + possessive (that my book). As language usage develops and becomes more sophisticated, Brown's semantic relationships become more difficult to apply. Another method that can be used for describing utterances of increased length and complexity is *case grammar*. Case grammar provides information about the meaning of the utterance that cannot be derived from Brown's semantic relationships. The cases shown in Table 5.8 are a combination of those proposed by Fillmore (1968) and their expansion by Goldberg (1989). By determining the percentages of each case in the child's spontaneous language productions, the clinician can develop an understanding of the child's relationships with the environment. For example, some children with cognitive impairments have few adverbs or adjectives in their speech. This might be indicative of their difficulty in perceiving the more abstract elements of their experiences, such as size or speed. Unfortunately, normative data regarding case grammar is unavailable.

Pragmatics. Just because children have knowledge of grammatical rules does not necessarily mean that they are used or used in all situations. It may not be appropriate for a child to use a complete sentence during play, yet it is expected in a classroom setting. Examining the relationship that environment has on the

Table 5.5
Transformation types

Transformation Types	Examples
Passive	He got tired.
	He was washed.
Negation	He isn't a good boy.
Question	Are you nice?
Contraction	He'll be good.
Inversion	Here is the toothpaste.
Relative Question	Where are you going?
Imperative	Don't use my dough.
Pronominalization	There isn't any more.
Separation	He took it off.
Got	I've got a lollipop.
Auxiliary *Be* Placement	He is not going.
Auxiliary *Have* Placement	I've already been there.
Do	I did read the book.
Possessive	I'm writing daddy's name.
Reflexive	I cut myself.
Conjunction	Peter is here and you are there.
Conjunction Deletion	I see a red book and a blue book.
If Conjunction	I'll give it to you if you want it.
So Conjunction	He saw him so he hit him.
Cause Conjunction	He ate it because it's good.
Pronoun in Conjunction	David saw the bicycle and he was happy.
Adjective	I have a pink dog.
Relative Clause	I don't know what he's doing.
Infinitival Complement	I want to play.
Participial Complement	I like painting.
Iteration	You have to drink milk to grow strong.
Nominalization	She does the shopping and cooking and baking.
Nominal Compound	The baby carriage is here.

Table 5.6
Restricted transformations

Restricted Forms	Examples
Verb Phrase Omission	This green.
Verb Phrase Substitution	He tries to take the knife from following.
Verb Phrase Redundancy	He'll might get in jail.
Noun Phrase Omission	Look at.
Noun Phrase Redundancy	I want it the paint.
Preposition Omission	He'll have to go the doctor's.
Preposition Substitution	He took me at the circus.
Preposition Redundancy	Take it off from here.
Article Omission	Daddy has new office.
Article Substitution	I want a milk please.
Article Redundancy	I like the Donny.
Particle Omission	Put the hat.
Particle Redundancy	The barber cut off his hair off.
Contraction Deletion *Be*	I going.
Contraction Deletion *Have*	I been thinking about that.
Double Negation	You can't put no more water in it.
Inversion Subject-Object	Crayons I want.
Inversion Verb number	Here's two clouds.
No Question	Take off it.
Pronominalization Substitution	It was snow yesterday.
No Separation	Take off it.

use of language is known as *pragmatics*. According to Duchan (1984), the study of pragmatics has undergone tremendous changes over the last 20 years and currently is practiced in a variety of ways:

> Like Buffalo chicken wings, pragmatics can be bought in its mild, medium, or hot versions. The mild version takes pragmatics as a new aspect of language which needs to be assessed along with our traditional assessment approaches. It is also the case that those who select the mild version would hope that the new area of pragmatics will soon give birth to formal tests, or standardized informal assessment procedures, which will offer them ways to determine which areas of pragmatics children show deficiencies in.
>
> Those with medium tastes see pragmatics as more pervasive, and a movement which requires them to evaluate their children's language in natural contexts, even when the language problem is one of phonology or syntax, or has as its source a cognitive deficiency. This group will willingly abandon their standardized procedures and look at the child's language in light of its intentions and listener and situational

Table 5.7
Brown's semantic relationships

Semantic Relation	Form	Example
Nomination	that + N	that book
Notice	hi + N	hi belt
Recurrence	more + N, 'nother + noun	more milk
Nonexistence	allgone + N, no more + N	allgone rattle
Attributive	Adj + N	big train
Possessive	N + N	mommy lunch
Locative	N + N	sweater chair
Agent-Action	N + V	Eve read
Agent-Object	N + N	mommy sock
Action-Object	V + N	put book

Source: From *PSYCHOLINGUISTICS* (p. 220) by R. Brown, 1970, New York: Free Press. Copyright 1970 by The Free Press, a Division of Macmillan, Inc. Adapted by permission.

appropriateness. However, they still hold to the idea that language is what they are studying, and context is what is influencing it.

The hot version of the pragmatics movement is forwarded by the movement's revolutionaries, who opt for overthrowing our previous conceptions that language is what we are assessing, and propose that we move toward a new conceptualization which examines communication and context, and if called for, the language within it. The hot view is the one that must be embraced if we are to take seriously what the literature in pragmatics has to tell us. (pp. 177–178)

According to Duchan, analyzing a child's language only in terms of its grammatical correctness produces a false picture of the child's linguistic abilities. Children adjust their verbal output according to the needs of the situation. Therefore, it is quite likely that the form and content of their utterances will sound very different when they are playing with a friend as opposed to conversing with a speech pathologist.

Duchan maintains that pragmatics should concentrate on four aspects of the communication: (a) interaction, (b) sensemaking, (c) intentionality, and only peripherally (d) the formal language system. In this section, behaviors related to interaction, sensemaking, and intentionality will be discussed.

Interactions involve complex processes, since the parties of the interactions define the situation through their verbal and nonverbal behaviors. The principles of the interaction are as follows:

1. The interaction is negotiated through *cooperation* and *rules of turn-taking*.
2. The interaction is affected by the *roles* of the interactants.
3. The interaction is affected by how well each interactant *listens* to the other person.

Table 5.8
Case grammar

Cases	Examples
Noun	
Noun-Objective	I see *you*.
Noun-Experiencer	*Adam* saw Eve.
Noun-Locative	The car is *there*.
Noun-Agent	*He* opened the door.
Noun-Instrument	That *screwdriver* screws.
Noun-Factitive	He made a *mess*.
Noun-Dative	He gave it to *me*.
Verb	
Verb-Preference	I *want* it.
Verb-Behavior	I *go*.
Verb-Notice	I *see* you.
Verb-Sensation	It *feels* soft.
Verb-Condition	I *live* there.
Adjective	
Adjective-Possessive	That's *mine*.
Adjective-Number	*Two* ball.
Adjective-Temporal	I did it *yesterday*.
Adjective-Size	It's a *big* ball.
Adjective-Color	That's a *red* ball.
Adjective-Quality	That's a *nice* dog.
Adverb	
Adverb-Qualification	He ran *fast*.

It has been suggested that the most important of these pragmatic skills for children to possess is conversational "turn-taking." The ability to appropriately take one's turn in speaking may be critical in integrating individuals with language disabilities within a nondisabled population. By assessing the child's ability to elaborate on the immediately preceding statements of a conversational partner, the clinician may be able to develop appropriate communicative goals. The identification of interaction behaviors involves a more subjective assessment than does syntactic analysis or the identification of case grammatical structures. According to Leonard (1984)

> The available evidence regarding children's developing turn-taking skills has implications for intervention. For example, children for whom conversational turn-taking is a clinical goal might first be encouraged to participate in a dyad. If a child

must interact with more than one other child at a time, as is often the case in some preschool language-stimulation programs, the child's conversations may amount to frequent and ill-timed interruptions—or the opposite extreme, a reluctance to actively participate. Triadic communication, then, might be reserved as a later goal of intervention. A child's ability to take conversational turns might be promoted by insuring that a number of the utterances initially directed his or her way have predictable responses whose formulation can be based on a small set of response alternatives, and where, in some cases, simple repetition or confirmation is appropriate. (p. 21)

Although it is not possible to script out in advance every instance of interaction behaviors, examples of their presence and absence may be instructive. These appear in Table 5.9.

Sensemaking involves how well the participants are making sense of what is going on in the interaction. It involves the ability to predict events based on prior experiences. If the child is able to make sense of the interaction, certain types of behaviors can occur:

1. The discourse will be *organized*.
2. The discourse will have *cohesion*.
3. There will be *topic comprehension* and *elaboration*.

Examples of the presence and absence of organization, cohesion, and topic comprehension and elaboration appear in Table 5.10.

Communication involves **intentionality**. In other words, people communicate for specific reasons. In analyzing an interaction, one must be cognizant of the communicator's intentions. Specifically, the clinician should determine the following:

1. What is the *purpose* of the communication?
2. Is the purpose *social* or *not social*?
3. What kind of *structure* is the person using for realizing the goal?

Table 5.11 provides an example of how an interaction can be described in terms of purpose and structure.

Duchan's argument for a "hot" approach to pragmatics is compelling. It is more realistic and not only provides a better assessment of linguistic ability but also allows us to understand communicative competency. *Communicative competency* is the ability of the individual to convey a message reasonably and accurately. It is not necessarily related to "correct" linguistics. For example, when children play, they often use linguistic structures that are either incomplete or not "age-appropriate" according to normative data. However, not only are the utterances correct within that setting, but the use of more complete, "proper" linguistic utterances might adversely affect their communicative competency.

❑ ❑ ❑ **ADULT LANGUAGE DISORDERS**

The largest category of adult language disorders encountered by clinicians are those associated with aphasia. The next largest category are language behaviors

Table 5.9
Examples of the presence and absence of interaction behaviors

Example:

Two children enter a room with all the materials necessary to simulate a grocery store. The only instruction given to the children is that they are to "play store." The clinician leaves the room and then observes the interaction.

Cooperation

Presence.

The materials for the store are randomly lying around the room. For the game to begin, the store has to be constructed. Both children help in arranging the materials, jointly and independently deciding where objects should go. If there is a disagreement, a discussion ensues and a decision is made.

Absence.

The materials for the store are randomly lying around the room. For the game to begin, the store has to be constructed. Only one child arranges the material. When the other child objects to the placement, he is ignored.

Rules of Turn-taking

Presence.

The customer brings his items for purchase to the storekeeper. The storekeeper asks if the customer wishes to purchase anything else. He says no. The storekeeper enters the amount in the cash register and tells the customer how much he owes. The customer pays the storekeeper, who then thanks the customer for shopping at her store.

Absence.

The customer brings his items for purchase to the storekeeper who is playing with the cash register. Despite repeated attempts to pay for his items, the storekeeper ignores them, remaining fascinated by the cash register's digital displays.

Roles

Presence.

The two children decide who will be the storekeeper and who will be the customer. Throughout the interaction, each maintains his or her role.

Absence.

The two children decide who will be the storekeeper and who will be the customer. The boy playing the customer frequently assumes the role of the storekeeper, even though it was agreed that he would remain the customer throughout the play period.

Listening

Presence.

The storekeeper asks the customer what he would like to purchase. The customer says that he would like a pound of ground meat, but only if it's fresh. The storekeeper says that it was just ground and that she guarantees he will like it. The customer says that he trusts her and will therefore buy the ground meat.

Absence.

The storekeeper asks the customer what he would like to purchase. The customer says that he would like a pound of ground meat, but only if it's fresh. The storekeeper says that she keeps the oranges in the refrigerator if he would like some.

Table 5.10
Example of the presence and absence of sensemaking behaviors

Example:

Two children enter a room with all the materials necessary to simulate a grocery store. The only instruction given to the children is that they are to "play store." The clinician leaves the room and then observes the interaction.

Cohesion and Organized Discourse

Presence.

The conversation between the two children appears to revolve around selecting, purchasing, and wrapping grocery items.

Absence.

Although the conversation between the two children appears to revolve around buying grocery items, the sequence of verbal interactions does not follow the expected sequence of purchasing behaviors.

Topic Comprehension and Elaboration.

Presence.

The storekeeper asks the customer what he would like to purchase. The customer says that he would like a pound of ground meat. The storekeeper asks what kind of meat the customer would like. He says "beef." The storekeeper asks if he would like sirloin or chuck.

Absence.

The storekeeper asks the customer what he would like to purchase. The customer says that he would like a pound of ground meat, but only if it's fresh. The storekeeper says that she just received an order of milk that spilled on the floor, and she must clean it up.

---

exhibited by adults who have been cognitively disabled since childhood. A rapidly increasing population of clients have suffered a brain injury that was not caused by a cardiovascular accident (stroke).

Aphasia

Aphasia refers to the loss or impairment of expressive or receptive language due to a brain injury, usually located in the left hemisphere. The most common cause of aphasia is stroke, a sudden disorder that usually occurs in older individuals and can be devastating to a person's emotional and psychological well-being. The following excerpts are from a book written by Helen Wulf (1973), a woman who became aphasic because of a stroke.

> [The brr-r-r- of the alarm clock sounds somewhere in my head . . . then it stops.]
> What is today? Oh yes! It's Tuesday, February third, and tomorrow I'm going all the way to the Valley with Hans. . . .
> How odd! My right arm feels so big I can't even move it! . . . And my head! . . . Surely the hurting should be over by now. Well, last week was awfully strenuous.

Table 5.11
Intentionality example

Example:

Two children enter a room with all the materials necessary to simulate a grocery store. The only instruction given to the children is that they are to "play store." The clinician leaves the room and then observes the interaction.

The materials for the store are randomly lying around the room. For the game to begin, the store has to be constructed. Both children help in arranging the materials, jointly and independently deciding where objects should go. If there is a disagreement, a discussion ensues and a decision is made.

The child acting the customer role brings his items for purchase to the storekeeper. The storekeeper asks if the customer wishes to purchase anything else. The customer says that he would like a pound of ground meat. The storekeeper asks what kind of meat the customer would like. The customer says "beef." The storekeeper asks if he wants chuck or sirloin. He says "sirloin." The storekeeper wraps the beef and asks if there is anything else she could get him. He says no. The storekeeper enters the amount on the cash register and the customer gives her some play money. Then the game ends.

Purpose of the Communication

The purpose of the communication was to facilitate the playing of a game involving a simulation of roles and activities occurring in grocery stores.

The communication was social.

Structure

The structure of the communication involved questions followed by answers and/or elaboration.

When you stop to think about it, it was the first hectic week since August. . . . How long is it going to take me to recoup my lost pep?

Hans is dressed and ready to go . . .

Where in the world have I been? . . .

How icky I feel . . .

Got to get to the office and tend to things . . .

Surely when I get up I'll feel better . . .

[I say something to Hans—I do not remember what, nor do I know that it is completely unintelligible.

I put on a robe and go to the bathroom. . . .]

I can't brush my teeth . . . I can't seem to do anything . . . I'll take a hormone pill . . . Maybe that's what I need . . . Here it is in your hand . . . you know you can't take it . . . Put it back . . . I can't get it back . . . Oh, just put it down . . .

[I feel a wall at my back—I have no inclination to go back to bed or to sit down—I seem unable to move, mentally or physically, but without anxiety.

Terrible nausea sweeps over me . . .]

Oh, don't worry—you haven't had anything to drink so probably there won't be much of anything to come up. . . .

[I feel myself slide quietly down the wall to the floor, my right leg going at right angles, and who knows where my left leg is. Then Hans is beside me. . . .]

Why, he's worried . . . goodness, this will be over soon . . . whatever it is.

[I can't say anything. . . . Then . . . I . . . remember . . . nothing . . . until . . . I I find myself in bed.] (pp. 20–21)

For Helen Wulf (1973), this was the beginning of her aphasia. Damage to the brain can cause a multitude of physical and linguistic problems. The problems can range from very mild with eventual and complete recovery to very severe and permanent damage. When observing clients with aphasia, focus on three areas of functioning: (a) motor behavior, (b) sensory behavior, and (c) communicative behavior.

Motor Behavior. The left hemisphere controls the behavior on the right side of the body, and the right hemisphere controls the behavior on the left side of the body. This is known as *contralateral behavior.* If you observe someone who has had a stroke with the resulting paralysis on the right side of the body, the damage occurred in the left hemisphere. Someone with a paralysis on the left side of the body suffered the stroke in the right hemisphere. Paralysis is not a necessary condition of a stroke, but it is usually present in some form. Two terms that are related to impairments of motor behavior are hemiplegia and dysarthria. *Hemiplegia* is also known as *hemiparesis,* or paralysis on one side of the body. It can be either a right hemiplegia or a left hemiplegia. *Dysarthria* is a motor speech disorder that may affect respiration, articulation, phonation, resonation, or prosody. Movements of the jaw and tongue may also be impaired.

Sensory Behavior. Whereas the motor control of one half of the body is completely controlled by the opposite hemisphere, vision and hearing for each eye and each ear are controlled by both hemispheres. Therefore, even if the portions of the left hemisphere that control the right eye and ear are damaged, sensations to these organs are not completely destroyed. Damage will be more extensive with vision than with audition. Half of the visual field of one eye may be lost. *Hemianopsia* is the loss of one half of the visual field for each eye. *Homonymous hemianopsia* is the loss of the same visual half field. Another type of sensory disorder is *apraxia,* a difficulty in programming the articulators for the correct use of phonemes within words.

Communicative Behavior. Aphasic disorders tend to be classified in terms of syndromes. A *syndrome* is a collection of behaviors that usually occur together. There are seven major aphasia syndromes, or classifications. They are (a) Wernicke's aphasia, (b) anomic aphasia, (c) conduction aphasia, (d) transcortical sensory aphasia, (e) Broca's aphasia, (f) transcortical motor aphasia, and (h) global aphasia. The differential diagnosis of aphasia is best left to a seminar on the disorder.

For purposes of observation, new clinical students should focus on six categories of behaviors: (a) conversational speech, (b) comprehension, (c) confrontational naming, (d) reading, (e) writing, and (f) ability to repeat an utterance. *Conversational speech* refers to the organization, structure, and flow of normal conversation. *Comprehension* involves the ability to understand various levels of abstractions. *Confrontational naming* is the ability to name an object, action, or idea when asked by the clinician to name it. Reading and writing are self-explanatory. Holland and Reinmuth (1982) have constructed an excellent table for identifying the aphasia syndrome based on these six behavioral categories (Table 5.12).

Table 5.12
Basic language characteristics of some major syndromes of aphasia.

Language Form	Wernicke	Anomic	Conduction	Transcortical Sensory	Broca	Transcortical Motor	Global
Conversational speech	Fluent, paraphasic	Fluent, empty	Fluent, paraphasic	Fluent, paraphasic, echolalic	Nonfluent	Nonfluent	Nonfluent
Comprehension of speech	Below normal to poor	Relatively good	Relatively good	Poor to extremely poor	Relatively good	Relatively good	Poor
Repetition	Predictable from comprehension	Good	Not predictable from comprehension, poor	Not predictable from comprehension, good to excellent	Predictable from comprehension, good	Predictable from comprehension, good to excellent	Predictable from comprehension, poor
Confrontation naming	Defective to poor	Defective	Usually defective	Poor	Defective to poor	Defective	Poor
Reading comprehension	Defective to poor	Usually moderately good	Usually good	Defective to poor	Not predictable	Not predictable	Poor
Writing	Poor	Moderately good, abnormal in substantive word finding	Moderately impaired	Poor	Moderately impaired	Moderately impaired	Poor

Source: From "Aphasia in adults" by A. L. Holland and O. M. Reinmuth, 1982, in G. H. Shames and E. H. Wiig (Eds.), *Human communication disorders* (pp. 426–452). Columbus, OH: Merrill/Macmillan. Copyright 1982 by Merrill/Macmillan. Reprinted by permission.

Traumatic Brain Injury

Traumatic brain injury (TBI) is defined as an injury to the brain caused by a physical trauma. Four major types of trauma can cause traumatic brain injury: (a) closed head injury, (b) open head injury, (c) coma, and (d) posttraumatic amnesia (Beukelman & Yorkston, 1991)

Types of Head Injuries. *Closed head injuries,* the most common cause of TBI, are injuries that usually occur when the skull is severely impacted without any penetration occurring. Injuries of this type are associated with blows to the head resulting from falls, assaults, and vehicle accidents. The type of damage occurring to the brain tends to be diffuse.

Open head injuries occur either when the skull is penetrated by an object or the skull is cracked. Gunshot wounds and skull fractures are the most commonly occurring causes of open head injuries. Unlike closed head injuries, the brain damage tends to be confined to the area of penetration.

Coma occurs because of damage or depression to the normal functioning of the central nervous system. It can be caused by neuronal or axonal injury, hypoxemia, or ischemia. The physiology of coma is still not completely understood. Descriptions usually involve its depth and an evaluation of performance on eye opening, motor responses, and verbal responses (Teasdale & Jennett, 1974).

Posttraumatic amnesia can occur following an injury. Memory loss can be limited to the events immediately preceding and following the injury or may be extensive, including loss of all memory. Names of people and events are often unretrievable. In time, access may return to some or all stored information.

General Behavioral Problems. Problems associated with TBI can range over the full spectrum of human behaviors, depending on the site and extent of the damage. They can affect an individual's functioning in the areas of cognition, language, and social integration. The greatest amount of impairment in each area occurs immediately after the injury. In time, some or all of the behaviors may return to their premorbid state. Twenty-four of the most commonly appearing behaviors are listed in Table 5.13.

Speech and Language Behaviors. Speech behaviors will be affected only if the areas in the brain that control speech are damaged. Of primary concern for speech production is the area known as the *motor strip*. Damage in this area can result in dysarthric speech similar to that found in clients with aphasia. The language of TBI clients tends to have fewer syntactic and retrieval problems and significantly more problems in the area of pragmatics.

❑ ❑ ❑ METALINGUISTIC ANALYSIS

The term *metalinguistics* has been used to refer to the study of the linguistic intent, or classification, of whole utterances rather than specific words or small combi-

Table 5.13
Problems associated with TBI

Cognition	Speech/Motor Control
Concentration	Elective mutism
Mental shifting	Apraxia
Learning	Dysarthria
Incomplete thoughts	Swallowing problems
Reasoning	Respiration
Problem solving	Writing
Planning and execution	
Memory	**Emotional/Social**
	Impulse control
Language	Use of social rules
Disorganization	Humor
Pragmatics	Confusion
Word retrieval	Initiation
Reading	Disorientation

nations of words. This type of linguistic analysis can provide the observer with a way of understanding either the flow of communication or how one person in the interaction views the other person. Although general methods of metalinguistic analysis can be used for assessing the communication of many children, a more specific method is required for others who have less sophisticated language.

Children's Metalinguistic Analysis

An excellent metalinguistic system for children was developed by McShane (1980). His five communicative function categories can be very useful for analyzing the intent of a child's communication. They can allow the clinician to classify the communicative intent of a child's early language. The categories appear in Table 5.14.

Adult Metalinguistic Analysis

Various methods have been devised for analyzing different types of interactions. Culatta and Seltzer (1976) developed a simple method of analyzing the interactions that occur between clinicians and supervisors. This method was later used to analyze client-clinician interactions. A modification of the Culatta and Seltzer system allows new clinicians to begin the process of metalinguistic analysis. The observer classifies all utterances into eight categories. These categories are identical for both client and clinician.

Demand	Asks for a verbal response or to perform a behavior
Description	Cites location or attribute of an object
Closed Question	Question requiring less than a two-word response

Table 5.14
Children's communicative function categories

Category	Definition	Example
Regulation		
Attention	An utterance that attempts to direct the attention of another person	*look,* as the child points to an object and looks up at the listener
Request	An utterance that requests that another person do something	*juice,* as the child holds out a glass to the mother
Vocative	An utterance that calls another person to locate him or her or to request his or her presence	*Mommy* (spoken loudly) as the child goes from room to room in search of mother
Statement		
Naming	An utterance that refers to an object or person by name only	*car,* as the child points to a car
Description	An utterance that makes some statement, other than naming, about an object, action, or event	*gone,* as the child arrives at the location where a desired object is usually found, but is unable to find it
Information	An utterance that makes a statement about an event beyond the "here-and-now", excluding acts that the child is about to perform	*chick,* as the child looks at the visitor. The mother then comments, "We saw some chicks at the farm yesterday, didn't we?"
Exchange		
Giving	An utterance spoken while giving or attempting to give an object to another person	*here,* as the child hands a doll to the father
Receiving	An utterance spoken while receiving an object from another person	*thank you,* as the child takes the offered cookie

Open Question	Question requiring more than a two-word response
Statement	Utterance that is neither a description nor a question
No Response	No verbal response (or desired behavior)
One- to Two-Word Answer	Made in response to a question
Long Answer	Made in response to a question

By using this method, even new clinicians can perform a simple form of metalinguistic analysis. With the use of these categories, an observer may be able to determine if a significant pattern of clinical interaction is occurring. For example, if closed questions are usually followed by one to two word answers, and

Category	Definition	Example
Personal		
Doing	An utterance describing an act the child is performing or has just performed	*down,* after the child has just put a box of blocks on the floor
Determination	An utterance specifying the child's intention to carry out some act immediately	*out,* spoken immediately before standing up and walking toward the door
Refusal	An utterance used to refuse an object or request to do something	*no,* as the mother hands the child a hat to put on the doll
Protest	A "high-pitched" utterance expressing the child's displeasure with an action by another person	*don't!* as the child's brother starts to take the play phone away from the child
Conversation		
Imitation	An utterance that imitates all or part of a preceding adult utterance with no intervening utterance on the child's part	*fish,* in response to the father's utterance, "What a big fish."
Answer	An utterance spoken in response to a question (excluding imitations)	*shoe,* in response to the mother's question, "What's this called?"
Follow-on	An utterance serving as a conversational response that is neither an imitation nor an answer	*yeah,* in response to the visitor's comment, "Let's see what's in the box."
Question	An utterance that requests information from another person	*what's that?* as the child looks first at a microphone, then at the visitor

Source: From *Learning to Talk* by J. McShane, 1980, Cambridge, England: Cambridge University Press. Copyright 1980 by Cambridge University Press. Reprinted by permission.

open questions are usually followed by long answers, the observer may have found a way of increasing the length of client responses.

Although some important information can be gained through this analysis, it is not sophisticated enough to provide the observer with many of the more subtle metalinguistic forms that occur during clinical interactions. Molyneaux and Lane's (1982) interview analysis format provides the sophistication necessary for an in-depth analysis. In their system, 20 categories are applied to interviewer utterances and 15 categories are applied to respondent utterances. Many of the categories can be applied either to the clinician or the client. Categories referring to the interviewer appear in Table 5.15 and respondent responses appear in Table 5.16. For coding purposes, interviewer utterances are numbered between 1 and 49, and respondent utterances are numbered between 50 and 99.

Table 5.15
Interviewer categories

01 Indirect Question: Does not require question mark punctuation yet encourages discussion of a particular topic
Example: Tell me about his stuttering problem.

02 Direct Question I: Requests specific externally verifiable statistic
Example: How old is she?

03 Direct Question II: Requests information, opinion, or conclusion other than an externally verifiable statistic
Example: Why do you think he does that?

04 Leading Question: Asks a direct question that indicates the specific answer is expected or preferred
Example: You wouldn't let him do that, would you?

05 Double Question I: Asks two questions, the second question identical or almost identical to the first
Example: What does he do? What job does he have?

06 Double Question II: Asks two questions, the second question dissimilar to the first or incomplete
Example: How old is he? Is he in school today?

07 Bombardment: Contains three or more questions of any type
Example: Do you read to him? Does he listen? How often?

08 MM-HM Response: Indicates that listener is "tuned in" and following conversation
Example: That's interesting.

09 Approval: Expresses agreement with or favorable judgment of respondent's statement, action, and/or reported behavior when respondent has not expressed a judgment
Example: You did the right thing.

10 Disapproval: Expresses negative evaluation of respondent's statement, action, and/or reported behavior
Example: You shouldn't really do that.

11 Forcing Client Responsibility: Immediately redirects respondent's question back to respondent
Example: I will tell you what I think, but how do you feel about it?

12 Information: Provides data
Example: I will be here Tuesday.

13 Reassurance: Confirms or validates respondent's stated information or supposition
Example: Most professionals would agree with you.

14 Restatement of Content: Repeats or summarizes actual material or data expressed verbally by respondent
Example: What you are saying then is that he's slow.

15 Reflection of Feeling: Attempts to verbalize current emotions expressed either verbally or nonverbally by respondent
Example: I can tell that this is important to you.

16 Structuring: Orients respondent to interview situation or procedure to be followed during interview
Example: During this interview we will talk only about your son's problems.

17 Interpretation: Suggests possible motivation (not verbally expressed by the respondent) to account for respondent's expressed action or feeling
Example: You said you were uncomfortable. Is that because I have insulted you?

18 Advice or Suggestion: Recommends a course of action to be followed by the respondent other than during the interview
Example: Listen to him only when he is fluent.

19 Nonpertinent Small Talk: Consists of irrelevant comments or social amenities
Example: What a lovely day it is today.

20 Other: Any utterance not defined above

Source: From *Effective Interviewing* by D. Molyneaux and V. W. Lane, 1982, New York: Allyn & Bacon. Copyright 1982 by Allyn & Bacon. Reprinted by permission.

Table 5.16
Respondent categories (I = Interviewer; R = Respondent)

50 Agreement: Confirms interviewer's statement
Example: I: Your daughter doesn't have much language.
R: Yes, she has only a few words.

51 Disagreement: Denies or differs with interviewer's statement
Example: I: You should require her to use words.
R: No, I don't think that is a good idea.

52 Request for Information: Seeks data from interviewer
Example: I: We have time to talk about his development.
R: What is it you want to know?

53 Information: Provides data for interviewer
Example: I: How did you hear about this program?
R: I read about it in the newspaper.

54 Indication of Problem Area: Identifies or indicates situation that is currently causing stress or concern
Example: I: How are things going at home?
R: Not well, I can't seem to control my children.

55 Insight: Expresses awareness of motivation or consequences of behavior that was not previously understood or verbalized
Example: I: You've expressed some real anger today.
R: You're right. For the first time I allowed myself to feel that kind of anger.

56 Planning: Verbalizes own planned future behavior
Example: I: It's difficult to organize activities with three children.
R: I know, but starting next week I'm sticking to my schedule.

57 MM-HM Responses: Indicates listener is "tuned in" and following conversation
Example: I: Our student clinicians are very competent.
R: I see.

58 Advice or Suggestion: Recommends course of action to be followed by the interviewer or the interviewer's agency
Example: I: After observing Jim, what did you think of his behavior?
R: I think the clinician let him get away with murder. Tell her to be more strict.

59 Agreement with Restatement, Reflection, Interpretation, or Leading Question Plus Asking for Information: Confirms interviewer's statement and seeks data from interviewer
Example: I: You sound worried about his language development.
R: Yes, I am. How will he function as an adult?

60 Agreement with Restatement, Reflection, Interpretation, or Leading Question Plus Giving Information: Confirms interviewer's statement and provides data
Example: I: So, he has always been slow in developing.
R: Yes, especially in the area of toileting.

61 Disagreement with Restatement, Reflection, Interpretation, or Leading Question Plus Asking for Information: Denies or differs with interviewer's statement and seeks data from interviewer
Example: I: I think he is very distractable.
R: No, he's not. Did you see him working with the puzzle?

62 Disagreement with Restatement, Reflection, Interpretation, or Leading Question Plus Giving Information: Denies or differs with interviewer's statement and provides data
Example: I: It sounds as if you think Bobby is unhappy.
R: No, not at all. He's just angry sometimes.

63 Nonpertinent Small Talk: Consists of irrelevant comments or social amenities
Example: I: Thank you for coming in today.
R: You're welcome. It was a nice day for a drive.

64 Other: Any utterance not defined above

Source: From *Effective Interviewing* by D. Molyneaux and V. W. Lane, 1982, New York: Allyn & Bacon. Copyright 1982 by Allyn & Bacon. Reprinted by permission.

SUMMARY

In this chapter the various components of language and their potential disruptions were presented. The ability to describe language accurately depends on the context in which language occurs. Language is communication, not merely a collection of linguistic components that can be understood without reference to the speaker, listener, and intent of the message. The importance of language to an individual's everyday functioning elevates it to a status that many believe is above all other communicative disorders. It probably is also the most complex behavior to describe accurately.

Since it is based on cognitive processes, language comprehension must often be inferred rather than objectively determined. For example, is a brain-injured individual unable to engage in conversations because of an inability to use appropriate pragmatic skills, or has the emotional trauma of being disabled resulted in a lack of desire to communicate? Ambiguities are also present in language productions. Does the child who uses verb phrases have a language disorder, or are verb phrases more appropriate than complete sentences in the situation in which the language sample was taken? What these questions exemplify is that language comprises many interrelated parts, some linguistic, some cognitive, and others situational. To describe language behaviors, a view of the "gestalt," or whole, must be kept in mind.

SUGGESTED READINGS

Beukelman, D. R., & Yorkston, K. M. (1991). *Communication disorders following traumatic brain injury.* Austin, TX: Pro-ed.

Brown, R. (1973). *A first language, the early stages.* Cambridge, MA: Harvard University Press.

Compton, C. (1990). *A guide to 85 tests for special education.* Belmont, CA: Fearon Education.

Darley, F. L. (Ed.) (1979). *Evaluation of appraisal techniques in speech and language pathology.* Reading, MA: Addison-Wesley.

Duchan, J. F. (1984). Language assessment: The pragmatics revolution. In R. C. Naremore (Ed.), *Language science,* (pp. 147–180). San Diego, CA: College-Hill Press.

Holland, A. L.; Swindell, C. S.; & Reinmuth, O. M. (1990). Aphasia and related adult disorders. In G. H. Shames and E. H. Wiig (Eds.), *Human communication disorders: An introduction* (3rd ed., pp. 424–461). New York: Merrill/Macmillan.

McShane, J. (1980). *Learning to talk.* Cambridge, England: Cambridge University Press.

Molyneaux, D., & Lane, V. W. (1982). *Effective interviewing.* New York: Allyn & Bacon.

Wulf, H. H. (1973). *Aphasia, my world alone.* Detroit, MI: Wayne State University Press.

❑ **Activity 5.1**
Language Observation

The analysis of linguistic disorders can be complex and require sophisticated diagnostic instruments. This section has provided the clinician with guidelines for focusing attention on specific aspects of language: lexicon, syntax, morphology, and pragmatics. Before analyzing a language sample, the clinician should follow these instructions:

1. Record a 15-minute segment of the speech of a client. Be sure to tell the child's clinician that you will be doing a language sample so that he or she can try to elicit speech from the child. Share your results with your clinician.
2. Transcribe the first 50 utterances of the child along with the clinician's statements. Use the transcription sheets that follow.
3. Analyze the child's constituent structure grammar.
4. Analyze the child's transformational grammar.
5. Analyze the child's case structure grammar.
6. Analyze the child's functional language categories.

Transcription Form

Measures of Sentence Length

1. Longest Utterance [ ]
2. Most Frequently Occurring Utterance Length [ ]
3. MLU [ ]

Lexicon

1. Total number of words spoken [ ]
2. Number of different words spoken [ ]
3. Percentage of different words for sample [ ]

Morphology

Check the appropriate boxes.	Not Heard	Present
Simple Present Progressive	[ ]	[ ]
Simple Future Progressive	[ ]	[ ]
Simple Past Progressive	[ ]	[ ]
Present Perfect Progressive	[ ]	[ ]
Future Perfect Progressive	[ ]	[ ]
Past Perfect Progressive	[ ]	[ ]
Plural	[ ]	[ ]
Past Irregular	[ ]	[ ]
Past Regular	[ ]	[ ]
Contractible Copula	[ ]	[ ]
Uncontractible Copula	[ ]	[ ]
Articles	[ ]	[ ]
Third Person Singular Regular	[ ]	[ ]
Third Person Singular Irregular	[ ]	[ ]
Contractible Auxiliary	[ ]	[ ]
Uncontractible Auxiliary	[ ]	[ ]

continues

Activity 5.1, continued

Syntax

	Not Heard	Present
Check the appropriate boxes.		

1. Phrase Structure Grammar

	Not Heard	Present
Article	[ ]	[ ]
Adjective	[ ]	[ ]
Adverb	[ ]	[ ]
Preposition	[ ]	[ ]
Verb	[ ]	[ ]
Noun	[ ]	[ ]
Conjunction	[ ]	[ ]
Verb Phrase	[ ]	[ ]
Noun Phrase	[ ]	[ ]
Sentence	[ ]	[ ]

2. Transformational Grammar

	Not Heard	Present

Appropriate Types

	Not Heard	Present
Passive	[ ]	[ ]
Negation	[ ]	[ ]
Question	[ ]	[ ]
Contraction	[ ]	[ ]
Inversion	[ ]	[ ]
Relative Question	[ ]	[ ]
Imperative	[ ]	[ ]
Pronominalization	[ ]	[ ]
Separation	[ ]	[ ]
Got	[ ]	[ ]
Auxiliary *Be* Placement	[ ]	[ ]
Auxiliary *Have* Placement	[ ]	[ ]
Do	[ ]	[ ]
Possessive	[ ]	[ ]
Reflexive	[ ]	[ ]
Conjunction	[ ]	[ ]
Conjunction Deletion	[ ]	[ ]
If Conjunction	[ ]	[ ]
So Conjunction	[ ]	[ ]
Cause Conjunction	[ ]	[ ]
Pronoun in Conjunction	[ ]	[ ]
Adjective	[ ]	[ ]
Relative Clause	[ ]	[ ]
Infinitival Complement	[ ]	[ ]
Participial Complement	[ ]	[ ]
Iteration	[ ]	[ ]
Nominalization	[ ]	[ ]
Nominal Compound	[ ]	[ ]

	Not Heard	Present
Restricted Forms		
Verb Phrase Omission	[ ]	[ ]
Verb Phrase Substitution	[ ]	[ ]
Verb Phrase Redundancy	[ ]	[ ]
Noun Phrase Omission	[ ]	[ ]
Noun Phrase Redundancy	[ ]	[ ]
Preposition Omission	[ ]	[ ]
Preposition Substitution	[ ]	[ ]
Preposition Redundancy	[ ]	[ ]
Article Omission	[ ]	[ ]
Article Substitution	[ ]	[ ]
Article Redundancy	[ ]	[ ]
Particle Omission	[ ]	[ ]
Particle Redundancy	[ ]	[ ]
Contraction Deletion *Be*	[ ]	[ ]
Contraction Deletion *Have*	[ ]	[ ]
Double Negation	[ ]	[ ]
Inversion Subject-Object	[ ]	[ ]
Inversion Verb Number	[ ]	[ ]
No Question	[ ]	[ ]
Pronominalization Substitution	[ ]	[ ]
No Separation	[ ]	[ ]

Semantic Relations

Check the appropriate boxes.	Not Heard	Present
Two-Word Combinations		
Nomination	[ ]	[ ]
Notice	[ ]	[ ]
Recurrence	[ ]	[ ]
Nonexistence	[ ]	[ ]
Attributive	[ ]	[ ]
Possessive	[ ]	[ ]
Locative	[ ]	[ ]
Agent-Action	[ ]	[ ]
Agent-Object	[ ]	[ ]
Action-Object		
Case Structures		
Noun-Objective	[ ]	[ ]
Noun-Experiencer	[ ]	[ ]
Noun-Locative	[ ]	[ ]
Noun-Agent	[ ]	[ ]
Noun-Instrument	[ ]	[ ]
Noun-Factitive	[ ]	[ ]
Noun-Dative	[ ]	[ ]

continues

Activity 5.1, continued

Verb-Preference	[ ]	[ ]
Verb-Behavior	[ ]	[ ]
Verb-Notice	[ ]	[ ]
Verb-Sensation	[ ]	[ ]
Verb-Condition	[ ]	[ ]
Adjective-Possessive	[ ]	[ ]
Adjective-Number	[ ]	[ ]
Adjective-Temporal	[ ]	[ ]
Adjective-Size	[ ]	[ ]
Adjective-Color	[ ]	[ ]
Adjective-Quality	[ ]	[ ]
Adverb-Qualification	[ ]	[ ]

Pragmatics

Check the appropriate boxes.   **Appropriate Inappropriate**

Interactions

Cooperation and Turn-Taking	[ ]	[ ]
Role Relationship	[ ]	[ ]
Listening	[ ]	[ ]

Sensemaking

Organization of Discourse	[ ]	[ ]
Cohesion of Discourse	[ ]	[ ]
Topic Comprehension	[ ]	[ ]
Topic Elaboration	[ ]	[ ]

Intentionality

Purpose of the interaction _____ (complete)

Was the interaction social?   yes   no   (circle one)

Structure for realizing goal _____ (complete)

❑ *Activity 5.2*
Aphasia Observation

When initially observing the behaviors of an aphasic client, new clinicians should not be concerned with identifying syndromes. It is more important to first identify all behaviors that may be associated with the aphasic condition. Additionally, we will use the subjective judgments of *moderate* and *poor* in our observations. These terms are used because many new clinicians may not have had an academic course in aphasia. When additional knowledge is acquired and formal diagnostic tests are used, these terms may be discarded for more objective measurements. Observe a client for at least 20 minutes. Use the following checklist to identify the behaviors you observe.

Aphasia

Check the appropriate boxes.

	No Problem	Problem Present
Motor Behavior		
Right Hemiplegia	[ ]	[ ]
Left Hemiplegia	[ ]	[ ]
Dysarthria	[ ]	[ ]
Sensory Behavior		
Right Hemianopsia	[ ]	[ ]
Left Hemianopsia	[ ]	[ ]
Apraxia	[ ]	[ ]

	No Problem	Mild Problem	Moderate Problem	Severe Problem
Language Behavior				
Conversational Speech	[ ]	[ ]	[ ]	[ ]
Comprehension of Speech	[ ]	[ ]	[ ]	[ ]
Repetition	[ ]	[ ]	[ ]	[ ]
Confrontation Naming	[ ]	[ ]	[ ]	[ ]
Reading Comprehension	[ ]	[ ]	[ ]	[ ]
Writing	[ ]	[ ]	[ ]	[ ]

Activity 5.3
Metalinguistic Analysis

In this activity you will be performing a metalinguistic analysis on a child-clinician interaction and an adult-clinician interaction. The first step is to transcribe the verbal interaction that occurs between a client and the clinician. Record the first 20 verbal interactions for your analysis on the form that appears at the end of this section. On both the child and the adult forms, spaces are provided for two different types of metalinguistic analysis. For children, use both the modified Culatta-Seltzer model and the McShane model. For adults, use the modified Culatta-Seltzer model and the Molyneaux-Lane model. Following the classification of utterances, summarize your findings in the last section of each form.

Reference Chart for Metalinguistic Categories

Modified Culatta-Seltzer Model	McShane Model	Molyneaux-Lane Model
Demand	**Regulation**	**Interviewer** / **Respondent**
Description	Attention	Indirect Question / Agreement
Closed Question	Request	Direct Question I / Disagreement
Open Question	Vocative	Direct Question II / Request for Information
Statement	**Statement**	Leading Question / Information
No Response	Naming	Double Question I / Indication of Problem Area
One- to Two- Word Answer	Description	Double Question II / Insight
Long Answer	Information	Bombardment / Planning
Information	**Exchange**	MM-HM Response / MM-HM Response
	Giving	Approval / Advice or Suggestion
	Receiving	Disapproval / Agreement with Restatement, Reflection, Interpretation, or Leading Question plus Asking for Information
	Personal	Forcing Client Responsibility
	Doing	Information
	Determination	Reassurance
	Refusal	Restatement of Content / Agreement with Restatement, Reflection, Interpretation, or Leading Question plus Giving Information
	Protest	Reflection of Feeling
	Conversation	Structuring
	Imitation	Interpretation / Disagreement with Restatement, Reflection, Interpretation, or Leading Question plus Asking for Information
	Answer	Advice or Suggestion
	Follow-On	Nonpertinent Small Talk
	Question	Other / Disagreement with Restatement, Reflection, Interpretation, or Leading Question plus Giving Information
		Nonpertinent Small Talk
		Other

CHILD METALINGUISTIC ANALYSIS

There are two lines for each set of utterances. Record a *T* next to the clinician's statement and a *C* next to the client's. If only one person speaks, place an X on the remaining line of the utterance set.

T/C/X		Modified Culatta-Seltzer	McShane
1. ( )	_____	_____	_____
( )	_____	_____	_____
2. ( )	_____	_____	_____
( )	_____	_____	_____
3. ( )	_____	_____	_____
( )	_____	_____	_____
4. ( )	_____	_____	_____
( )	_____	_____	_____
5. ( )	_____	_____	_____
( )	_____	_____	_____
6. ( )	_____	_____	_____
( )	_____	_____	_____
7. ( )	_____	_____	_____
( )	_____	_____	_____
8. ( )	_____	_____	_____
( )	_____	_____	_____
9. ( )	_____	_____	_____
( )	_____	_____	_____
10. ( )	_____	_____	_____
( )	_____	_____	_____
11. ( )	_____	_____	_____
( )	_____	_____	_____
12. ( )	_____	_____	_____
( )	_____	_____	_____
13. ( )	_____	_____	_____
( )	_____	_____	_____
14. ( )	_____	_____	_____
( )	_____	_____	_____
15. ( )	_____	_____	_____

continues

Activity 5.3, continued

	T/C/X	Modified Culatta-Seltzer	McShane
	( ) _____	_____	_____
16.	( ) _____	_____	_____
	( ) _____	_____	_____
17.	( ) _____	_____	_____
	( ) _____	_____	_____
18.	( ) _____	_____	_____
	( ) _____	_____	_____
19.	( ) _____	_____	_____
	( ) _____	_____	_____
20.	( ) _____	_____	_____
	( ) _____	_____	_____

CHILD METALINGUISTIC SUMMARY DATA

Indicate the number and percent of utterances for clinician and client.

Modified Culatta-Seltzer Model

	Client		Clinician	
	Number of Utterances	Percentage of Utterances	Number of Utterances	Percentage of Utterances
Demand	[ ]	[ ]	[ ]	[ ]
Description	[ ]	[ ]	[ ]	[ ]
Closed Question	[ ]	[ ]	[ ]	[ ]
Open Question	[ ]	[ ]	[ ]	[ ]
Statement	[ ]	[ ]	[ ]	[ ]
No Response	[ ]	[ ]	[ ]	[ ]
One- to Two-Word Answer	[ ]	[ ]	[ ]	[ ]
Long Answer	[ ]	[ ]	[ ]	[ ]

Note any patterns of interaction that occurred.

McShane Model

	Client	
	Number of Utterances	**Percentage of Utterances**

Regulation
Attention   [   ]   [   ]
Request   [   ]   [   ]
Vocative   [   ]   [   ]

Statement
Naming   [   ]   [   ]
Description   [   ]   [   ]
Information   [   ]   [   ]

Exchange
Giving   [   ]   [   ]
Receiving   [   ]   [   ]

Personal
Doing   [   ]   [   ]
Determination   [   ]   [   ]
Refusal   [   ]   [   ]
Protest   [   ]   [   ]

Conversation
Imitation   [   ]   [   ]
Answer   [   ]   [   ]
Follow-On   [   ]   [   ]
Question   [   ]   [   ]

Totals   Number   Percentage
Regulation   [   ]   [   ]
Statement   [   ]   [   ]
Exchange   [   ]   [   ]
Personal   [   ]   [   ]
Conversation   [   ]   [   ]

Note any patterns of interaction that occurred.

continues

Activity 5.3, continued

ADULT METALINGUISTIC ANALYSIS

There are two lines for each set of utterances. Record a *T* next to the clinician's statement and a *C* next to the client's. If only one person speaks, place an X on the remaining line of the utterance set.

T/C/X	Modified Culatta-Seltzer	Molyneaux-Lane
1. ( ) _____	_____	_____
( ) _____	_____	_____
2. ( ) _____	_____	_____
( ) _____	_____	_____
3. ( ) _____	_____	_____
( ) _____	_____	_____
4. ( ) _____	_____	_____
( ) _____	_____	_____
5. ( ) _____	_____	_____
( ) _____	_____	_____
6. ( ) _____	_____	_____
( ) _____	_____	_____
7. ( ) _____	_____	_____
( ) _____	_____	_____
8. ( ) _____	_____	_____
( ) _____	_____	_____
9. ( ) _____	_____	_____
( ) _____	_____	_____
10. ( ) _____	_____	_____
( ) _____	_____	_____
11. ( ) _____	_____	_____
( ) _____	_____	_____
12. ( ) _____	_____	_____
( ) _____	_____	_____
13. ( ) _____	_____	_____
( ) _____	_____	_____
14. ( ) _____	_____	_____
( ) _____	_____	_____
15. ( ) _____	_____	_____
( ) _____	_____	_____
16. ( ) _____	_____	_____
( ) _____	_____	_____
17. ( ) _____	_____	_____
( ) _____	_____	_____
18. ( ) _____	_____	_____
( ) _____	_____	_____
19. ( ) _____	_____	_____
( ) _____	_____	_____
20. ( ) _____	_____	_____
( ) _____	_____	_____

Molyneaux-Lane Model

	Number of Utterances	Percentage of Utterances		Number of Utterances	Percentage of Utterances
Clinician			**Client**		
Indirect Question	[ ]	[ ]	Agreement	[ ]	[ ]
Direct Question I	[ ]	[ ]	Disagreement	[ ]	[ ]
Direct Question II	[ ]	[ ]	Request for Information	[ ]	[ ]
Leading Question	[ ]	[ ]	Information	[ ]	[ ]
Double Question I	[ ]	[ ]	Indication of Problem		
Double Question II	[ ]	[ ]	Area	[ ]	[ ]
Bombardment	[ ]	[ ]	Insight	[ ]	[ ]
MM-HM Response	[ ]	[ ]	Planning	[ ]	[ ]
Approval	[ ]	[ ]	MM-HM Responses	[ ]	[ ]
Disapproval	[ ]	[ ]	Advice or Suggestion	[ ]	[ ]
Forcing Client			Agree and ask for		
Responsibility	[ ]	[ ]	information	[ ]	[ ]
Information	[ ]	[ ]	Agree and give		
Reassurance	[ ]	[ ]	information	[ ]	[ ]
Restatement of Content	[ ]	[ ]	Disagree and ask for		
Reflection of Feeling	[ ]	[ ]	information	[ ]	[ ]
Structuring	[ ]	[ ]	Disagree and give		
Interpretation	[ ]	[ ]	information	[ ]	[ ]
Advice or Suggestion	[ ]	[ ]	Nonpertinent Small Talk	[ ]	[ ]
Nonpertinent Small Talk	[ ]	[ ]	Other	[ ]	[ ]
Other	[ ]	[ ]			

Note any patterns of interaction that occurred between the client and the clinician.

ADULT METALINGUISTIC SUMMARY

Indicate the number and percentage of utterances for clinician and client.

Modified Culatta-Seltzer Model

	Client		**Clinician**	
	Number of Utterances	Percentage of Utterances	Number of Utterances	Percentage of Utterances
Demand	[ ]	[ ]	[ ]	[ ]
Description	[ ]	[ ]	[ ]	[ ]
Closed Question	[ ]	[ ]	[ ]	[ ]
Open Question	[ ]	[ ]	[ ]	[ ]
Statement	[ ]	[ ]	[ ]	[ ]
No Response	[ ]	[ ]	[ ]	[ ]
One- to Two-Word Answer	[ ]	[ ]	[ ]	[ ]
Long Answer	[ ]	[ ]	[ ]	[ ]

Note any patterns of interaction that occurred.

Chapter 6
Nonverbal Observation

STUDY GUIDE

- ❏ Classify descriptions of various behaviors using appropriate terminology.
- ❏ Given nonverbal terminology, describe the behaviors to which they refer.
- ❏ Describe a unit of behavior known as a nonverbal act/position.
- ❏ Vocalic behaviors are divided into prosody and paralanguage. Given examples, classify them using appropriate terminology.
- ❏ Shown a videotape or given a description of an interaction, identify each of the five different types of contexts that are present.
- ❏ Nonverbal behaviors can have various functions. How are these related to verbal behaviors?
- ❏ Describe the rank ordering of body parts in their ability to send other-directed messages and also be sites of self-directed adaptive behaviors. How are these findings related to clinical situations?

Clinicians engaged in therapeutic interactions tend to rely heavily on verbal communication as a means of understanding their clients' problems. Communication, however, is a multidimensional process that depends on both verbal and nonverbal behaviors. Clinicians should be able to describe and classify the nonverbal behaviors they observe. Through the careful study of nonverbal behaviors, a fuller description and understanding of clinical interactions will be possible.

LEVELS OF ANALYSIS

Nonverbal behaviors can be analyzed at three different levels: prekinesics, microkinesics, and social kinesics. Prekinesics is the most basic nonverbal behavior, involving only physiology. Microkinesics involves individual communication, and social kinesics examines the behaviors within societal boundaries (Eisenberg & Smith, 1971).

Prekinesics

Prekinesics is the study of what movements the body is capable of making. For example, a study of the maximum physical extension of a wrist would be included in prekinesics. The observation and recording of prekinesic behaviors is a task best left to other disciplines. It has clinical usefulness only in so far as it describes the physical limitations of an individual's other- and self-directed nonverbal communicative behaviors as a result of a physical or neurological problem. For example, an aphasic client who is unable to move her right hand and foot may transfer other-directed behaviors to her left side while minimizing the display of self-directed behaviors.

Behaviors such as tics, torticollis, and fine tremor-like behaviors would be studied at the prekinesic level. These behaviors are thought to indicate a possible disorganization of the central motor coordinating mechanisms. An example in therapy would be tremors observed in an aphasic client's weakened arm or the inappropriate squealing associated with a neurological condition known as Gilles de la Tourette's syndrome.

Microkinesics

Microkinesics studies only expressive movements. This would include an examination of the hand movements made by a speaker attempting to emphasize his point nonverbally, as well as the repetitive leg movements of a client during a discussion of responsibility. Clinically, microkinesics is the starting point of nonverbal observation. It attempts to develop a behavioral repertoire of the client and relate it to the verbal interactions that are occurring. The person most responsible for developing the study of both prekinesics and microkinesics is Ray L. Birdwhistell. He contends that before we can ascribe meaning to any behavior, we must first observe and describe its smallest units (Birdwhistell, 1968). To achieve this task, he constructed a complex system of analysis similar to the systems that linguists use to describe the phonetic, phonemic, morphological, and syntactic aspects of language. As important as his system is to the general study of nonverbal behaviors, it may be too complex for new clinical students. A more effective way of studying clinical nonverbal behaviors is to divide the body into its major units and describe the behaviors that occur in each area. For analysis, the body observations are divided into face, arms/hands, feet/legs, posture, and vocalic.

Facial Behaviors. In most Western cultures, the area most often observed during interactions is the face. With hundreds of muscles, the face is capable of conveying a multitude of visual messages. These behaviors may regulate the interaction or be related to the verbal message.

Regulators are the behaviors that regulate the rate and flow of interactions between two or more people. In American culture, they consist mainly of head nods and eye movements. In a clinical interaction, a clinician's head nod often indicates agreement with the client's verbalization and is also interpreted as the message, "Continue talking. This is information I think is important."

The use of the face is more important in its relationship to verbal messages than in its use as a regulator. It is the part of the body most often used to convey a message intentionally. The speaker can easily control it since awareness results from kinesic feedback and listener reactions. Because the face is so visible and controllable, it becomes the principal nonverbal avenue for displaying both truthful and deceptive messages. The husband of an aphasic client who feels hostile towards the clinician because of her suggestions may continue to smile throughout the interaction to convey a sense of civility. The mother who was taught not to show her emotions yet is deeply troubled by her Down syndrome child's need for supportive services may present a neutral facial display when discussing her son's future. Of all nonverbal behaviors, these are the ones to which clinicians are most attuned, since this is the area of the body people feel most comfortable observing during interactions.

One should not view all facial displays with skepticism. Most are genuine and are often used to elaborate or emphasize what is being communicated verbally. However, clinicians should not rely solely on facial behaviors to confirm the intent of a client's verbal message.

Arms/Hands. Because the arms and hands are less visible than the face, they have less communicative ability (Bull, 1987). Since they are used less to convey messages, they become more available for self-directed behaviors. The arms and hands, therefore, differ from the face in that they display less communicative information but more self-directed behaviors. Intentional or other-directed behaviors can be divided into emblems and illustrators.

Emblems are behaviors that have been assigned an arbitrary meaning and function as pictures, sometimes conveying to listeners complex messages. For example, spinning the index finger around the side of one's head while looking at a person may indicate that the person is not making any sense or is acting in a crazy manner. The hitchhiker's extended thumb indicates that here is a person who needs a ride, does not have access to his own car, and possibly is without much money. The clinician giving the client a thumbs up sign at the end of a session may be indicating that the session went extremely well and she is proud of the client. Because emblems can be used instead of words, they may at times be substituted for them by clients who have certain types of communicative disorders. This is especially prevalent with clients who are aphasic or are stutterers. Some aphasic clients have vast repertoires of emblems that allow them to convey information where words cannot be retrieved. Stutterers will also use emblems when a verbal response may involve words on which they believe they will stutter.

Illustrators are behaviors directly related to verbalizations and either emphasize what is being said, point to objects, or visually construct thoughts or objects (Feyereisen & de Lannoy, 1991). An example would be an aphasic client who, unable to remember the word *comb*, pantomimes the action of combing his hair and says, "Ya know, it's this, like this." Illustrators can also provide information about the intensity of a verbalization. Imagine a session between a parent and a clinician where the discussion involves a particularly disturbing interaction the parent observed between her child and the clinician. The child refused to listen to the clinician and physically accosted her when asked to sit down. The mother is now directing the clinician on how to prevent this episode from occurring again. Imagine that the clinician and parent are sitting comfortably on two couches at right angles to each other. Without any movement, the mother says, "I was very upset when I saw how he hit you. If he ever does that again, grab hold of his shoulders very tightly and tell him to sit down or you will come get me." Now imagine the same scenario with the following changes. The mother is leaning forward and when she says, "Grab hold of his shoulders very tightly," she holds her two tightly clenched fists in front of her and shakes them violently. She has increased the intensity of the verbal message by adding illustrators.

Self-directed movements such as nail-picking, scratching, hair preening, leg rubbing, and finger tapping are called *adaptive*, since they provide a means for individuals to adapt to stress or to emotional or environmental demands. The term *autistic* is sometimes used to classify these behaviors. Since the term also refers to the communicative behaviors of individuals with severe language disorders, it is recommended that *autistic* not be used to describe nonpathological self-directed behaviors. Self-directed behaviors are usually beyond the awareness of the individual and therefore provide an opportunity for the observer to have insights into the nature of an interaction. The behaviors are habitual and routinized, having been formed early in the person's developmental history. By carefully observing a client's self-directed behaviors, the clinician may be able to predict a client's receptivity to an activity or statement. For example, when faced with stressful tasks, some children may begin random hand movements as an attempt to calm themselves. When bored, other children may engage in finger tapping.

Specific self-directed behaviors do not mean the same thing for every client. There is a tremendous diversity in self-directed behaviors and their possible meanings. It is fallacious to assume that something like repetitive finger rubbing means "anxiety" for all people. The importance of self-directed behaviors is derived from their association with other nonverbal behaviors and verbal behaviors. For example, suppose that a 5-year-old child consistently begins swinging his arms 5 to 10 minutes prior to becoming uncooperative during language therapy. The behavior could have meant that he was bored, unable to focus, unable to comprehend the task, or just tired. Regardless of what it meant, the occurrence of the behavior was a prognostic indicator that, if the current activity persisted, the child would become uncooperative. Once the association was observed, the occurrence of arm swinging, regardless of what it meant, became a signal to switch activities. Looking for associations between specific self-directed behaviors and other aspects of the clinical session is more important than trying to determine what the "true" meaning of a nonverbal behavior may be.

Feet/Legs. The feet and legs are the parts of the body that have the least amount of visibility, the least amount of communicative ability, and the greatest percentage of self-directed behaviors. The range of behaviors is limited when compared with the face and the arms/hands area. There are three major types of behaviors associated with the feet/legs area. The first is repetitive movements, such as a rapid up and down movement of a leg. The second involves the degree of muscular tension observed in the upper and lower portions of the leg. The third involves leg-crossing positions that actually could be considered to be a posture behavior.

Posture. Postural configurations are reliable indicators of three aspects of communication (Scheflen, 1967):

1. *Interaction components.* They demarcate components of individual behavior that a person contributes to group activities.
2. *Relates contributions.* They indicate how individual contributions are related to each other.
3. *Interaction steps.* They define the steps and order in an interaction.

Postures cannot be viewed by themselves as distinct meaningful units of behavior. They must be related to the overall interaction. In an early study that examined postures in 480 cultures, Hewes (1957) found that the human body could assume approximately 1,000 steady postures, some of which are universal. It appears that posture is a complex entity that is determined by many factors, serves numerous functions, and can be analyzed in terms of its component parts.

Vocalic Behaviors. All vocalic phenomena can be divided into two categories: (a) prosody and (b) paralanguage. *Prosody* includes the qualities of intensity, pitch, register, tempo, duration, and tension. These are the same behaviors described in Chapter 4 where no attempt was made to relate these vocal behaviors to other nonverbal or verbal behaviors. Yet these behaviors also serve important functions in understanding the communicative intent of verbal messages. Attending to elements such as intensity, pitch breaks, and tension can provide information on the connotative aspects of a verbal communication. For example, a clinician noted that the only time abnormal tension and pitch breaks occurred in an adolescent client's speech was when he explained to the clinician that he was not bothered by people teasing him about his stuttering. The regularity of the association alerted the clinician that the client was probably considerably more upset than his verbal message indicated.

Paralanguage can be divided into identifiers and characterizers. *Identifiers* are isolated phonemes or combinations of phonemes that are not words. These include such sounds as *uh-uh, ah,* and *um.* Sounds of these types are often used by stutterers as ways of initiating speech. Characterizers are sounds that can stand by themselves. These include laughing, crying, yawning, belching, swallowing, coughing, yelling, whispering, sneezing, snorting, and groaning. Except for laughing and crying, these nonverbal behaviors are relatively unimportant in clinical settings.

Social Kinesics

Social kinesics is the study of the meaning of specific movements in a particular culture. Two researchers who have studied nonverbal behaviors within a social kinesic context are Ekman and Friesen (Ekman, 1985; Ekman & Friesen, 1968, 1971, 1974). They contend that meaning can be ascribed to certain behaviors if the unit of analysis is the *nonverbal act/position.* An act begins when one movement is no longer apparent or when another visually distinctive type of movement begins. For example, when two people meet, the hand-shaking sequence would be an example of an act. A still position begins and ends when movement stops or begins. The nonverbal act is a movement within any single body area or across multiple body areas that is visually distinct from another act. In discussions of clinical sensitivity to cultural differences, the nonverbal act/ position is the basic unit of analysis and may be one of the few areas in which a catalog of cultural differences makes any sense within a clinical setting. This would be especially true for greeting patterns, acknowledgment rules, role-related behaviors, and departure customs. For example, when conveying information that directly affects the interaction patterns of a family in a matriarchal culture, the clinician should be addressing the mother and directing her posture towards her.

CONTEXT

It is difficult to analyze a behavior in isolation. Since nonverbal behaviors tend to be ambiguous, the use of context may clarify the meaning of a behavior. Five different types of contexts may be used: (a) linear-temporal, (b) multidimensional, (c) individual behavioral repertoire, (d) environmental, and (e) cultural.

Linear-Temporal Context

This is the context in which behavior is viewed as a function of time. That is, if a designated behavior occurs at time t, the observer should be aware of what behaviors occur at $t-1$ and $t+1$. This context allows the clinician to examine communication as an ongoing, dynamic process. For example, if a child throws a temper tantrum, it is clinically important to identify what immediately preceded it (t−1) and what follows it (t+1). Contextualists have argued that by abstracting the behavior from the events that precede and follow it, the behavior cannot be understood because the surrounding events are partially responsible for assigning meaning to the behavior (Berlo, 1960). The same argument has been presented for the analysis of verbal communication (Lund & Duchan, 1988).

Multidimensional Behavior Context

In this context we examine all the behaviors that occur in a given unit of time for a specific interactant. For example, an observer may wish to identify all the behaviors that a mother uses when she brings her child into the room. The duration of the observation unit will depend on the purpose of the study. An investigation of prekinesics may involve units in milliseconds, whereas a social kinesic analysis might use minutes as units of measurement.

Individual Behavior Repertoires

This context deals with the quantitative and qualitative range of individual behaviors. A contextual analysis on this level would examine the range and speed of a behavior and the number of times it occurs in relation to its past occurrence by the same individual. For example, a clinician may know that when a particular young client becomes frustrated, he starts moving his head back and forth, kicks his legs, and taps his fingers. The more intense the behaviors, the greater the frustration. Compiling individual behavioral repertoires has been useful in clinical situations in assessing affective moods and therapeutic progress (Kupfer, Maser, Blehar, & Miller, 1987; Gotlib, 1982). Since the use of this context requires extensive contact with the subject, it should be limited to the observation of ongoing clinical situations. Multiple observations of the same client may be necessary before a reliable behavioral repertoire can be developed.

Environmental Context

The environment is often directly responsible for the occurrence, shape, and meaning of behaviors. Environmental influences are often in the form of physical structures. For example, experiments on seating arrangements and physical designs have been shown to influence nonverbal behaviors directly. The interaction that occurs when the clinician and client are separated by a large table will probably be different from the interaction that would occur when they are sitting on the same side of the table or sitting facing each other with nothing between them. The other environmental influence that has been extensively researched is referred to as "stressful" or "anxious" situations. Investigators have found that the degree of stress present during an interaction directly affects the type and number of behaviors produced by the subject (Ekman, 1964; Frankel & Frankel, 1970). For example, a client coming to the clinic for the first time may be naturally apprehensive. The behaviors displayed during this first meeting may not occur during subsequent, more relaxed clinical sessions. The literature indicates that any attempts to assign meaning to a behavior produced during an interaction should be accompanied by a reference to the environment in which it was produced.

Cultural Context

Much has been written about the overriding importance of culture as a primary determinant of the type and meaning of nonverbal behaviors (Hall, 1959; Hodge & Kress, 1988). The findings of cross-cultural studies offer conclusive evidence that many behaviors are culturally determined. Few researchers would insist otherwise. Researchers do not agree, however, on whether there are any nonverbal behaviors that are not culturally bound. Birdwhistell (1968) has always insisted that no gestures have universal meaning. All gestures, he insists, are culturally linked both in shape and in meaning. However, some doubt has been cast on this position by experiments examining facial behaviors (Ekman & Friesen, 1971). Members of a preliterate culture who had no previous contact with members of literate Western and Eastern cultures participated in the experiment. The subjects were shown three pictures simultaneously while a story was read to them. They were then asked to point to the picture in which the person's face showed the emotion described in the story. The faces were those of adults from literate cultures. The stories read were about six emotions: (a) happiness; (b) sadness; (c) anger; (d) surprise; (e) disgust; and (f) fear. Accuracy scores were significantly better than chance levels, and the results of the test given to the preliterate subjects were positively correlated with the results of the identical test given to subjects from literate cultures. Although this experiment does not conclusively prove that certain facial expressions are universal, it does offer strong evidence in its favor. Quite possibly there may be innate neural programs and learning experiences that are common to human development regardless of culture.

FUNCTIONS OF NONVERBAL BEHAVIORS

The claim is often made that an analysis of nonverbal behavior contributes little to the understanding of clinical interactions that cannot be supplied by an analysis of the linguistic portion of the interaction. Such an assertion is made without fully understanding the functions of nonverbal behaviors. Their functional importance can be appreciated by examining how they affect verbal behaviors in four different ways: (a) amplifying, (b) contradicting, (c) qualifying, or (d) sending an unrelated message.

Amplify the Message

A verbal message can be amplified or strengthened by nonverbal behaviors. The use of illustrators or facial expressions can emphasize how strongly people feel about what they are saying. The client who explains in a monotone that she understands the point the clinician was making is conveying a different message than the client who says the same thing but emphasizes each word in a slow, precise manner.

Contradict the Message

Nonverbal behaviors can negate what is being said. For example, a client may be commenting on how relaxed and good he is feeling at the same time he is clenching his fists and holding his body in a stiff position. Since many clients resist examining their feelings honestly, an apparent contradiction between a verbal and a nonverbal behavior can become the vehicle for discussing emotions. Frederick Perls (1965) in a classic filmed interview noted that even though the client said she was afraid of him, she laughed. He commented that "frightened people don't laugh." His observation and comment became the starting point for examining the woman's use of a manipulative role that was negatively affecting her life.

Qualify the Message

Often when someone is expressing a verbal message that involves feelings, desires, or commitments, the connotative aspects of the message may be less intense than its denotative aspects. An example would be a farewell scene in which a person says, "I really will miss you a lot" but barely touches the other person during a hug. In therapy, clients who have been led logically to an important conclusion by the clinician may say that they realize its importance without fully understanding it. This lack of understanding may become evident by the use of an emotionless speech pattern while saying, "Yes, you are right. I can see how that is the core of my speaking problem."

Sending an Unrelated Message

Nonverbal behaviors are not always related to the verbal message. At times, a person can engage in an interaction while thinking about something else at the same time. The parent, for example, who is explaining how she is using the generalization procedures at home may be exhibiting self-directed behaviors not because of any concern with the procedures but rather because she is worried about the health of another child.

CLINICAL IMPLICATIONS

Speech pathologists need to be aware of nonverbal information that their clients are sending them. By tending to rely predominantly on the client's verbal output in formulating a diagnosis or designing therapy strategies, interviewers may be ignoring important information that the client is sending through nonverbal behaviors.

Most speech pathologists have not been trained in nonverbal observation. Therefore, it is not surprising that in most therapy situations a table is placed between the client and clinician, thereby effectively blocking the clinician's observation of some arms/hands and most feet/legs behaviors. Both of these observational factors tend to reduce the amount of awareness clinicians have of their client's nonverbal behaviors. The therapy situation may partially explain the rank order of the reported behaviors. That is, the areas of the body that are most visible are those which are most observed.

Sending Ability and Rank Order

Visibility is not sufficient for explaining the sending ability of various parts of the body. Besides visibility, it is necessary to examine the average transmission time and the number of discriminative stimulus patterns that can be emitted. Since the face has the shortest transmission time, the greatest number of discriminative stimulus patterns, and the greatest visibility, it is the best sender (Ekman & Friesen, 1968). The worst sender would be the feet and legs because their transmission time is slow, they possess a limited number of discriminative stimulus patterns, and generally have poor visibility. In terms of visibility, transmission time, and the number of discriminable stimulus patterns, the rank order of sending ability would therefore be

1. face
2. arms/hands
3. feet/legs

Factors Affecting the Sender

When trying to relate nonverbal behaviors to specific messages it is necessary first to record the behavior. It seems plausible that the subject who is engaging in many behaviors offers the observer more raw data than the subject who is engaging in relatively few behaviors. Baxter, Winters, and Hammer (1968) found that the number of gestures a subject engaged in depended on how well differentiated the subject was and how well he knew the topic discussed. Well-differentiated subjects discussing familiar topics (conditions for maximum number of gestures) not only produced the greatest number of gestures but also had more vigorous and extended movements.

Communication studies have shown that people use different parts of their body differently in the transmission of messages. Some attempts have been made to relate the patterns of gestures displayed to the portrayal of specific emotions. Much of the early research in nonverbal behavior attempted to do this by examining facial cues. It was found that happiness and love were judged more accurately than disgust, suffering, fear, anger, and contempt. These results would imply that identifiable displays of emotion exist for only certain emotions.

SUMMARY

Communication involves complex processes that are both verbal and nonverbal. To focus on only one channel may result in the loss of information that may be crucial for therapeutic planning or providing appropriate responses to the client. Observation of nonverbal behaviors should be used to supplement the clinician's understanding of the affective messages being sent by clients. Interpreting the meaning of these behaviors is significantly more difficult than determining the meaning of verbal behaviors due to their idiosyncrasy. Although certain expressions and postures are unambiguous, many more have personal meanings that cannot be reliably interpreted without understanding the person's behavioral repertoire and the verbal messages coexisting with the nonverbal behaviors.

Although the task of using and interpreting nonverbal behaviors is formidable, it can add an extra dimension to therapy. By understanding how nonverbal behaviors are interpreted, the clinician may avoid conveying an unintentional message to the client or may be able to reinforce one that should be emphasized. By understanding how nonverbal behaviors are related to verbal behaviors, the clinician may obtain insights not only into the client's espoused beliefs and feelings but also into those that the client does not feel comfortable sharing or finds too difficult or painful to acknowledge.

SUGGESTED READINGS

Bull, P. E. (1987). *Posture and gesture.* New York: Pergamon Press.
Ekman, P., & Friesen, W. (1971). *Emotion in the human face.* New York: Bobbs-Merrill.
Ekman, P. (1985). *Telling lies.* New York: Norton.
Feyereisen, P., & de Lannoy, J. (1991). *Gestures and speech: Psychological investigations.* New York: Cambridge Press.
Hall, E. T. (1959). *The silent language.* Garden City, NY: Doubleday.
Scheflen, A. E. (1967). On the structuring of human communication. *American Behavioral Scientist, 10,* 8, 8–12.

❏ **Activity 6.1**
Individual Behavior Repertoires

If possible, observe the same client for each of the activities in this chapter. Each activity requires a separate 15-minute observation. For the first activity, observe the client for 15 minutes and record only self-directed behaviors. When focusing only on nonverbal behaviors it is helpful to eliminate the client's verbalizations. If you are observing through a one-way observation booth, turn off the audio monitor, use earplugs, or listen to nondescript music through earphones. To acclimate yourself to observing only nonverbal behaviors, you might wish to watch a television show for 15 minutes with the audio portion turned off.

1. Self-Directed Behaviors

Facial Area

1. _____   5. _____
2. _____   6. _____
3. _____   7. _____
4. _____   8. _____

Arms/Hands

1. _____   5. _____
2. _____   6. _____
3. _____   7. _____
4. _____   8. _____

Feet/Legs

1. _____   5. _____
2. _____   6. _____
3. _____   7. _____
4. _____   8. _____

Observe the client for 15 minutes and record only the other-directed behaviors.

2. Other-Directed Behaviors

Facial Area

Displays   Regulators

1. _____   5. _____   1. _____
2. _____   6. _____   2. _____
3. _____   7. _____   3. _____
4. _____   8. _____   4. _____

Arms/Hands

Emblems	Illustrators	
1. _____	1. _____	5. _____
2. _____	2. _____	6. _____
3. _____	3. _____	7. _____
4. _____	4. _____	8. _____

Feet/Legs

Emblems	Illustrators	
1. _____	1. _____	5. _____
2. _____	2. _____	6. _____
3. _____	3. _____	7. _____
4. _____	4. _____	8. _____

Observe the client for 15 minutes and note the various postures the client assumes.

3. Posture

Position

		Check if Present	**Approximate Time**
Leaning Forward	(relaxed)	[ ]	_____
Leaning Forward	(tense)	[ ]	_____
Erect	(relaxed)	[ ]	_____
Erect	(tense)	[ ]	_____
Leaning Back	(relaxed)	[ ]	_____
Leaning Back	(tense)	[ ]	_____

❏ **Activity 6.2**
Linear-Temporal Context

Observe the client for 15 minutes. Identify the nonverbal interactions that are occurring and how they may be related to the verbal interactions.

First, identify all the behaviors that are occurring during the first four nonverbal act/positions. An act begins when one movement is no longer apparent or when another visually distinctive type of movement begins. When two people meet, the hand-shaking sequence would be an example of an act. A still position begins and ends when movement stops or begins. The nonverbal act is a movement within any single-body area or across multiple-body areas that is visually distinct from another act. Write whatever conclusion you can make based on your analysis.

Act/Pos	Person on the Left	Person on the Right
1.		
2.		
3.		
4.		

Conclusions

Nonverbal Interactions

Verbal Interactions

Nonverbal/Verbal Interactions

❑ *Activity 6.3*
Observation of Environmental Context

Observe the interaction for 15 minutes. Identify how the physical structure of the room in which the client is observed may be affecting therapy.

Furniture

Positions of the Interactants

PART III
Clinical Intervention

> ... *the aim of therapy is to make the patient* not *depend upon others, but to make the patient discover from the very first moment that he can do many things,* much *more than he thinks he can do. (p. 29)*

A critical concept for understanding the next four chapters is contained in the preceding quote from Perls' (1969) thoughts on the aim of therapy. Clinical relationships, by their very nature, start with dependency. If clients knew how to solve their communication problems, they would not seek guidance from clinicians. Although the relationship begins with dependency, Perls maintains that it should rapidly progress to independence, in which clients become their own therapists. In the next four chapters, various techniques are presented for effecting the change. Central to these techniques is structuring therapy to provide clients with strategies for problem solving.

Therapy that does not emphasize the development of problem-solving strategies fosters dependency relationships. For example, teaching carrier phrases may provide children with many stock communications but will not facilitate the development of unique, spontaneous productions. Having aphasic clients memorize standard greetings may enable them to begin conversations but will not result in the retrieval of the many names to which they no longer have access. Having stutterers practice speaking fluently in a quiet clinic room will allow for normal fluent communication with the clinician but will not prevent them from stuttering during the endless other situations they encounter daily. In each of these examples, the client must continue to rely on the clinician for developing new behaviors.

Therapy should be a facilitative process in which clients become their own therapists by first learning communicative strategies and then applying them in nonclinical settings. It is a unique relationship in which compassionate, scientifically oriented clinicians guide communicatively impaired individuals from other- to self-directed support.

Chapter 7
Principles of Learning

STUDY GUIDE

- There are two continua on which learning occurs. Given a sample learning situation, determine its location on each continuum.
- State the ethical arguments for using and not using operant conditioning.
- Operant terminology is very precise. Define each concept and cite examples.

*C*linical intervention involves more than simply applying appropriate operant techniques. Speech-language therapy is, above all else, teaching, and teaching requires an understanding of how people learn. Although the complexities of cognitive psychology and neurology are beyond the scope of this text, it is important to provide some information about the principles of learning.

❏ ❏ ❏ *LEARNING CONTINUA*

Clinicians should conceive of learning as occurring on two continua; one involving the complexity of the task to be learned and the other involving the steps required to learn a behavior, concept, or rule. Table 7.1 presents a matrix of these two continua. As you read through this section, you will notice frequent number-letter combinations (e.g., [A2] or [C6]). These refer to specific cells of the matrix in Table 7.1. By frequently referring to this matrix the reader will be better able to understand the various types of learning and how the process is achieved.

Stages in Learning and Retrieval

A widely held model of learning is one that divides the processes into four stages: apprehending, acquisition, retention, and retrieval (Gagné, 1970).

Apprehending. *Apprehending* refers to an individual's ability to be aware of a particular stimulus configuration. For example, when teaching a child to dis-

Table 7.1
Learning continua

	Stages in Learning and Retrieval			
Levels of Learning	**A Apprehending**	**B Acquisition**	**C Retention**	**D Retrieval**
1. Signal Learning	A1	B1	C1	D1
2. Stimulus-Response	A2	B2	C2	D2
3. Chaining	A3	B3	C3	D3
4. Verbal Association	A4	B4	C4	D4
5. Discrimination Learning	A5	B5	C5	D5
6. Concept Learning	A6	B6	C6	D6
7. Rule Learning	A7	B7	C7	D7
8. Problem Solving	A8	B8	C8	D8

criminate between a correct and incorrect production of /r/, the child must apprehend differences before she can acquire an understanding of the differences.

Acquisition. *Acquisition* refers to the process by which the components of a new behavior or idea are recognized. In the preceding example, the child may now understand the distinctive features of /r/ and therefore be able to apply this knowledge to differentiate between correct and incorrect productions of /r/.

Retention. *Retention* refers to the memory processes that result in information being stored in a manner that allows for retrieval at a later time. It is hypothesized that retention involves two memory processes: short-term and long-term. When the child learned the distinctive features of the /r/ phoneme, the initial knowledge involved short-term memory. After being processed in short-term memory, the information was transferred into long-term memory, where storage involved electrochemical processes.

Retrieval. *Retrieval* is the ability to recall information that will allow an individual to produce a previous learned behavior. Retrieval is the best method available for determining whether the information was learned. Until the child is asked to differentiate between correct and incorrect productions of /r/, it can never be known whether she learned the discrimination.

Levels of Learning

Gagné and his associates (1970, 1988) maintained that learning occurs at eight hierarchical levels, each one being dependent on the one that preceded it. His model of learning provides clinicians with a framework for understanding some of the cognitive problems clients have. The acquisition of a behavior that requires a higher level of learning assumes that the individual is able to use all of the lower, sequentially ordered levels of learning. Understanding Gagné's levels of learning can help the clinician not only to identify a client's cognitive deficits but also to construct intervention protocols.

Learning Type 1: Signal Learning. Another term for *signal learning* is *reflexive conditioning*. The most well-known example of how it occurs is the salivation condition Pavlov achieved in his dog experiments. Three steps are involved in signal learning: (a) eliciting an unconditioned response; (b) pairing a neutral stimulus with an unconditioned stimulus; and (c)transforming the neutral stimulus into a conditioned stimulus. Pavlov's classic experiment illustrates how the process occurs.

> *Step 1:* Food powder is placed in a dog's mouth, and he salivates. This would be an unconditioned response [A1].
>
> Food Powder   >   Salivation
> (unconditioned stimulus)   (unconditioned response)

Step 2: A few seconds before the food powder is placed in the dog's mouth, a bell rings. The dog will eventually associate the bell with food. Until that happens, the bell is called a neutral stimulus [B1].

Bell	+	Food Powder	>	Salivation
(neutral stimulus)		(unconditioned stimulus)		(unconditioned response)

Step 3: If the dog has associated the bell with the presentation of food powder, we should be able to ring the bell—without any food powder present—and create the salivating response [C1]. If this occurs, then the bell is now called a conditioned stimulus and the salivation a conditioned response [D1].

Bell	>	Salivation
(conditioned stimulus)		(conditioned response)

The preceding example is one that illustrates the process involved in learning an involuntary behavior. This type of learning does not occur when the behaviors are voluntary, such as learning to write or speak specific sounds.

Learning Type 2: Stimulus-Response Learning. *Stimulus-response learning* differs from signal learning in that it involves precise voluntary responses. A person or animal produces a behavior, with or without help, and is then reinforced. The behavior is produced as a consequence of being reinforced. An animal example would be teaching a dog to shake hands. A human example would be teaching a child to produce a combination of phonemes. Four conditions are usually associated with stimulus-response learning.

1. *Gradualness of the Act.* The act is learned gradually [B2]. Initially the person does not perform it perfectly, and repetitions of the presentation and reinforcement are necessary [C2]. For example, a child who has a lateral lisp will not immediately produce /s/ correctly on her first attempt when provided with an appropriate model [D2]. Most likely, it may sound like a distorted /s/ with less lateralized sounds than were produced prior to instruction.
2. *Increasing Proficiency of the Act.* The behavior that is performed becomes more refined with practice. The behavior is "shaped" by aiding the person with various types of cues. Gradually, the cues are reduced. This process is known as *successive approximations.* In our example, the child may have been instructed with the use of a mirror in which she observed herself and the model. The clinician may also have used her fingers to reduce the child's lateralizations.
3. *Increasing Strength of Controlling Stimulus.* Initially, the response may have occurred not only in the presence of the controlling stimulus but of others as well. With increased presentations, the response is elicited only in the presence of the controlling stimulus.
4. *Reinforcement.* The person will be reinforced when a correct response is emitted. He will not be reinforced when an incorrect response is emitted.

This type of learning, originally explored by B. F. Skinner, is commonly referred to as operant conditioning. Skinner (1957) contended that this type of learning can account for all of linguistic acquisition, a position strongly disputed by many linguists (Chomsky, 1972; Huxley & Ingram, 1971; Kausler, 1974; Naremore, 1984). Although operant conditioning may not be able to account for language learning, it is an important technique for the acquisition of new behaviors and will be extensively examined later in this chapter.

Learning Type 3: Chaining. *Chaining* occurs when two or more previously learned stimulus-response events are sequenced together. An example of this would be some of the very early naming activities of children. At some time in the past a child has learned that a doll is used for hugging, kissing, and cuddling. Whenever the child's parents give him the doll, the above activities occur. This is the first part of the chain. Also in the past, the child has been reinforced for imitating the mother's production of the word *doll*. This is the second part of the chain. The child is now lying in his crib, which he associates with doll playing. The doll is seen outside of the crib [A3]. He points to the doll, looks at his mother, and says the word *doll* [B3] [D3]. The child has just exhibited an example of learning type 3. Three conditions are necessary for chaining to occur.

1. *Previously Learned Behaviors.* Each link of the chain must have been previously learned.
2. *Contiguity of Links.* Each new link of the chain must follow the preceding link.
3. *Immediate Acquisition of Behavior.* If the two previous conditions are met, the acquisition of a chain is not a gradual process, but rather occurs on a single occasion.

Learning Type 4: Verbal Association. *Verbal association* is a subvariety of chaining that involves associating one word with another, for example in learning the French word for *match*. Four conditions must be present for verbal association to occur.

1. *Previously Learned Behaviors.* Each link of the chain must have been previously learned [B4]. In our example the person must know what a match is and know the English word for it [C4].
2. *Production of Verbal Associate.* The person must be able to correctly pronounce the French word for *match* [D4].
3. *Available Coding Connection.* The English and the French words for the object must be connected by a code that would be visual.
4. *Contiguity of Links.* Each new link of the chain must follow the preceding link.

Learning Type 5: Discrimination Learning. In *discrimination learning* two or more previously learned chains are juxtaposed. The individual is now expected to identify each type of chain correctly when in the presence of other previously learned chains. Two conditions are necessary for learning discriminations.

1. *Prior Learned Responses.* Each of the chains with their identifying responses must have been previously learned [B5]. If the responses have been learned,

it is assumed that the stimulus that elicited them can also be readily identified [C5] [D5].
2. *Interference Must Be Reduced.* If the stimuli of two or more chains or the responses of two or more chains are similar, it will become more difficult to differentiate between the chains. This is known as *interference*. Specific procedures need to be undertaken that will reduce interference.

Learning Type 6: Concept Learning. *Concept learning* depends on the neural processes of representation and involves classifying stimulus situations in terms of abstracted properties, such as color, shape, position, number, and others. In concept learning, the individual learns to classify objects or events according to specific discriminative stimuli, or critical attributes. For example, if a child uses the word *table* to refer only to one specific piece of furniture in his house even when other "tables" are present, he is using the word in the context of learning type 3: chaining. However, if he appropriately uses the word *table* to correctly identify various types of table, he is operating at the level of concept learning. Three necessary conditions must be present for concept learning to occur.

1. *Prior Learning of Stimulus.* The stimulus portion of the chain must have been previously learned, as must the response [B6] [C6].
2. *Variety of Stimulus Situations.* The concept that is to be learned must be presented in various ways. By doing this, the learner can identify the critical attributes of the concept when it appears in objects or events that have differences but are still occurrences of the concept.
3. *Gradual Learning.* The concept may be learned gradually over a period of time [D6].

Learning Type 7: Rule Learning. A *rule* is a chain of two or more concepts. In its simplest form, a rule would have the structure of "If A, then B." Rule learning is more than just the memorization of verbal facts. Otherwise, rule learning would be identical to stimulus-response chains. In rule learning, the individual is expected to apply the rule to a variety of situations. For example, a simple early linguistic rule that children use in describing objects and people is "color + object." A child who understands this rule can apply it in a multitude of ways, such as "red ball," "black doggie," and "blue car." Three conditions must be present for rule learning to occur.

1. *Previously Learned Concepts.* The concepts that are linked in the rule must have been previously learned [B7] [C7].
2. *Simple Application.* Understanding the rule results in its application to a variety of situations involving previously learned concepts.
3. *Immediate Learning.* The learning of a rule takes place on a single occasion [D7].

Learning Type 8: Problem Solving. Problem solving involves the combination of two or more previously learned rules to address a problem not previously solved by the individual. For example, let us assume that a child has learned two basic linguistic rules that are appropriate for describing objects. Rule 1 is "color + object". Rule 2 is "size + object". In the past, the child has said "blue ball" and "big ball." As he is sitting in the living room, he notices a very large blue ball that is out of his reach. He would like his father to give it to him and is about to formulate the verbal request. Since there are other balls of various shapes and colors next to the big blue ball, the application of either his previously learned rules would not assure him of receiving the big blue ball. He now combines the two rules into a new one having the formula "size + color + object," and he says "big blue ball." The child has solved a problem by chaining and synthesizing two previously learned rules. Four conditions are essential for problem solving to occur.

1. *Identification of Essential Features.* The person must identify the essential features of the response before he produces it. In other words, he must know what the activity's goal is [A8].
2. *Recall of Past Rules.* All past rules that will be relevant to solving the problem must be recalled [B8] [C8] [D8].
3. *Combining Recalled Rules.* The rules that have been recalled are combined to formulate a new rule.
4. *Sudden Solution.* The processes involved in combining rules may be lengthy and complex, but the solution appears suddenly. Repetition plays no part in problem solving.

COGNITION AND LEARNING STYLES

In the early 1960s American educators began questioning their form of education with the advent of innovative approaches to teaching children. The tedium of rote memorization of meaningless facts became viewed as a primary factor in the "dulling" of American youth. Open classrooms, experiential learning, and alternative educational formats became the standard in many school settings. The child became an active learner, involved in deciding what was to be learned. The philosophy was best summed up by John Holt (1964) when he wrote:

> The alternative—I can see no other—is to have schools and classrooms in which each child in his own way can satisfy his curiosity, develop his abilities and talents, pursue his interests, and from the adults and older children around him get a glimpse of the great variety and richness of life. In short, the school should be a great smorgasbord of intellectual, artistic, creative, and athletic activities, from which each child could take whatever he wanted, and as much as he wanted, or as little. (p. 108)

Teaching practices had swung 180 degrees. Whereas before the 1960s children had little control or input in their education, during the 1960s they were given a multitude of options. In open classrooms, learning centers were established where children could choose to go and learn about science, read books, and engage in creative arts. By the late 1960s it became apparent to even the most progressive educators that this new, more open system of education was not working as they thought it should. The very bright children were no longer bored; nor did they fail. But other, less intellectually endowed or motivated children were failing in large numbers. Significant research on learning began. In 1977 a major book on the state of the art in learning was published (Cronbach & Snow, 1977). The authors examined all of the available relevant research on aptitudes and instructional methods. Their conclusions were shocking to many. The open system of education was appropriate only to very bright or motivated children. Children who did not fit into either of these two categories did significantly better in more structurally closed educational systems where the parameters of their actions were defined by others. The bright and motivated students did well in either setting.

The studies demonstrated that good values and a humane philosophy were not sufficient for meeting the needs of children who had heterogeneous learning styles. The lesson for the speech pathologist is clear. The degree of direction and guidance we offer to our clients should depend on the client's cognitive ability and motivation. It would make little sense to allow the Down syndrome child to determine if language was an important behavior to acquire or to allow a 5-year-old who does not care how he sounds determine whether the /r/ phoneme should be learned. Although Cronbach and Snow's book contained many specific findings, these three are the most applicable to the speech pathologist:

1. The greater the cognitive problem of the client, the fewer the choices they should be allowed. Always provide choices, but the parameters should be narrowed with clients who have cognitive impairments.
2. Clients who are not motivated to learn new behaviors should be given minimal choices in the structure and control of the therapy program.
3. Insight and self-discovery are appropriate for clients who have at least normal intelligence. Guided instruction is more appropriate for clients of normal or below normal intelligence.

❑ ❑ ❑ OPERANT CONDITIONING

The words *operant conditioning* and *behavior modification* tend to generate strong reactions from both proponents and opponents of the technique. The use of this approach has been called manipulative and anti-humanistic by some, whereas others believe that it constitutes the only scientific methodology of behavior change. The truth, as is the case with all maps of reality, falls somewhere in the middle.

History

Operant conditioning in the field of psychology was pioneered by the animal research of B. F. Skinner. Although Skinner had been publishing his research since the 1930s, the most vehement opposition to his work started in the mid-1950s after the publication of his book *Science and Human Behavior* (1953). There were various reasons for the initial adverse reactions. Since Skinner had developed his theories of behavior from experimentation on animals and birds, many people believed that his laws of behavior did not apply to human beings. After all, we not only have vastly greater cognitive abilities than rats and pigeons but also possess free will. Also, his experiments were conducted within a laboratory under controlled conditions with all extraneous variables eliminated. His critics maintained that since human beings interact within continually changing conditions, extraneous variables could not be controlled, and it would therefore not be possible to state scientific laws regarding human behaviors. Succinctly put, the argument was presented that "pigeons are not people." Throughout the 1950s and 1960s researchers in all areas of human behavior began testing the scientific laws developed by Skinner. What they found was startling, even to those who opposed Skinner's view. In many ways, the behaviors of human beings could be controlled and predicted with the same degree of certainty as could the behavior of pigeons. With their findings, the attack became two-fold, one practical and the other ethical.

The argument from practicality was that the sterility of an experimental condition does not lend itself to the everyday settings in which practitioners in psychology and speech-language pathology must function. It may be possible to reinforce a child's attention within a therapy room with an M&M candy, but this would not work in a classroom of 35 students. Proponents of operant conditioning countered that the introduction of independent variables does not negate a law of human behavior, but rather the variables require the practitioner to account for them in the development of intervention strategies. The opponents of operant conditioning were left with few persuasive arguments when the application of operant clinical strategies began resulting in successes. Shames and Sherrick (1963) demonstrated that stuttering could be minimized or eliminated by the use of operant techniques. Holland and Matthew's (1963) article on the use of teaching machine concepts in speech pathology and audiology introduced the field to the scientific application of operant principles in various areas. Sufficient research had been done by the mid-1960s that Sloan and MacAulay (1968) were able to provide specific operant techniques that could be used in the areas of speech and language therapy.

With the conclusive evidence that operant conditioning could be applied effectively to human beings, it became a panacea for solving all behavioral problems in the 1960s and 1970s. Some proponents believed that the techniques were in and of themselves sufficient for remediating everything from self-destructive behaviors to complicated linguistic constructions (Lovaas, 1965, 1966). People with little or no training in linguistics applied operant procedures to teach language, which resulted in children who could produce long and complex sentences by rote, but rarely, if ever, produced a unique utterance. Within institutions for the retarded and emotionally disturbed, poorly trained care givers viewed operant conditioning as a way of changing behaviors through the application of aversive stimuli. Many people became outraged by the use of confining time-out boxes and sensory-deprivation rooms. The adverse notoriety these institutions gained through the inappropriate use of punishment created a public outcry against operant conditioning. Even the use of reinforcement in humane, noninstitutionalized settings was criticized. Many parents, clinicians, and educators believed that children should not produce behaviors simply to receive a tangible reward. They were afraid that children would begin expecting rewards for behaviors that "children ought to do just because it's right." The irrational fear of operant conditioning was best exemplified in Skinner's novel *Walden Two* (1948), when a member of the operant society was explaining its principles to a visitor:

> It's a little late to be proving that a behavioral technology is well advanced. How can you deny it? Many of its methods and techniques are really as old as the hills. Look at their frightful misuse in the hands of the Nazis! And what about the techniques of the psychological clinic? What about education? Or religion? Or practical politics? Or advertising and salesmanship? Bring them all together and you have a sort of rule-of-thumb technology of vast power. No, Mr. Castle, the science is there for the asking. But its techniques and methods are in the wrong hands—they are used for personal aggrandizement in a competitive world or, in the case of the psychologist and educator, for futilely corrective purposes. My question is, have you the courage to take up and wield the science of behavior for the good of mankind? You answer that you would dump it in the ocean! (pp. 256–257)

Skinner was maintaining that operant conditioning is not something that we have a choice in applying. It is, always has been, and always will be prevalent in all forms of social organizations and interactions. Operant conditioning is no more than the scientific application of the laws of human behavior. The laws "are." They are not created by practitioners. Practitioners can use them for good or for evil. The members of the society in the novel presented a compelling argument for using them for good.

Ethical and Moral Conditions of Behavior Change

Right Behavior Without Rewards. The popular concept that one should engage in activities without wanting to be rewarded concerned Kanfer (1968). He believed that the destructive notion that one should do the "right" thing without the hope of being rewarded stemmed from an underlying value of our society and government. Kanfer maintained that our societal structure is based on the use of coercion, not reinforcement, for maintaining order. Coercion is in the form of adverse contingencies for noncompliance or nonperformance. For example, laws are created to specify what actions need to be taken to avoid a punishment. For example, if you don't stop when the traffic light turns red, you will receive a ticket and must pay $20; if you commit a violent crime, you will go to jail if caught; if you do not pay your taxes by April 15, you will pay a fine and may go to jail. In *Walden Two* the visitor receives a lesson on the use of positive reinforcement rather than punishment (Skinner, 1948):

> We are gradually discovering—at an untold cost in human suffering—that in the long run punishment doesn't reduce the probability that an act will occur. We have been so preoccupied with the contrary that we always take *force* to mean punishment. We don't say we're using force when we send shiploads of food into a starving country, though we're displaying quite as much power as if we were sending troops and guns. (p. 260)

The notion of not reinforcing children for "good" behavior is illogical. It is unreasonable to expect children to do certain behaviors when nothing is rewarding about the behavior or its completion. As college students you are reading this book with the hope of being reinforced. Either the material is sufficiently interesting that you are reading it for the sheer joy of accumulating knowledge, or you are anticipating eventually applying the techniques presented, or you will be tested on its contents and receive a grade related to the information you have acquired. It is doubtful that you would be reading this text if none of these reinforcements were present. In fact, some of you would probably not be reading it unless your grade depended on it. Why should children be different? Learning must be reinforcing or it will not continue.

Unethical and Incompetent Applications. One may reasonably conclude that operant conditioning suffered from "bad press" and incompetent applications throughout the 1960s and 1970s. Initially, practitioners expected too much of the procedure. Instead of viewing it as a technique that could result in the efficient application of content knowledge, it became its substitute. Poorly trained individuals applied the techniques without really understanding the technical complexities of operant conditioning and its limitations. An inappropriate application of a principle is not sufficient evidence to damn it. If, for example, a mentally deranged individual was seen attacking another person with a teaspoon, it would be ludicrous to label spoons as weapons that should be banned. Few people would be so incensed as to form a "Citizens Against Spoons" movement. Yet, this is exactly what happened in the 1960s with operant conditioning.

The argument has also been made that it is not enough to blame only the practitioners of a procedure rather than indicting the procedure. After all, was this not the line of reasoning so popular during World War II? "I only make the rockets go up. There is nothing wrong with that. Punish the people who are responsible for making them go down; they are the evil ones." If operant conditioners were similar to the "up-rocket" men, the argument could be valid. However, the opposite is true. Individuals who clearly understand operant procedures and appropriately apply them believe in the very positive ethical values associated with operant conditioning. The use of positive reinforcement to establish new behaviors is a good example. What better, more humane way is there to establish new behaviors than by providing individuals with "strokes" for their accomplishments? What is immoral or unethical about using successive approximations to give people the feeling that they can succeed? Is it immoral to use aversive stimuli to stop the physically self-destructive behaviors of an autistic child?

The End Justifies the Means. Even if one accepts the ethical nature of the goals of operant conditioning, many people are still uncomfortable with the methods that are employed to achieve those goals. The "end justifies the means" principle is the most common ethical criticism encountered by operant conditioners. Simply put, it states that in behavior modification any degree of punishment or unethical behavior is appropriate if the end goal is sufficiently important. The underlying assumption is that aversive stimuli will usually be the "means." In fact, a competent operant conditioner will initially try to use positive reinforcement to teach a new behavior or eliminate a maladaptive one. Only under extremely rare situations would punishment be used to develop a new behavior, because research has shown that it is not very effective. However, the application of aversive stimuli is effective in eliminating behaviors. Since the operant conditioner must continually face the dilemma of when to use aversive stimuli, the decision is not made lightly. One principle is to use the lowest possible strength of an aversive stimulus to change the behavior. The strength of an aversive stimulus may need to be increased if the behavior is interfering with the acquisition of a new, desirable behavior.

Although the "end justifies the means" argument is an important one, it should not be made in a vacuum. The disorder, parental feeling, and societal norms are all considered in the decision to use aversive stimuli. The problem of weighing the means and ends of therapy is one that is constantly present, regardless of the clinician's orientation. By continually facing it, the operant conditioner may in fact be acting more ethically and in the better interests of the client than the supposedly more "humane" practitioner who refuses to deal with the issue.

Operant conditioning is a very positive helping approach. It views the individual as responding better to positive reinforcement than to punishment. It tries to develop procedures that allow even the most severely involved individual to experience feelings of success. Operant conditioning is not the incursion of experimentally contrived procedures for controlling human behavior. It is the application of techniques that are directly related to how human beings function, regardless of what is or is not done in the laboratory. Operant conditioning is simply an understanding of the laws of human behavior. The decision to not use operant procedures is really a choice to ignore the reasons we behave as we do. To ignore information that can be helpful in allowing our clients to achieve their greatest potential is unethical. It is not the operant conditioner who faces the greatest moral dilemma, but rather "humanitarians" who prevent their clients from achieving their maximum.

Role of the Clinician. Operant conditioners are often portrayed as cold, unfeeling extensions of mechanical M&M dispensers. This image often results from clinicians subverting their own values for the benefit of the client. There may be times when it is important to appear to be unemotional with your client or to standardize clinical procedures. Of primary concern is what will be therapeutically beneficial to the client. Of secondary importance is the clinician's need to assume a desirable role or be the object of client admiration. A good operant clinical session can be exciting, warm, and interesting both for the client and the clinician. If these elements are important for clinical growth, then they should be applied.

Operant Conditioning as a Technique. Operant conditioning is a technique, not a clinical approach. The distinction is similar to that between a transmitting medium and the message being transmitted. For example, television is an effective learning medium for young children. However, one would be foolish to talk about the value of television in teaching without referring to the specific shows being broadcast. "Sesame Street" would hardly be lumped in the same category as a Saturday morning cartoon show that emphasizes violence. Operant conditioning, therefore, cannot stand by itself; it is the medium for applying clinical principles.

If practicality was no longer a viable argument against operant conditioning, ethics still was. Clinicians who used operant conditioning were viewed as seductive manipulators of their clients. The issue of free will and the client's right to choose became a paramount concern. The most elegant and convincing proponents of this belief were Carl Rogers (1965) and followers of his counseling approach, called client-centered therapy. Rogers maintained that clients can best solve their own problems if they are allowed to define the problem and then derive its solution. According to Rogers, the role of the clinician is one of a facilitator, not a manipulator. Clinicians should not specify what they think is best for the client. By doing this, clinicians are merely imposing their values on the client. The result may be that clients never solve their real problems but rather concentrate on the clinicians' conception of them.

Mediation

Operant conditioners are often referred to as "those people who know what goes in and what comes out, but they don't care what happens in the middle." The objection has some validity. Operant conditioners maintain that they do not need to be concerned with how a person mediates incoming stimuli. If they can identify stimulus-response relationships, the desired results can be achieved without spending much time examining the client's feelings.

Those who object to the approach would also maintain that by only examining what goes in and what comes out, the true causes of a problem can never be identified. However, in many situations the identification of a cause may not be important. For example, if I know that a person's feelings of alienation are causing him to be violent, the identification of the cause is not sufficient to change the behavior. Conversely, I may not need to know that he feels alienated in order to help him become less violent. Operant conditioners are not maintaining that feelings do not exist. Rather, they maintain that they are not important in changing behavior.

The discarding of "inner states" is not accepted by all operant conditioners. Many believe that the mediation that occurs after a stimulus is presented is critical for understanding the effect the stimulus has on the individual (Meichenbaum, 1977). By understanding the individual's cognitive processing skills, clinicians may be able to develop more efficient and effective methods of presenting stimuli.

Basic Concepts

One must understand a set of basic definitions and concepts if effective operant programs are to be developed for the remediation of speech and language disorders. That will be the function of this section. Terms are precise and refer to specific events or objects that are operationally defined. For each definition or concept an example will be provided.

Reflexive Behavior. *Reflexive behavior* occurs as a result of the contraction of the smooth muscles and does not involve any volitional action. An example would be the knee-jerk movement when a physician taps a knee. Although reflexive behavior does not involve any learning, the behavior can be conditioned through association with a stimulus. The classic example is Pavlov's experiment in which a bell elicited the response of salivation in a dog. Three steps are involved in conditioning a reflexive behavior. These steps are outlined in Gagné's Learning Level 1: Signal Learning, described previously.

Some theorists believe that stuttering involves conditioned reflexive behavior. Brutten and Shoemaker (1967) maintained that primary stuttering results when the speech mechanism physically breaks down under stress. It involves no learning and is therefore a reflexive behavior. However, associating specific people or situations with stress does involve learning. After a sufficient number of pairings, the mere presence of certain people or situations can create the stress, which causes the speech mechanism breakdown to occur. If one adhered to Brutten's position, then therapy would involve deconditioning the learned reflexive behavior (primary stuttering) by changing the eliciting stimulus to a neutral stimulus.

One method of doing this is called *systematic desensitization*. It involves reducing the eliciting stress of the stimulus through initially presenting the stimulus at a very low level of eliciting power and gradually increasing it. For example, if it was determined that a client became very disfluent when he had to speak in front of a group of strangers, we might have him practice speaking in the following situations, in the order that they are listed.

1. Speaking alone in a room
2. Speaking alone in a room with a friend outside the door
3. Speaking in a room with a friend
4. Speaking in a room with two friends
5. Speaking in a room with two friends and a stranger outside the door
6. Speaking in a room with two friends who can hear you and a stranger who has his ears covered
7. Speaking in a room with two friends and one stranger
8. Speaking in a room with one friend and one stranger
9. Speaking in a room with one stranger
10. Speaking in a room with two strangers
11. Speaking in a room with three strangers
12. Four, five, six (and so on) strangers.

As you can see, the process involves many small steps. By increasing the strength of the stimulus only slightly when the client has become accustomed to the preceding stimuli, the eliciting power of the stimulus is reduced or eliminated. Approaches of this type have also been used in voice therapy for spastic dysphonia (Boone, 1983).

Another method of deconditioning reflexive behavior is *relaxation therapy*. Clients are usually asked to assume a prone position with their eyes closed. The clinician then suggests that various parts of their body are becoming relaxed. When the client is in a state of physical relaxation, the eliciting stimulus is introduced. By continually pairing the eliciting stimulus with a state of deep relaxation, the strength of the eliciting stimulus is reduced and hopefully eliminated. This approach is limited to certain forms of stuttering therapy and voice therapy.

Operant Behaviors. *Operant behaviors* are behaviors whose rates of occurrence can be controlled by the consequences of the behaviors. This definition will become clearer in the example that follows. Operant behavior differs from reflexive behavior in terms of volitional action. In other words, operant behavior involves decisions. Also the order of events is different. When conditioning reflexive behavior, a stimulus is presented first, and then the response occurs. In operant conditioning, a response appears first, and then a reinforcing stimulus is presented. According to Bandura (1969)

> In most real life circumstances the cues which designate probable consequences usually appear as part of a bewildering variety of irrelevant events. One must, therefore, abstract the critical feature common to a variety of situations. Behavior can be brought under control of abstract stimulus properties if responses to situations containing the critical element are reinforced, whereas responses to all other stimulus patterns lacking the essential elements go unreinforced. (p. 24)

In the clinic we may wish to have a client correctly produce /p/ at the beginning of a word. Every time he correctly produces the behavior, we may give him a point that he can apply towards the purchase of a toy. The /p/ is the response, and the point is the reinforcing stimulus. This type of event sequence would also be applicable in all other communicative disorders, although the complexity of the response and the form of the reinforcing stimulus may be different.

Positive and Aversive Stimuli

New clinicians often are confused about the differences that exist between positive reinforcers, positive reinforcement, negative reinforcement, aversive stimuli, and punishment. Table 7.2 is a grid that can make the distinctions between these terms more obvious. There are two rows and two columns. The rows represent what one can do with a stimulus. One can present it or withdraw it. The columns represent a positive or a negative stimulus. With a 2 × 2 grid, four combinations are possible. If one presents a positive stimulus it is called positive reinforcement. If one presents an aversive stimulus, this is known as punishment. If one withdraws a positive stimulus, it is called punishment, or response cost. If an aversive stimulus is withdrawn, it is called negative reinforcement. A positive reinforcer is a specific stimulus, such as a piece of fruit, a token, a toy, or a specific number of minutes at a pleasurable activity. A positive reinforcer is simply something that a person receives for doing a desired behavior. If the stimulus increases the likelihood that the desired behavior will occur again, it is a positive reinforcer.

Table 7.2
Reinforcement and punishment

	Positive Stimulus	**Aversive Stimulus**
Administering	Positive Reinforcement	Punishment
Withdrawing	Punishment (Response cost)	Negative Reinforcement

If it does not increase the likelihood that it will occur again, we call it a neutral stimulus. Therefore, our definition of what is a positive reinforcer depends on its effect on the client.

Reinforcement refers to the entire event during which a positive reinforcer was given or a negative reinforcer withdrawn. For example, a child is asked to produce the phoneme /s/ when the clinician raises her hand. If the child produces it correctly, the clinician gives him a small piece of an apple. The positive reinforcer is the apple. The reinforcement would be the presentation of the apple contingent on the production of a correct response. There are many ways of classifying reinforcers and reinforcements. The major classifications appear in the following sections. Often it is possible for a positive reinforcer or reinforcement to be classified in more than one way.

Unconditioned and Conditioned Reinforcers. These are also known as primary and secondary reinforcers. An *unconditioned* or *primary reinforcer* is something that reinforces without the necessity of any prior learning. It consists of stimuli that involve fulfilling a basic need, such as hunger, thirst, warmth, and sleep. Within the clinic, food is the most often used unconditioned reinforcer. It can be easily presented to children who may have severe cognitive deficits, understand little language, or have little motivation to engage in clinical activities. Since the strength of a primary reinforcer depends on the state of a client's need deprivation, its value may be limited. For example, if pieces of an apple are used to reinforce a client's vocalizations, the apple will be effective only as long as the client remains hungry or likes the taste of the apple. Of course, we could increase the reinforcing power of the apple by increasing the client's hunger. Andrews and Ingham (1971) effectively used primary reinforcers in a voluntary program for adult stutterers. The amount of food each stutterer received was dependent on the percentage of fluent words he would use during controlled and uncontrolled activities. A state of need deprivation can be ethically used by engaging in the activity immediately prior to a designated snack time or meal. In cases such as these, the clinician is practicing "good timing" rather than unethically increasing a primary need. This type of procedure is usually limited to very low functioning children, with the goal of developing a conditioned or secondary reinforcer.

A *conditioned* or *secondary reinforcer* requires prior learning before it can be successful. The procedures required to establish a conditioned reinforcer are similar to the procedures involved in establishing a conditioned stimulus in reflexive behavior. A neutral stimulus (NS) is paired with an unconditioned reinforcer (UR). For example, with autistic children, a clinician may pair the verbalization "good boy" (NS) with a piece of fruit (UR) when the child emitted a desired response. With each pairing the child will hopefully associate the reinforcing properties of the apple with the verbalization. In time, the verbalization alone may be sufficient to develop the desired behavior. These types of conditioned reinforcers are also known as *social reinforcers*. Obviously with many clients the conditioning has taken place prior to their interaction with the clinician. The greater the amount of language that the client understands, the more likely that conditioned reinforcers can be effective without the necessity of using primary reinforcers.

Generalized Reinforcer. A *generalized reinforcer* is a special type of conditioned reinforcer that can be effective regardless of how clients feel at the time of the activity or their desire for verbal praise. In nonclinical settings, money is the best example of a generalized reinforcer. Regardless of how terrible a person may feel while doing a job, the knowledge that he is acquiring money that can be used at a later date may be sufficient to make the experience rewarding. In a clinical setting, tokens can serve the same function. For a designated number of correct responses the client can receive a token. When the client has amassed a given number of tokens, certain items or activities can be purchased.

Intrinsic/Extrinsic/Extraneous Reinforcement. When designing intervention programs, the clinician should be concerned not only about providing a specific generalized reinforcer at the end of the activity but also about the reinforcing qualities of the activity. The clinical activity can be divided into three units, each presenting an opportunity for the clinician to apply reinforcement procedures.

The first unit is the activity itself. An activity can be *intrinsically reinforcing*, that is, people will engage in certain activities because of the pleasure involved in the activity itself. Accomplished musicians may cry with pleasure as they play a passage in a violin concerto that is especially moving. Or the Saturday morning softball player may feel euphoric as he reaches high in the air to catch a ball. Everyone's life is hopefully filled with these types of activities—activities that are pleasurable in and of themselves. In a clinical setting, the clinician must find or construct intrinsically reinforcing activities. In some types of disorders, such as stuttering, the production of an appropriate speech or language behavior is intrinsically reinforcing. For most stutterers, speaking fluently is very rewarding. Not having to repeat or block on words can be more reinforcing than anything given to the stutterer because he was fluent. At the other end of the continuum would be the young child with a minor articulation problem who does not find it reinforcing to produce /r/ rather than its substitute, /w/. For this child, the intrinsically reinforcing event has to be the activity, not the correct speech behavior. In a later chapter, material design elements will be discussed that are related to intrinsic reinforcement.

When the completion of an activity is reinforcing, regardless of the reinforcing quality of the activity itself, the activity is *extrinsically reinforcing*. An example might be cleaning one's kitchen. A person may hate the drudgery involved in cleaning a kitchen following a party. If the cleaning depended on the reinforcing qualities of the activity itself, many kitchens would probably become breeding grounds for as yet unknown diseases. Why then should one engage in an unpleasant activity such as cleaning? It is the completion of the activity that is reinforcing. The extrinsic reinforcement in this example would be a clean kitchen. To have it, the person would be willing to engage in the activity of cleaning. In therapy the client is often involved in similar situations. Hopefully, the activities are not aversive but merely neutral. For example, if a young child is being taught to combine single-word utterances to produce action + object constructions, he may not feel anything rewarding in the actual production of the phrase "push car." However, if at the completion of the utterance the clinician then pushes a car that the child wanted in his direction, the child is being extrinsically reinforced for the verbal production of "push car."

If neither the activity nor its completion is reinforcing, then an *extraneous reinforcer* is necessary for the person to continue to engage in the activity. For example, an automobile worker's responsibility might be the production of bumpers. To produce a bumper, a button must be pressed to engage a computerized operation. The worker finds nothing reinforcing about the pushing of the button. Nor does he get any pleasure from seeing hundreds of shiny bumpers made every day. Why then should he continue working in the factory? Because he is being extrinsically reinforced. That is, he is receiving enough money every two weeks to make his job acceptable, even though he might hate it. In the clinic, two types of extraneous reinforcer can be used. One is verbal praise and the other involves a token system. It would be nice to believe that our clients would work hard and produce correct responses just because they wanted our praise. Unfortunately, not all children believe that their clinician's praise is that important. For these children, a token system can be very effective, especially if the activities they are engaging in are neither intrinsically nor extrinsically reinforcing. Since extraneous reinforcers are also generalized reinforcers, they should be effective regardless of the present condition of the client or his feeling towards the clinician.

When one thinks about reinforcement, more often than not it is extraneous reinforcement that receives the attention and criticism. The last form of reinforcement that the clinician should concentrate on should be extraneous reinforcement. First design an intervention program that is intrinsically reinforcing. Then have the completion of the activity be extrinsically reinforcing. Finally, have an extraneous reinforcer available if all else fails. Although desired behaviors may be elicited merely by having the child engage in an intrinsically reinforcing activity, it is often not sufficient. The most powerful intervention program involves intrinsic, extrinsic, and extraneous reinforcers.

Negative Reinforcement. If you examine the grid in Table 7.2, it is apparent that the activities involved in negative reinforcement are different from those that involve punishment. Negative reinforcement involves the termination of an aversive stimulus contingent upon emitting a desired behavior. In *negative reinforcement,* the aversive stimulus precedes the behavior. This is very different from punishment, where the aversive stimulus follows the behavior. In the area of communicative disorders, negative reinforcement has been used only in very special circumstances, and then with much controversy. Lovaas (1966) used it to develop and enhance autistic children's physical contact with adults. The child was placed in a narrow hallway whose floor was lined with a metal grid and emitted a mild but uncomfortable electric shock. The child entered at one end of the hallway and the door was closed. At the other end was an adult with open arms who stood immediately beyond the electrified floor of the hallway. As the child entered the hallway he received a shock, which was an aversive stimulus. The shock stopped only when he left the hallway and went into the arms of the adult. The child terminated the aversive stimulus (shock) when he performed the desired behavior (touching the adult). Within a relatively short time, the autistic child was nonverbally interacting with the adult without having to be placed on the electrified grid. Although the procedure may have been effective, it was questionable to those who found the use of electric shock objectionable. Negative reinforcement has also been used to reduce or eliminate stuttering behavior. Goldiamond (1965) terminated a loud noise contingent upon the stutterer's speaking fluently. Negative reinforcement is used rarely in speech pathology, since it requires sophisticated instrumentation and the application of continuous aversive stimuli.

Punishment.   According to the grid in Table 7.2, punishment can involve either the administration of aversive stimuli or the withdrawal of positive reinforcers. Punishment has been used both to establish new behaviors and to extinguish maladaptive ones. A *maladaptive behavior* is any behavior that interferes with learning. The administration of an aversive stimulus should not be used to establish a new behavior for three reasons. The first is that when the aversive stimulus is eliminated, the behavior is likely to be extinguished (Skinner, 1953). Human conditions within prisons parallel the laboratory experiments done by Skinner. In prisons where there is little training in or reinforcement of new, socially acceptable behaviors, the threat of continued aversive stimuli is effective in minimizing antisocial behavior only as long as the threat continues. This is evidenced by the very high recidivism rate associated with prisons that are little more than holding cells for criminals. Within clinical situations, it is not effective to use aversive stimuli to establish a behavior that the client does not know how to perform.

The second reason that aversive stimuli should be avoided is that the clinician is committed to increase the strength of the aversive stimulus when the client does not respond appropriately. People can and do adapt to the strength of an aversive stimulus. The abused child who initially may have been terrified of a parent's slap across the face eventually learns to tolerate severe beatings. Within a clinical situation a clinician may decide to say "No" in an angry tone whenever the child does not respond correctly during a vocal imitative activity. If the aversive quality of "no" is effective in increasing vocal imitation, then the clinician can feel comfortable in the decision to use aversive stimuli. But what happens if the utterance has no effect or loses its effect after a few presentations? The clinician who is committed to using aversive stimuli must now increase the strength of the stimulus. What would be more aversive—yelling, grabbing, or a slight slap on the child's bottom? Possibly all would have to be tried as each loses its punishing effects.

The third reason that aversive stimuli should not be used to teach a new behavior is that the usage presents a model of teaching that is antithetical to the values of our profession. If we are committed to the humane development of a person's maximum potential, then it is inappropriate to rely on punishment to accomplish it. The clinical setting becomes a place to which the client no longer enjoys coming, a place where punishment will be applied if the client cannot perform adequately.

If aversive stimuli should not be used to teach a new behavior, does the usage have a place within clinical practice? Yes. It can be used to reduce or eliminate maladaptive behaviors. In eliminating maladaptive behaviors, the clinician is not teaching the client a new behavior but rather is suppressing one that the client already knows how to do. Inattention, excessive physical movement, and abusive and aggressive behaviors are types of behaviors that respond favorably to punishment. If the clinician decides to administer an aversive stimulus, all of the problems associated with the adaptation to punishing situations are again encountered. In severely disturbed children or children having significant cognitive deficits, the clinician may be limited to the presentation of aversive stimuli. In studies done by Lovaas et al. (1965), it was shown that administering aversive stimuli was the most effective way of rapidly eliminating the self-destructive behavior of psychotic children.

Punishment may instead involve the removal of a positive reinforcer. This is usually done through two clinical procedures: time out and token cost. *Time out* is a procedure that was developed by Ferster (1957) and refers to the removal of a child from a reinforcing setting to one that contains no reinforcers. Typically, a child who was acting out was placed in a bare, windowless room or small enclosure, often with the lights turned off. The assumption was that this form of punishment not only was more humane than the administration of aversive stimuli but also was easy for parents and trainers to use. Time out is effective only if it is viewed by the child as the removal from a reinforcing situation. Unfortunately, being moved from a classroom that the child views as aversive to a setting where no demands are made is not punishing but rather reinforcing. Eventually the child conditions the teacher. Whenever the situation becomes too demanding or too unpleasant, the child knows that if he acts out, he will be placed in the calmer, less demanding room, where he can rest or be entertained by his own fantasies. Time out can also be very inefficient. During that period of time when the child is isolated, no learning of new behaviors can take place. With some children time out may need to last an extensive amount of time to be effective.

The use of *token cost* or *response-cost* in many situations may be more effective than time out to eliminate maladaptive behaviors, because the procedure is coupled with a schedule of positive reinforcement. Typically, a token or positive reinforcer is removed whenever the child either does a maladaptive behavior or responds inappropriately. The relationship between response-cost and positive reinforcement is exemplified by the following example. A child is given one token for every 5 correct productions of the phoneme /r/. If at the end of the session he has accumulated 10 tokens, he can cash them in for a very desirable prize. With 15 minutes left in the session, the child has accumulated 9 tokens. With 5 additional correct responses, the prize is his. However, he realizes that with 15 minutes left, he can produce a large number of incorrect responses and still have time to receive the token. Worse, he can even act out, deliberately ignoring the clinician for a good portion of the 15 minutes. The clinician now faces a dilemma. She realizes the importance of honoring the commitment to reinforce correct productions, regardless of the number of incorrect productions. But she also realizes that the child is using this fact to manipulate her behavior. If she decides to administer aversive stimuli or institute a time-out procedure, the consequences of the punishment may not be effective since the child is so close to receiving the positive reinforcer for the acceptable behavior he has already displayed. In this case, punishment may not be effective in increasing the likelihood that appropriate behavior will increase. The child may stop the maladaptive behaviors even with no punishment to have enough time to produce just the right amount of responses to receive the positive reinforcer. The situation is changed dramatically if a response-cost is introduced. The clinician may explain to the child that since the child knows how to produce the /r/ phoneme, he not only will get a token for every correct response but also will lose one for incorrect responses or inattention. When response-costs are introduced, the effects are quite dramatic on maladaptive behaviors if the client views the positive reinforcer as something that is very desirable. The clinician must be careful, however, in coupling incorrect responses with a response-cost. This could be equivalent to using aversive stimuli to teach a new behavior if the child did not already know how to perform the behavior. Response-costs for incorrect behaviors are appropriate only if the clinician believes that the incorrect behaviors are the result of inattention or contrivance rather than of not knowing the specifics involved in correctly producing the behavior.

Reinforcement Schedules

The reinforcement of desired behaviors can occur after a specific number of responses or after a specified amount of time.

Ratio Schedules of Reinforcement. Reinforcement schedules that are related to the number of correct responses are called *ratio schedules of reinforcement.* If the client is reinforced after every response, a 1:1 or continuous schedule of reinforcement is used. A 1:1 schedule of reinforcement may be necessary with clients who have severe cognitive deficits, are very young, or are not used to having contingencies following their behaviors. In each of these cases, the 1:1 schedule of reinforcement is necessary to establish a reinforcing paradigm. After the association is made between the behavior and the reinforcer, the schedule of reinforcement is changed, requiring additional amounts of correct behaviors to be exhibited before a reinforcer is given. If it is established that the reinforcer is given after a specific number of correct behaviors, such as 3 or 5, then the reinforcement schedule is a *fixed ratio schedule of reinforcement*. This is also known as an intermittent schedule of reinforcement. In these cases it would be a 3:1 or 5:1 fixed ratio schedule of reinforcement. Under certain circumstances, we may require a variable number of correct responses to receive a reinforcer. The number of responses required could change from 2 to 4 to 3 to 8 and back again to 2. These are called *variable ratio schedules*. The changes can be random or determined prior to the clinical activity. In either case, the client does not know how many responses will be required, only that the amount will keep changing. Although variable ratio schedules are harder to administer, they do have some advantages over fixed ratio schedules. With fixed ratio schedules the client may become inattentive if he knows that he is getting close to receiving a reinforcer. However, when the number of correct responses required for reinforcement continually changes, the client must remain attentive at all times.

Interval Schedules of Reinforcement. *Interval schedules of reinforcement* involve the administration of a positive reinforcer after a specified amount of time. It is not related to the number of correct behaviors. If the reinforcer is given after a specific amount of time, the client is on a fixed interval schedule of reinforcement. If the amount of time varies, the client is on a variable interval schedule of reinforcement. As was the case with the variable ratio schedule, variable interval schedules can be determined prior to the clinical interaction or can be random. Interval schedules are less effective in teaching new behaviors than are ratio schedules. However, they can be very effective in eliminating maladaptive behaviors. For example, a child is told that after he sits quietly for 5 minutes he will receive a token. This would be a 5:1 fixed interval schedule of reinforcement. If the amount of time is variable, then the child would be on a variable interval schedule of reinforcement.

Mixed Schedules of Reinforcement. In a clinical session it is possible to use multiple reinforcement schedules to achieve various results. For example, a clinician could use (a) 5:1 fixed ratio schedule of reinforcement for correct productions of personal pronouns within sentences; (b) 2:1 fixed ratio schedule if the sentence had at least five words; (c) 3:1 fixed ratio schedule if the sentence dealt with future relationships; and (d) a variable interval schedule that reinforced quiet sitting.

Response Differentiation

"Think small" is one adage that clinicians should continually say to themselves. Most clients enter into clinical situations with a history of communicative failures. On a general level, one can attribute their failures to an inability to master one or more communicative behaviors. Since the client has been unable to develop the behaviors "normally," a remedial approach is required. The remediation should be designed to accomplish two goals: (a) affirm or re-affirm the client's belief that he or she can be successful, and (b) provide a technology that facilitates learning. Both of these goals can be accomplished through the use of response differentiation. *Response differentiation* involves shaping a response in one of two different ways. The clinician may select a series of target responses that successively approximate the final goal or may hold the final goal constant and successively reduce the cues that are provided to the client for successful completion of the behavior. The first procedure is known as *successive approximations* and the second as *multiple cuing*.

Successive Approximation. In attempting to teach a client a new behavior, the clinician should first dissect the behavior into its smallest component units. For each unit, a separate therapy program is written, specifying criterion levels, stimulus presentations, and reinforcing contingencies. The simpler the unit of behavior, the more likely it can be quickly and easily mastered by the client. Not only is a necessary behavior mastered, but also the client can begin to feel a sense of accomplishment. Also, if the transition between one step and the next does not involve many new behaviors, the probability of success will be enhanced. In the following example, the goal of therapy will be to have an 8-year-old child spontaneously correctly produce the phoneme /s/ in all contexts. Prior to therapy, he consistently substitutes /θ/ for /s/. If the clinician believed that auditory discrimination was important for the successful production of /s/, eight specific therapy steps would be required to achieve the goal. If the clinician did not believe that auditory discrimination was necessary, then the first three steps would be eliminated. As you examine each of these steps you can see that the acquisition of a behavior at one step depends on acquiring a behavior at the step that immediately precedes it. With each successive step, the client comes closer to approximating the goal.

1. *Distinguishing Between /s/ and Gross Sounds.* This would be the lowest level of the program. The client is asked to differentiate the /s/ phoneme produced in isolation from easily distinguishable sounds such as grunts and moans, which are naturally occurring sounds.
2. *Distinguishing Between /s/ and Phonemes Other Than /θ/.* At this step all phonemes other than the substitution would be juxtaposed to the /s/.
3. *Distinguishing Between /s/ and /θ/.* The child is taught how to auditorially distinguish between two sounds that have only one distinctive feature difference.
4. *Correct Production of /s/ in Isolation.* The child would be taught to produce /s/ in isolation. This may presuppose that he can distinguish between /s/ and his substitute phoneme /θ/.
5. *Correct Production of /s/ in Phonemic Contexts.* The child would be taught to produce /s/ when it is surrounded by various other phonemes. However, this presupposes that the child can produce /s/ in isolation.
6. *Correct Production of /s/ in All Words.* The child would be required to correctly produce the /s/ when various /s/ cards or objects are presented to him. However, this presupposes that he can produce the /s/ in various phonemic contexts.
7. *Correct Production of /s/ in Structured Situations.* The child would be required to produce specific words in sentences, under clinical conditions. However, this presupposes that the child can produce the /s/ in all words.

8. *Spontaneous Correct Production of /s/ in All Contexts.* This step would involve the spontaneous correct production of /s/ whenever it is used in sentences. However, spontaneous usage implies that the child has mastered the task in structured situations.

In this example, what appeared to be a relatively minor articulation problem was divided into eight separate program steps, with each step coming closer to approximating the final goal.

Multiple Cuing. Not all behaviors are amenable to the type of reduction displayed in the preceding example. Often, the behavior is one that would be difficult to simplify. In situations such as these, the target behavior is kept constant, but a series of cues are provided to the client that will enable him to produce the correct behavior. The cues are arranged in a hierarchy, so that they may be systematically eliminated, starting with the most concrete cue and ending with the most abstract one. In the following example, a clinician wishes to teach a client the linguistic rule Actor + Action + Object (A+A+O). The client is already producing Action + Object constructions, so it would be difficult to think of a series of target behaviors falling between A+A+O and A+O. However, the transition from a two-word rule to a three-word rule may not be as easy as it would appear, even though there do not seem to be any successive approximations of the behavior between A+A+O and A+O. Rule understanding and formation involve abstract processing, an ability that is impaired in clients with cognitive deficits. Therefore, various cues are provided that can enable the client to effect the transition. In the following example, multiple cues are provided in the first step, then each is eliminated in subsequent steps.

1. *Production of A+A+O with Modeling and Three-Card Pointing.* The clinician produces the utterance, "Jim push ball." With the production of each word, she touches a small blank card. The shape of each blank card is different. Touching each card conveys the idea that each word is separate and connected in a specific way. The clinician then takes the child's hand and places it on each card as the child says the appropriate word.
2. *Production of A+A+O with Three-Card Pointing.* Step 1 is repeated, but this time the clinician does not provide a model.
3. *Production of A+A+O with Independent Three-Card Pointing.* The clinician now requires the child to tap on the cards independently as he produces each of the words.
4. *Production of A+A+O with Tapping and No Cards.* The cards are now removed, but the child is required to tap out the three-word sequence.
5. *Production of A+A+O with No Tapping.* In this final step the child is now required to produce the three-word sequence without any aids.

Criteria for Advancement. In response differentiation the client is progressing through a set of sequential program steps, with the acquisition of behaviors at each step dependent on the behaviors acquired in the preceding steps. It is critical therefore that the clinician is reasonably certain that the client has acquired the prerequisite behaviors. A specified number of behaviors or percentage of correct responses is known as the *criteria for advancement,* or *criterion level.* Prior to beginning the therapy program, the clinician should specify what the criteria for advancement will be. We can be absolutely sure a client has acquired a behavior if he produces it correctly 100% of the time. However, this level of advancement may be too stringent in that it does not allow for inattention or other interfering variables.

It is generally agreed that a 90% criterion level for advancement is sufficient for guaranteeing that the client has mastered the task. Some research indicates that an 80 to 85% criterion level may be sufficient (Diedrich & Bangert, 1980). Until more research is available, it is advisable to use the 90% criterion level as a standard from which slight downward deviations can be made so that the child does not become bored with the activities through endless repetition. When expressing criterion levels, some clinicians refer only to a percentage figure. Although this does provide some information to the listener or reader, a significant element is missing: the number of items in each trial. Therefore, when specifying criterion levels, always refer to the number of items. For example, "Criterion for advancement in each stage of the program is 90% for trials containing 20 items."

Operant Principles of Therapeutic Intervention

Clinical intervention involves complex interactions and processes. Clinicians must prepare for various contingencies, anticipate many possible outcomes, and always weigh decisions based on the therapeutic benefit to the client. In this chapter we have examined some basic operant concepts. In the following sections, these concepts are now used to develop operant principles of intervention that are applicable to all communicative disorders.

Do Not Assume Anything. One should begin therapeutic interventions with a healthy dose of skepticism. In other words, if something is not in writing, on audiotape, visually observed, or verbally attested to, assume that it does not exist. The 18th century philosopher Hume presented and developed an approach to the study of knowledge known as empiricism (Flew, 1961). The empiricist relies only on externally verifiable data. In designing intervention strategies, the clinician must function as an extreme empiricist. This form of clinical blindness may appear to be an overreaction. However, it is always better to err on the side of caution rather than to assume that a task has been performed or a condition exists. The following example will emphasize this point.

At a center for children with multiple disabilities, an 8-year-old child was observed sitting in a wheelchair for an entire day. He had no verbalizations, did not respond to verbal or signed requests, and in general appeared oblivious to the people around him. His records indicated that he had been diagnosed as severely mentally retarded. He had spent the last six years of his life at a large institute for the retarded. Although confined to a wheelchair, he appeared to have a significant amount of leg movement. While producing a guttural sound, he would move his legs alternately in a rapid up and down movement for as long as 20 continuous seconds. At other times, normal lateral movement could be observed. Muscle tone appeared to be normal and the child reacted appropriately to pin pricks on both legs. Movement in all other parts of his body appeared to be normal. However, when taken out of the wheelchair and forced to stand without support, he would always immediately collapse onto the floor.

The speech-language pathologist who was consulting for the center was confused by his observations. In his discussions with the staff, they informed him that since the child arrived at the center in a wheelchair, they assumed that he was not physically capable of standing or walking. Their conclusion was affirmed on many occasions when they pulled him out of his wheelchair and he collapsed onto the floor. The consultant examined the child's medical records and found no indication of any physical problems. Subsequent conversations with the staff at the institute resulted in similar findings. The staff had all assumed that since the child was not walking when he came in contact with them, he obviously was unable to walk. The consultant decided that the proper assumption was that the child *could* walk but for some reason either had not been taught to or was not allowed to. Through an operant program involving successive approximations of normal walking movements and differential reinforcement of desired behaviors, the child was walking independently after 5 hours of training. One would like to think that this example is an extreme case of making a wrong assumption. However, similar tragic occurrences often result from such a simple oversight.

Perform Audiological Screening on All Children. The loss of hearing, even if minor and of short duration, can affect children's ability to learn and can adversely affect interactions with both peers and adults. An audiological screening is a relatively easy and quick procedure to perform. It is especially important for children who have never had a hearing test, who have had hearing or articulation problems, or who appear to be mentally retarded. Essentially, all children who come for speech or language therapy should be screened. The following example taken from the center cited in the previous section illustrates this principle.

The center had contracted with a noted hospital to perform a complete diagnostic workup on all of their children. The assessment was to include a hearing evaluation. After examining 35 files, the consultant found that audiological screening was mentioned in only three of the files. The wording of the hospital's contract was "audiological testing when indicated." The hospital was assuming that audiological testing was appropriate only for those children who had "obvious" hearing problems. On the insistence of the consultant, hearing screenings were performed for the rest of the children. Seven of the 32 failed the screening. On subsequent testing, three were found to be within normal limits, one had a unilateral hearing loss of 30 db, one had a bilateral hearing loss of between 20 and 35 db, and two had bilateral hearing losses of greater than 90 db. The two with the 90 db losses would be classified as profoundly deaf. One child was 13 and the other was 8. Neither child had ever been previously tested, and both had resided in an institution for the retarded for most of their lives. It is quite possible that their only initial problem was hearing, and both may have possessed normal intelligence. However, being treated as if they were profoundly retarded over a period of many years resulted in a substantial environmental deprivation, possibly causing the ensuing mental retardation. Misdiagnosing hearing loss as mental retardation can still occur, however infrequently, when audiological testing is not routinely performed.

Start With the Behaviors the Client Can Perform. Clients come into clinical sessions with a history of communicative failure. If this was not the case, there would be no reason for therapy. It is crucial for clinicians to understand this point. One's self-image will have a direct and substantial effect on the outcome of therapy. Clients who view themselves as failures will assume that therapy will be of limited success. If the tasks clinicians ask clients to perform are beyond their capability, the negative self-image is confirmed. For this reason, it is imperative that clinicians begin with a behavior that is sufficiently simple to guarantee success.

For example, one would not ask a client with spastic dysphonia to speak for 10 minutes. Rather the first goal might be to speak in an "easy" voice for 1 or 2 minutes. The child with an articulation problem would be taught to produce the target phoneme either in isolation or within a phonemic context that allows for correct production. To assure success, the stutterer who is using prolonged speech would start using the method for 30 to 60 seconds.

Emphasize Progress Toward Desired Behaviors. Clinical intervention should be viewed as a way of facilitating the growth process. In growing, one is moving toward a desired goal. Therefore, it seems reasonable to emphasize the goal one is attempting to achieve rather than the behavior one is trying to eliminate. Take, for example, the aphasic client who during past therapies was having word-finding difficulties. In the past on most activities he was able to recall the names of 60% of the pictures or objects presented. During the current session he knew the names of 80% of them. The clinician can present this information to the client in the following way:

> That was pretty good. You only missed 20% of the cards. Last week you missed 40% of them!

It appears that the clinician is giving the client a sincere compliment. However, examine carefully what actually is being said. "Last week you erred 40% of the time. This week you erred 20% of the time." This is like telling someone that in the past they were "very boring," but now they are only "slightly boring." Backhanded compliments have no place in therapy, whether they are intentional or unintentional. A better way to convey the client's progress to him would be to say:

> That was pretty good. Last week you had 60% of the cards correct. This week you had 80%!

By using slightly different words, the focus of therapy is shifted. Instead of focusing the client's attention on the problems he is having, the clinician has shifted the focus to the progress made.

Reinforce Positive Behaviors. Research has shown that the best way to develop new behaviors is to reinforce their occurrence positively. However, this does not mean that clinicians are limited to reinforcing only the final target behavior. For example, if a clinician is attempting to teach a child to produce /s/ without lateral or excessive frontal air emission, approximations of the target should be reinforced. If in the past the child had both types of lisps but he now produces the /s/ with only a slight frontal lisp, his productions should be reinforced as approximations of the target sound. Always reinforce positive changes in a client's behavior, regardless how small they may appear.

The idea of reinforcing any positive change should be emphasized with parents and other adults who may be involved in the therapy. Persons who have not been trained in the areas of speech-language pathology may not be able to see the small differences. The clinician should spend whatever time is necessary with the parents in training them to notice differences.

Punishment should never be used to develop a new behavior. Research has shown that this is the most inefficient way of developing new behaviors. Usually, after the aversive stimulus is removed, the behavior is extinguished.

Eliminate Maladaptive Behaviors Through Negative Reinforcement, Punishment, or the Development of Incompatible Behaviors. A *maladaptive behavior* is any behavior that interferes with the learning process. It can range from head banging to inattention. As long as a maladaptive behavior is present, the individual's growth will be impeded. Three methods can be used to eliminate these behaviors: negative reinforcement, punishment, and the development of incompatible behaviors.

Negative reinforcement occurs when an aversive stimulus is eliminated contingent upon a desirable response. For example, a loud, high-pitched tone is emitted whenever a child walks around a room. The tone, which is the aversive stimulus, is terminated whenever the child sits in a chair.

Punishment involves either the administration of an aversive stimulus or the withdrawal of a positive reinforcer, contingent upon the performance of an undesirable behavior. An example of the administration of an aversive stimulus would be a short blast of noise administered as soon as the child stands up. An example of the withdrawal of a positive reinforcer (response cost) would be taking away a token if the child was not in his seat when the clinician began the activity.

Creation of an *incompatible behavior* involves having the client engage in an activity that is incompatible with an undesirable behavior. In our example, something could be placed at the table that was so intrinsically reinforcing that the child would of his own accord come to the table, sit down, and engage in the activity.

During therapy, any of these three methods of eliminating maladaptive behaviors may be appropriate. The use of negative reinforcement is often technically difficult to accomplish. The administration of aversive stimuli may not be allowed or may involve basic ethical issues. The use of a response cost is simple, easy, and effective. Creating an incompatible behavior poses the fewest difficulties for the clinician, is positive, and may be the most effective method of eliminating maladaptive behaviors.

To create the incompatible behavior, the clinician must discover things that will be intrinsically reinforcing to the client. Anything that is intrinsically reinforcing tends to produce attending behavior and positive results. Additionally, since the incompatible behavior is also a component in the training of a new behavior, there is an efficiency of effort.

Develop Problem-Solving Strategies. A client who comes to speech or language therapy not only has a specific problem but also does not know how to solve it or cope with it. If they could, they would either not have the problem or would be able to solve it on their own. Therefore, clients need to be viewed as having two distinct problems. The first obviously is that they have a communication problem. The second is that they do not have a strategy for solving the problem.

With this perspective, clinicians must develop a two-part therapy program. The first part involves correcting the specific problem. The second is to teach the client a strategy to solve similar problems independently. For example, take the child who is functioning only at a one-word level. Not only does the child have a basic communication problem, but he also has difficulty determining the rules of language usage. Merely teaching the child to combine a large number of words into two-word utterances is not enough. Although this instruction will give the child some basic tools for communicating with people in his environment, it may not be sufficient for teaching him the rules of language. Without looking at language as a set of rules, the child will require assistance to learn all new utterances. If he can be taught how to use rules to produce unique structures, the child is learning a strategy for solving problems, and he thereby becomes his own therapist.

Incorporate Decision-Making Activities into Therapy. Children with severe communicative problems often are not given the opportunity to control their environment and understand the consequences of their actions. This also is true for many adults. When viewed in this context, people with communicative disorders may be treated as less than responsible functioning individuals. If children have trouble communicating their needs, the parents will intercede for them, often making their decisions. Many of these children grow up never really understanding the importance of controlling their own environment.

Within a clinical context, the ability to make meaningful decisions can be taught to children in an easy, systematic way. Initially clinicians can give children a choice of one of two activities that will be engaged in during the session. Gradually, the number of items from which an activity can be chosen can be increased. This process places an extra burden on the clinician. Most clinicians enter the session with a set of specific goals that hopefully will be arrived at through specific activities. If decision-making activities are to be incorporated within the session, clinicians must be able to achieve the same goals regardless of the activity the child chooses. This is known as *contingency planning*. Contingency planning allows clinicians to achieve desired effects while providing children the freedom to choose within set parameters.

The right to chose or to make decisions carries the responsibility of accepting consequences. If children choose a certain activity, they should understand that the selection requires them to perform specific behaviors. Further, noncompliance results in the application of aversive contingencies or the withholding or removal of positive reinforcers. The relationship between the control of one's environment, the right to make meaningful decisions, and the acceptance of consequences for one's actions is central not only in therapeutic relationships but also in life. When doing therapy with communicatively disabled individuals, clinicians should not forget this delicate balance. Therapy is a facilitative process that should be used to help disabled individuals gain or regain their maximum capability as independent, responsible human beings.

Consistency. Clinicians need to be consistent in their approach and procedures. This does not imply that they should be rigid. Rather, unless a clinician consistently engages in a recurring activity, it will be difficult to determine what caused success or failure. Consistency can also be a problem in a clinician's overall approach. Often a clinician will attempt a specific procedure. If the procedure fails, another approach will be tried, and then another and another. One might argue that if a procedure fails, it makes little sense to stay with it. Rather, something different is warranted. This may be true in many instances. However, by too rapidly changing an approach to something that is vastly different, clients may develop an inappropriate view of their problem.

For example, a clinician was working with an adolescent stutterer who had undergone many years of therapy. To facilitate fluent speech, the clinician first tried having the client use single-word utterances. When this did not produce the desired effect after 20 minutes, the clinician had the client begin relaxation exercises. After completing 12 exercises the client still was very disfluent. At the next session the clinician asked the client to whisper the first part of each word and then phonate on the remainder of the word. When this did not produce satisfactory results after 30 minutes, the clinician asked the client to practice his stuttering pattern until he felt no anxiety. In this example, the client may begin to experience two negative feelings. The first is that "My problem is so severe that no matter what technique is used, it doesn't help." The second feeling is that "My stuttering problem could be cured if only the right technique could be found." The first feeling reinforces the client's negative image of himself, while the second absolves the client of all responsibility for positive behavioral change.

Changes in therapeutic procedures and techniques should be done slowly and carefully. The clinician should start with the assumption that the approach is basically correct but in need of a "fine-tuning adjustment." Major changes in therapeutic procedures and techniques should be contemplated only after adjustments do not result in the desired change.

Clinical Progress Should Be Assessed Continuously. Speech-language pathology is a clinical science. As such, it relies on objective data for assessing and remediating communicative problems. The clinician should always keep this in mind. The collection of objective data does not rule out the use of subjective inferences. However, the clinician should be aware that decisions based on subjective inferences have a higher probability of being wrong than decisions based on objective data. Additionally, unless everyone who comes in contact with the client has the same semantic system and inferential skill as the clinician, there is the likelihood that the clinician's inferences will be misunderstood.

Clinicians should at all times be able to specify clearly how well a client is doing and relate progress to the therapeutic program. To do this, the clinician must regularly collect objective data. It is not sufficient for a clinician to say "He is doing much better this week." *Much* means very little in a clinical sense. A supervisor was observing a clinician engaging in therapy with an adult aphasic. During the 20- minute session, the clinician did not take any notes or record the client's responses. After the session, the bewildered supervisor asked the clinician how she could tell if the client was improving. The clinician responded that she remembered the type of correct and incorrect responses made by the client, and "just knew" when the client was ready for the next step in therapy. Fortunately, the supervisor had recorded all responses. When questioned, the clinician was unable to remember accurately (a) the pictures the client was asked to identify; (b) which pictures were correctly identified; (c) the number of times each picture was presented; or (d) the type of errors the client had made. Since the supervisor questioned the clinician immediately after the session, it is likely that the clinician's memory would have been even hazier a few days after therapy.

Too much occurs during a clinical session for the clinician to rely on memory. By doing this, one is left only with vague judgments like "much better" or "improved significantly." It is impossible to fine-tune a client's therapy if data is collected only once a month or at other long intervals. Clinicians must keep a running count of the variables that will determine when a client should progress to the next stage and what works and what fails in the therapy program.

Involve Parents, Teachers, and Staff When Appropriate. As great as many clinicians might be, they are with the client for only a limited amount of time each week. Significant behavioral changes require not only a compassionate and competent clinician and a motivated client but also other individuals who are willing to reinforce newly acquired behaviors. This is especially true with young children, who often do not see any intrinsic benefit in changing a behavior. Why should a 6-year-old child be concerned with a frontal lisp if all of his friends can understand him and nobody makes fun of him? How do you convince a 6-year-old that he will be glad 10 years from now that he practiced the speech exercises you instructed him to do. You don't!

It is absurd to assume a child has the same value system as his parents or the clinician. Because of this, extraneous reinforcement is often necessary for new behaviors to be established in the child's repertoire. If the behaviors can be reinforced in various settings, then stimulus and response generalization will be facilitated.

Giving Homework. Behaviors need to be practiced in various settings if stimulus generalization is to occur. Unfortunately, this is often translated into "speech homework," such as cutting "/s/ words" out of magazines and pasting them into a homework book. The child brings the book to the next clinical session and receives a star for every five pictures. How this facilitates stimulus generalization is anyone's guess. Activities should be performed by the client between clinical sessions. Significant behavioral change will not occur without it. However, the clinician should not describe the activities as a "homework assignment." Generalization of desired behaviors involves the use of normal activities. The homework should be restricted to recording responses, either by the client or the client's parents.

For example, a child has finally been able to produce /t/ in all phonemic contexts. The clinician would like to see the behavior generalized at home. A program is developed that requires the child to produce five sentences each with at least one /t/ sound, five times each day. The sets of sentences must be produced during the following activities: eating dinner, watching television, doing school work, driving in a car, and playing basketball. Either the child or the child's parents record the number of correct responses the child makes.

Continually Reinforce New Behaviors in Various Settings. A new behavior is a fragile item. One of the best ways to strengthen a behavior is to reinforce it whenever it occurs. The clinician needs to be aware of this and provide "strokes" to the client. Often, since the behavioral changes are so small, the clinician may be the only person who is aware that change has occurred. For generalization to occur, the behavior should be practiced and reinforced in as many settings as possible.

Clients may forget behaviors and also have them extinguished. Since most clinical programs are sequentially ordered with the development of one behavior being the base for the next, the loss of a previously learned behavior can have a serious effect on a current aspect of therapy. For these reasons it is important to reassess quickly the previously learned behaviors at the beginning of the therapy session. Obviously not all behaviors have to be continually reassessed, but those that will be critical for the development of the current goals should be reevaluated.

Supplement Standardized Tests with Analyses of Conversational Speech. Diagnostic test batteries should include both standardized and nonstandardized testing procedures. The standardized tests provide diagnosticians with an objective basis for categorizing the client's problems. However, with many children, a formal testing situation may prove to be too threatening. If children feel insecure or frightened, their verbal performance can be affected. Through the use of informal methods, such as conversation and play therapy, a language sample can be taken that may provide important information unavailable through normal testing procedures.

SUMMARY

Therapy should be based on the principles of learning. All therapy requires clients to change something about themselves. These changes may involve simple motor patterns such as a slight shifting in the position of the tongue to produce an /r/ or complex behavioral changes such as having the wife of an aphasic client understand why her husband is reluctant to engage in sexual activities with her. Although the therapeutic approaches for these examples would be different, the principles on which they are based are similar.

In this chapter we discussed how people learn new behaviors and attitudes and how they subsequently retrieve and use them. Understanding these principles allows the clinician to construct efficient clinical activities that minimize client frustration and feelings of failure while maximizing opportunities for success. By realizing that learning involves both stages and levels, clinicians can construct activities that are cognitively appropriate for the client.

And finally, the uses and misuses of operant conditioning were discussed. Operant conditioning should be viewed as a technique that is based on the principles of human behavior. It is neither ethical nor unethical. Rather, moral attributions are related to its applications. The ethical application of operant techniques has been shown to offer the clinician the best and most efficient manner of structuring therapy.

SUGGESTED READINGS

Bandura, A. (1969). *Principles of behavior modification.* New York: Holt, Rinehart & Winston.
Cronbach, L. J., & Snow, R. E. (1977). *Aptitudes and instructional methods.* New York: Irvington Publishers.
Gagné, R. M.; Briggs, L. J.; & Wager, W. W. (1988). *Principles of instructional design.* New York: Holt, Rinehart & Winston.
Meichenbaum, D. (1977). *Cognitive-behavior modification.* New York: Plenum Press.
Skinner, B. F. (1948). *Walden two.* New York: Macmillian.
Skinner, B. F. (1953). *Science and human behavior.* New York: Macmillian.
Skinner, B. F. (1957). *Verbal behavior.* New York: Appleton-Century-Crofts.

❑ *Activity 7.1*
Identification of Learning Continua

Below you will find the learning continuum matrix described in Table 7.1. Observe a client with a speech or language disorder for 30 minutes. During this time, provide examples of as many stages and learning levels as you can identify. If the client is having difficulty with learning a task, identify at what level the problem is occurring and describe it.

| | Stages in Learning and Retrieval ||||
Levels of Learning	**A** **Apprehending**	**B** **Acquisition**	**C** **Retention**	**D** **Retrieval**
1. Signal Learning				
2. Stimulus-Response				
3. Chaining				
4. Verbal Association				
5. Discrimination Learning				
6. Concept Learning				
7. Rule Learning				
8. Problem Solving				

Activity 7.2
Operant Procedures

Observe a client and clinician for 30 minutes. During this time, identify all incidents of operant procedures being applied. A list of procedures is on the left side of this sheet. On the right, provide examples.

Reflexive Behavior	
Positive Reinforcement	
Punishment	
Negative Reinforcement	
Ratio Reinforcement Schedule	
Interval Reinforcement Schedule	
Intrinsic Reinforcement	
Extrinsic Reinforcement	
Extraneous Reinforcement	
Unconditioned Reinforcer	
Successive Approximations	
Multiple Cuing	
Criteria for Advancement	

Chapter 8
Principles of Group Therapy

STUDY GUIDE

- ❏ The use of group therapy is often determined by the requirements of the work-setting. Briefly describe the four settings in which group therapy is the primary form of intervention.
- ❏ Group therapy can serve four functions, each of which requires specific procedures and techniques. Identify the procedures and techniques associated with each function.
- ❏ Describe the qualities of an effective group leader.
- ❏ How can cultural variables both enhance and hinder group therapy?
- ❏ What should be the relationship between support groups and formal speech-language therapy?

*C*lients may be treated both individually and within group settings. The term *dyadic* is frequently used in reference to individual therapy. The decision to work in a dyad or with a group depends on many factors, including work setting, financial resources, disorder, and time commitments. While many of the strategies and techniques used with dyads can be directly applied within a group setting, others require modifications. Some techniques, such as principles of group interaction and leadership strategies, are applicable only in group therapy. In this chapter, the techniques and strategies of group therapy will be presented.

❑ ❑ ❑ SETTING REQUIREMENTS

Often one's employment setting dictates the parameters of therapy, setting limitations on both the type and extent of services to be offered (Cornett & Chabon, 1988; Flower, 1984). In certain settings dyadic therapy may be financially prohibitive; in others, a sufficient number of speech-language pathologists may not be available. Although group therapy can be found as an adjunct to dyadic therapy in virtually all settings, there are four employment settings in which group therapy is the primary form of intervention. They are public schools, senior centers, preschools, and community centers.

Public Schools

Public schools seem to be continually under financial assault because they often lack adequate money or personnel to provide the services demanded by parents and mandated by state and federal laws. Traditionally, speech-language therapy in the public schools has been practiced in less than ideal circumstances. It is arguable whether the problem is the result of the expense of treating communicative disorders in comparison to other services or of administrators not realizing the importance of the services provided by speech-language pathologists. At one time in the history of the profession, most therapy was conducted in the public schools. For the last 10 years the employment trend has shifted from public school placement to hospitals, rehabilitation centers, and private facilities. In 1991 only 60% of ASHA-certified speech-language pathologists listed "public school" as their place of employment (ASHA, 1992). Twenty years ago, it was 90%. This decrease is due to an ever-increasing range of employment opportunities. Because of a lower percentage of new speech-language pathologists choosing to work in the public schools and the increase in children requiring services (Hanson, 1990), many public schools find that the only way they can meet the mandated needs of their children is through group therapy. When possible, children with similar disorders are treated in a group whose membership can range from two to five individuals. Rarely are more than five children seen together. When children with similar disorders cannot be scheduled together, they are often grouped by age. When this is not possible, children who have time available within their schedule are grouped together.

With the implementation of Public Laws 94-142 and 99-457 guaranteeing appropriate services to disabled children, many parents of children with communicative disorders have refused to accept inappropriate groupings of their children. Faced with potential grievance procedures, many administrators are reluctant to require their speech-language pathologists to form therapy groups of children with very dissimilar disorders.

Recently, some school districts have begun using a "consultative model" with mixed results (Sailor, Gee, & Karasoff, 1991). The model places the speech-language pathologist in the role of a consultant either to the classroom teacher or the special educator. The speech-language pathologist develops classroom activities that are used by other professionals or teaching aides. In many instances the speech-language pathologist will also provide the staff training necessary for implementing the intervention program. The model was designed for two purposes: (a) to provide special services within the least restrictive environment and (b) to compensate for shortages in personnel. Groupings of children in the consultative model can range from a manageable number to an entire class.

Senior Centers

Senior centers tend to function as social organizations where senior citizens can engage in socially or personally rewarding experiences with individuals their own age. These centers are ideal settings for conducting classes for the hearing impaired and offering aphasia group therapy for seniors and their families. The centers also provide a setting where students can learn about the problems associated with aging.

Preschools

Preschools often establish speech and language enrichment programs for their children. Because this service is provided at the expense of the school, it has financial limitations. Most of the children in preschools function within normal limits, and activities within a group setting are aimed at speech and language stimulation. In many large cities, increasing numbers of children are entering preschools with either limited or no proficiency in English (California Department of Education, 1991). These children present a special problem to the speech-language pathologist who can work with them only in a group setting. An even greater problem is children who have been prenatally exposed to drugs or alcohol. Even though they may require intensive special services, the speech-language pathologist must often provide them with the same amount of attention given to a child who is developing normally.

Community Centers

Community centers can provide the speech-language pathologist with a unique opportunity to offer services to individuals who either are not aware of services or could not afford them in other settings. In large cities these centers tend to serve newly arrived immigrants (Gollnick & Chinn, 1990). Therapy is often conducted within a group setting, but the speech-language pathologist must also rely on an interpreter. Group therapy within community centers can be viewed as a way of determining appropriate services for new citizens.

FUNCTION OF GROUPS

Not only are there significant differences between the communicative styles exhibited in dyadic and group settings (Gladding, 1991), but individuals with communicative disorders may display their disorders differently in each setting. Albertini et al. (1983) for example, compared the speech intelligibility and articulation skills of deaf young adults who were receiving individual and group therapy. Although there was no significant difference between the subject groups in terms of these communicative behaviors, there were differences in the number and type of utterances used. Albertini concluded that although group therapy was cost effective for the acquisition of articulation skills and improvement of speech intelligibility, it fell short of what could be accomplished in individual therapy in terms of the number and type of utterances used.

The advantages of group over dyadic therapy were emphasized in another study on an aphasic population. The study found that the use of group therapy activities significantly eased depression and anxiety, eliminated unfavorable reactions to disability, shaped everyday activities, and helped the aphasic clients become active and self-dependent (Pachalska, 1982). These positive changes resulted primarily from the support and interaction of the group. Although some of these changes may have been possible solely through dyadic therapy, it is unlikely that the results could have been achieved as effectively or as rapidly.

Clinicians should not have to choose between dyadic and group therapy, since each can provide the client with skills and behaviors that can be generalized to a variety of situations outside the clinic.

The techniques used within a group setting depend on the purpose of the group. Groups can serve four purposes. They can (a) change speech and language behaviors, (b) provide a safe environment where new speech and language behaviors can be practiced, (c) provide an opportunity for clients and parents to discuss the effects of the communicative disorder on their lives, and (d) allow the speech-language pathologist an opportunity to observe, without interference, an individual's communicative behaviors. Quite often a group has more than one function, alternating between various activities when they are appropriate. Although a group can serve various functions, it is important to realize that the strategies used for each function differ.

Changing Speech and Language Behaviors

Many believe that the use of a group setting is probably less efficient in teaching a new behavior than dyadic therapy (Cornett & Chabon, 1988). The argument may be irrelevant if speech-language pathologists find themselves in a setting that only provides group therapy. The speech-language pathologist can use specific strategies to maximize the efficiency and effectiveness of the group setting to teach new behaviors. These are presented in the following sections.

Appropriate Groupings. Although the ideal group usually occurs only within one's imagination, the variables that are associated with it are ones that should be used as guidelines for group formation. The more homogeneous the group is in terms of disorder, severity, and age, the greater the ease in using the group as a vehicle for changing behaviors (Gladding, 1991). Rarely, if ever, is the ideal encountered. The usual situation is that group members share a general disorder. It is not unlikely that children with articulation disorders will be grouped together, regardless of what phonemes are misarticulated. A stuttering group may contain individuals whose stuttering ranges from 50% disfluency to monitored normal fluent speech. Voice groups may contain cases of hypernasality and vocal abuse. The acuity of a hearing impaired group may range from a unilateral 40 db hearing loss to total deafness. Within school settings attempts are made to group children not only by disorder but also by grade. Selection by grade is usually limited to a spread of three grade levels.

Time Management. One of the most difficult problems encountered when teaching new behaviors within a group setting is the management of time (Corey, 1990). It goes without saying that time spent with one individual is time not spent with everyone else. The task for the speech-language pathologist is to construct activities for each member of the group to minimize unproductive time. This can be accomplished in three different ways when the individual is not working directly with the speech-language therapist: (a) practicing the newly acquired behaviors, (b) monitoring someone else's production of appropriate behaviors, and (c) engaging in reinforcing activities.

When waiting one's turn, the client can spend time most productively in *practicing* new behaviors. For example, if a child is working on the production of /r/ in isolation, his task between turns might be to produce the sound a given number of times. If two or more children are working on the same behavior, they could practice together until it is their turn to work with the clinician. An example from an adult stuttering group would be the practice of prolonged speech with another group member who is also waiting his turn to interact with the speech-language pathologist.

Monitoring by a "waiting" individual of an "active" individual's behavior may be an appropriate use of time, especially if both individuals are working on the same behavior. The role of "monitor" could be switched, giving each client an opportunity to practice the behavior and also monitor the correct production of that behavior. This approach has been used effectively with adult groups of stutterers (Shames & Egolf, 1976) and aphasics (Hill & Carper, 1985).

If it is not appropriate or possible to use the time between turns for practice or monitoring, the time could be used to reinforce the child for correct productions. *Reinforcement* for children and young adolescents should involve an activity that can be continued throughout the session, such as drawing or constructing an object. Reinforcement for adults and older adolescents would not be an appropriate use of this time.

Competitiveness. There is a natural inclination within a group setting to compete. Competition may take various forms, ranging from a desire to win at a game to seeking the approval of the clinician for correct responses. Competition is a natural feeling of children and adolescents (Gardner, 1982). Regardless of the value the clinician places on competition, it is a variable within group settings and as such should not be ignored. If it is ignored either because the clinician is not aware of it or because the clinician chooses not to acknowledge and use it, it can become a destructive element within a group. If it is addressed, it can be used in a positive manner to facilitate the development of new behaviors. Group competitiveness should not be confused with an individual's striving to better his or her own past performance, a characteristic that is always positive and should be continually reinforced by clinicians. Group competitiveness relates to an individual's need to best other members of the group, regardless of the quality of his or her own performance. Competitiveness can be an acceptable feature of the group activity as long as it does not negatively impact on the group members. Constructing activities that account for both individual and group performance will test the creativity of the clinician. The following example shows one way this can be accomplished in articulation therapy.

- *Group Membership.* The group consists of three 7-year-olds, each having an articulation problem. Jim is just beginning to correctly produce /r/ in isolation. Marge had a frontal lisp that has now been corrected and is beginning to generalize into her unmonitored speech. Elizabeth is beginning to correctly produce /dr/ blends in initial positions.
- *Group Activity.* A board game is being used in which the correct production of a speech behavior results in movement of the child's piece. What is defined as a "correct production" differs for each child. For this session, Jim is required to produce 10 consecutive /r/ phonemes correctly. During the last session he was required to produce five consecutive /r/ phonemes. Marge must produce two sentences, each containing at least one sound on which she had lisped in the past. During the last session she was required to produce only one sentence. Elizabeth must choose two words containing the /dr/ blends and produce each five times correctly. During the last session she was required to produce only one word five times.
- *Goals of the Activity.* The child who reaches the end of the game first will win an inexpensive toy. Every child who does better this session than last session will win a special sticker.

Control. Issues of control are different for child, adolescent, and adult groups. Control within groups of children tends to center around appropriateness of behaviors (Myrick, 1987). New clinicians are especially prone to lose control with children, often not recognizing the gradual slippage until it is too late. Maintaining control within groups poses more difficulty than in dyadic settings. To maintain control, the speech-language pathologist can use three specific strategies: (a) establish clearly defined parameters of acceptable and nonacceptable behavior, (b) allow choices within established parameters, and (c) establish consequences for both appropriate and inappropriate behavior. Although each of these strategies can be used for both individual and group therapy, they are especially important to use with groups.

Children have a natural tendency to push at the outer limits of acceptable behaviors (Walker, 1979). It is the rare child who does not test limits. By clearly establishing what is acceptable and not acceptable, the clinician provides parameters of behavior for the child. Usually, a new clinician allows too much freedom for the group, eventually finding it necessary to reduce the parameters of acceptable behavior. A better method of maintaining control is to begin with very narrow parameters and gradually increase them as the behavior of the children warrants it. Initial parameters may involve choosing between two activities, such as practicing vocal volume control while either playing a game or constructing a play figure. With acceptable group behavior, the choices can be expanded gradually to include other activities.

The freedom to choose within specified parameters can develop either a cohesiveness for the group or can divide it. Problems with splits in voting can be avoided by allowing the "losing side" to choose the activity for the subsequent session. As was stated in Chapter 7, the element of choice is important for developing a sense of commitment on the part of clients. The sensitivity displayed by the clinician to the needs of "outvoted" group members is important in establishing the notion of fairness. An alternative method of developing cohesiveness is by using a consensus model. Within this model of group activity, there are no winning or losing sides. Decisions require the agreement of all members. Although this form of group decision making may take longer, some believe that it results in cohesiveness and commitment on the part of all group members and therefore significantly reduces problems of control (Rogers, 1965).

Imposing consequences for actions establishes a model for behavior within a group by building on the concept of personal responsibility, not only for the development of speech and language behaviors but also for behaviors in general. This is especially important for children, who are in the process of establishing lifelong patterns. When one child engages in a behavior that has been clearly identified as inappropriate and then faces the consequences, a powerful model for the other children is established. Three important canons should be remembered when imposing consequences. The first is that any consequence for a behavior should be clearly stated prior to its imposition. To do otherwise suggests an arbitrariness or capriciousness that is not conducive to therapy. The second is that a consequence should never be chosen that the clinician is not prepared to impose. The clinician who says, "If you aren't going to get back to practicing, we will sit here and do nothing," should be prepared to do nothing for the remainder of the session. By not imposing a threatened consequence, clinicians reduce their credibility and may lose control over the group. The third canon is that consequences should be consistently imposed.

Although some control issues for adolescent and adult groups may be similar to those of child groups, most problems of control involve task orientation (Piercy & Sprenkle, 1986). Group members may tend to stray off the assigned task or to spend more time than is desired on a given task. In adult stuttering groups, for example, the clinician may require the participants to talk about instances when they were fluent, using an exaggerated form of fluency called prolongation. Although some members may wish instead to present instances of disfluency, it is the responsibility of the clinician to keep them on task. The clinician's leadership qualities become important for keeping the group focused.

Orientation. Probably the most successful approach to changing specific, observable behaviors within a group setting is behavioral group therapy (Corey, 1990). In groups using this orientation the focus is on the modification, elimination, and substitution of behaviors, not underlying causes. In these groups the focus of therapy is primarily on behaviors that can be observed, measured, and precisely transformed. While they support a behavioral orientation, some authors believe that thoughts are also acceptable behaviors to manipulate within a group setting (Beck, 1976; Meichenbaum, 1977). Thoughts for some therapists are viewed as integral parts of communicative disorders, often being a key variable necessary for changing a communicative disorder such as vocal abuse, aphasic speech, or stuttering. Egolf, Shames, and Seltzer (1973), for example, were able to shift the focus of group discussion from talking about how it felt to stutter to how it felt to speak fluently. The shift in thinking resulted in a reduction in disfluency and a greater willingness to engage in fluency-enhancing activities.

Generalization of Behaviors

Groups can serve as safe environments in which new speech and language behaviors can be practiced under the guidance of a speech-language pathologist and with individuals who may be more tolerant of communicative failure than nongroup members. Three types of activities can be engaged in that facilitate the generalization of new behaviors: (a) formalized clinician-directed activities, (b) simulations, and (c) unstructured communicative activities.

Formalized Clinician-Directed Activities. When a new behavior is learned, the clinician often will want the individual to produce it in a highly structured activity that results in the best possibility of its correct production and also facilitates its generalization. An example would be teaching a child to use the word *in* when any object was placed in a container. During individual therapy, the clinician would hold various objects over a box and ask the child, "Where should it go?" If the child said *in*, the object would be dropped into the box with a loud bang, delighting the child. After the child has consistently produced the word *in,* the clinician introduced the child into a "communication-centered" group that consisted of six other children at various stages of language therapy. The function of communication-centered groups is to provide a less clinically structured environment in which children engage in new behaviors (Molyneaux & Lane, 1992). In this group another child is now given an object and asked to hold it over a box until the first child says *in* when asked the question. Various clinicians and children could then alternate placing objects into different containers.

An adult example of a formalized clinician-directed activity is the generalization of esophageal speech. Once an individual learned how to produce esophageal speech correctly, he could enter a communication group consisting of other esophageal speakers. His first activity might be to practice producing very short utterances with each member of the group.

Simulations. A *simulation* is an approximation of an event that contains the most relevant aspects of the event. Although these events are contrived, they can be an important component of therapy. Simulations serve as a bridge between highly structured activities and normal nonclinical activities. The following example of a simulation for a child involves teaching lip-reading skills. A moderately hearing-impaired child has been learning to lip read. Her instructor first taught her individually the skills that she would be required to use during everyday activities outside of the clinic. Then, within a group setting, the child practiced reading the lips of the children as they read a sentence or said predetermined words. In preparation for the child entering a non-hearing-impaired class, the speech-language pathologist developed a simulation in which the teacher is giving instructions to the whole class. The key elements of the simulation are that (a) the teacher modulates her voice from loud to soft, (b) the teacher occasionally turns toward the chalkboard when talking, and (c) a few children are talking during the teacher's instruction. Although the activity is contrived, it contains the variables that will most likely interfere with the child's successful reading of lips.

The following adult example is taken from a fluency group. Each member of the group has been taught a form of fluent speech production. Although the speech sounds normal, it requires the client to expend a tremendous amount of energy in its production. An activity is designed to simulate a nonclinical situation in which an individual is placing a food order in a restaurant. Key elements in the simulation are that (a) the waiter will interrupt the order if there is any hesitation on the part of the client, (b) everyone at the client's table will be intently listening to the client, and (c) the client will be surrounded by other tables, each filled with people. In this example, three variables are present that many stutterers indicate interfere with their ability to use fluency-enhancing techniques.

Unstructured Communicative Activities. The group can help generalize behaviors through the use of unstructured activities. This allows both the clinician and client to assess the degree to which the new behavior is becoming automatic, since during unstructured activities the careful monitoring of behaviors is less likely to occur. Many researchers have emphasized the importance of using activities that facilitate the transformation of newly learned behaviors to automatic behaviors (Goldberg, 1981; Shames & Florence, 1980). One example is a child's correct production of targeted phonemes. After learning how to produce certain phonemes in isolation, within words, and during simulated activities, the children within an articulation group are told that they can engage in a game that requires each of them to talk. They are not asked to produce any specific words or sounds, just to play the game. The clinician, however, notes both the correct and incorrect productions of each child's target phonemes. Children who consistently produce correct productions become candidates for dismissal from therapy.

Another example is an adult aphasic client who has been taught how to structure her language so that it is simplified, direct, and communicative. In the group, she is asked to have a casual conversation with other group members about any topic of interest. The clinician analyzes her verbalizations to see if the response patterns she has been taught are becoming a part of her verbal repertoire.

Discussion Groups

Speech-language pathologists are not expected to be group counselors, competent to lead in-depth discussions on the entire spectrum of human emotions and problems. They are, however, expected to help individuals examine the impact that communicative behaviors have on their lives. Counseling courses both within and outside communicative disorders departments can help clinicians accomplish this goal. The purpose of this section is to set acceptable goals for groups directed by speech-language pathologists and to specify some of the basic techniques that can be used to accomplish these objectives. Techniques are related to the focus of topics, orientation, and age of the groups.

Focus of Topics. Group discussions are thought by many to be vehicles for individuals to present problems and develop solutions for their remediation or acceptance (Rogers, 1965). Other clinicians use the group setting to refocus attitudes about speech and language (Rubin, 1986). A good example is a cognitive rehabilitation program for patients with head injuries developed by The Greenery Rehabilitation Center in Boston (Hill & Carper, 1985). The program focuses on the development of a positive attitude toward rehabilitation by both patients and staff. In this program and others addressing various communicative disorders, clinicians refocus the group's orientation on discussing their feelings when they are successful in communicating rather then spending time continually discussing the negative aspects of the disorders. The move is positive, reinforces successful communication, and acts as an incentive for continued work.

Orientation. Some orientations are better suited for groups focusing on communication problems than others. For example, many people find the person-centered group therapy orientation of Carl Rogers easily adaptable to communications groups (Frank, 1961). *Person-centered therapy,* also known as *client-centered therapy* or *nondirective therapy,* involves the therapist's reflecting what group members have said within a framework that clarifies each individual's thoughts, without making any judgments (Rogers, 1965). The value of this orientation is that it focuses on the unconditional acceptance of the individual by the group. For many group members, this is a unique experience, one that can lead to reinforcing positive changes in their speech or language.

Almost the complete opposite of person-oriented therapy is *rational-emotive therapy*, developed by Albert Ellis (1962). Whereas group leaders using Rogers' approach allow the group to formulate goals, therapists using rational-emotive therapy use a highly structured, logical format to lead group participants to a more rational way of thinking and behaving (Wessler, 1986). A variation of this form of therapy for stutterers was developed by Rubin and Culatta (1971). The advantage of using a rational-emotive type of therapy is that it focuses the client's attention on understanding a specific problem and deriving the means for its solution.

The orientation that most closely follows the training of speech-language pathologists is that of *behavioral group therapy*. In this form of therapy, underlying symptoms are not examined (Wilson, 1989). Emphasis is on learning and modifying behaviors. The group is used as a vehicle for monitoring and reinforcing positive behaviors and occasionally for punishing inappropriate behaviors (Hollander & Kazaoka, 1988).

Other orientations to group therapy, while as legitimate as the three just described, require training beyond that normally derived from graduate courses in speech-language pathology. Many clinicians have found that the acquisition of these advanced skills has significantly improved their group therapy effectiveness. These orientations are Gestalt group therapy (Latner, 1973), Adlerian group therapy (Corsini, 1988), traditional psychoanalysis (Wolf, 1963), transactional analysis (Berne, 1966), and Jungian therapy (Rollin, 1987).

Children's Groups. The impact a communicative disorder can have on a child can range from none to devastating. The 5-year-old child whose /w/ for /r/ misarticulation goes unnoticed by other children may not even realize that a problem exists. Another 5-year-old child who is unmercifully teased by his classmates because of his stuttering is daily traumatized by his problem. These two very different examples point out the necessity of first determining how a communicative disorder is affecting the child before assuming that he or she needs to discuss it. The old adage, "If it's not broken, don't fix it," is very applicable. Not all children need to talk about their communicative problem, especially those who do not view it as a problem.

Discussing a child's problem directly may be too threatening. The use of puppets, stories, or plays is often less threatening and can allow children to discuss problems openly by attributing the problem to the puppet, the child they are talking about in the story, or the character being portrayed in the play.

Adolescent Groups. Adolescence is a difficult developmental stage. The individual is generally more affected by a communicative disorder than a child is. The adolescent also has a greater capacity to discuss feelings. Accompanying this greater awareness may be a reluctance to discuss personal problems in the presence of other adolescents (LeCroy, 1986). The use of puppets or other indirect methods of discussing feeling about their communicative disorder may be inappropriate. A less threatening way to discuss feelings may be to focus the discussion on what they are feeling while experiencing communicative successes.

Adult Groups. The topics of discussion for adult groups can range from the specific disorder to how the group members feel about their communicative ability and its relationship to their lives. Discussions of communicative ability can be focused on specific areas of functioning, such as at work, in social settings, and with significant others.

Baseline Data Through Group Observation

Speech-language pathologists are continually gathering data so they can assess their clients' progress. Usually, clinicians gather data in a dyadic session prior to and at the end of therapy. A group setting provides a unique opportunity for gathering additional data. While contrived in terms of membership and focus, it does offer a more natural environment to observe clients' developing communicative abilities. When gathering data, it is important for clinicians not to engage in any communicative behavior. Their role is that of an observer. Data can be gathered through the use of check-off forms and audio or videotapes.

Regardless of the age range of the group, the clinician can focus on some specific areas, most important of which are, for each client, (a) percentage of correctly produced target behaviors, (b) number of target behavior productions, (c) evidence of generalization of the behavior, (d) reaction to correct/incorrect productions by the group, (e) awareness of and reactions to own correct/incorrect productions of the target behaviors, and (f) extent of communication with other group members as a function of communicative ability.

Percentage of Correctly Produced Target Behaviors. The goal of speech and language therapy is the generalization of new behaviors. Once a behavior is learned within a structured setting, it gradually replaces the incorrect behavior. By observing the percentage of time the new behavior is produced, the clinician can begin to gauge the extent to which the behavior is becoming a part of the client's behavioral repertoire.

Number of Target Behaviors Produced. For a new behavior to be established, the individual must be given ample opportunity to produce it (Bandura, 1969). If the opportunity is not present, the conditioning that is so necessary for the establishment of behaviors will not occur. For example, although a child may be able to consistently use the question marker *where,* she may take longer than necessary to generalize it if she is not given any practice opportunities. If during the observational group session, the clinician notices that opportunities to ask questions are not given to the client, it would be appropriate to structure the sessions so that questions could be asked.

An example for adolescents and adults of providing an opportunity to establish a new behavior would be the reduction of vocal abuse. During the individual session the goal of therapy could be the modulation of vocal intensity so that vocal nodules would not reoccur after their surgical removal. The client may have been taught how to engage in conversation at a reduced volume level, even when surrounding noises make it difficult. If the level of conversation and the ambient noise levels in the group are low, the client would not have an opportunity to practice the new speaking skill. However, if the clinician could have a radio playing music while the group members were engaging in unstructured activities, the client would have an opportunity to practice her newly learned skill.

❑ ❑ ❑ QUALITIES OF THE GROUP LEADER

Various authors have presented lists of what they believe to be the essential qualities of a group leader. Since these qualities are usually related to the counseling orientation of the author (Corsini, 1988), they tend to reflect specific approaches to therapy. Although a comparison of different viewpoints of leadership qualities is beyond the scope of this text, characteristics common to most approaches will be examined.

General Competency

Regardless of the orientation that is used in group therapy, it is critical that the client perceive the clinician as competent. Clinicians should be aware that their attitudes, values, and behaviors become a model for emulation to clients (Dinkmeyer, Dinkmeyer, & Sperry, 1987). The clinician who is unprepared and disorganized for the group session with language-disordered children presents a very different picture from the clinician whose presentation of activities to a similar group is logically structured, systematic, and clear.

Empathic

Empathy involves the ability of a therapist to understand the emotion a client is experiencing and display sensitivity toward it. It does not require the clinician to have had an identical experience. The pain associated with the inability to communicate effectively may differ little from the pain associated with the humiliation experienced with being fired from a job. Not being empathic can seriously affect clinical interactions. The clinician, for example, who shows little regard for the nonspeech concerns of her elderly hearing-impaired group engenders a very different feeling in her clients than the clinician who, while focusing the group discussion on hearing impairments, is very concerned about the life issues of the group members.

Multidimensional

Clinicians change many things other than the specific speech-language behaviors they are charged to address. Some of these changes are direct, such as suggesting to a stutterer that he confront his parents about their attitude toward his speech.

Others are indirect, such as watching a depressed aphasic client modeling the hopefulness seen in her clinician. As clinicians develop their clinical skills, the interrelationship of problems becomes more understandable (Murphy, 1982). Within group settings, the importance of being multidimensional may be critical for addressing the myriad of problems that clients present (Scheuerle, 1992).

Age-Specific Characteristics

Most groups contain members in the same age ranges. The behavior of the group leader should be adjusted to meet the needs of the group. The characteristics needed to lead child, adolescent, and adult groups are different. Within each group the qualities displayed by the group leader will be related to the function of the group.

Child Groups. Leaders of children's groups should act as facilitators who provide strategies and instructional techniques for the development of specific communicative behaviors. If the function of the group is to provide ways to explore and discuss emotions, the leader becomes a teaching facilitator who encourages self-exploration (Gladding, 1991). The methods used to encourage self-exploration will depend on the counseling orientation (Long, 1988).

Adolescent Groups. Adolescent groups present special challenges to the group leader. Whereas childhood growth tends to be steady and somewhat predictable, adolescence is a developmental period when tremendous psychological and social changes occur, often in uneven progressions (George & Dustin, 1988). During this period, individuals begin struggling with the issues of both identity and sexuality. Behind a tough, uncaring, facade, teenagers may actually be confused and vulnerable, not fully able to understand the changes occurring in their lives. The reality of a communicative disorder may already be too difficult to confront in a dyadic setting. The openness necessary to modify a behavior publicly or discuss the problem in the presence of other adolescents may be too threatening for the individual. One of the qualities necessary for a group leader of adolescents is to have good judgment regarding the appropriateness of certain topics. Behaviors and discussions of disorders that even remotely address a teenager's sexuality are best examined within single-sex groups (Myrick, 1987). Since communication is such a central feature of an adolescent's identity, the group leader needs to be careful that the communicative disorder does not become the primary identifying feature of the group member, either in his or the other group members' eyes. Myrick (1987) lists six behaviors that leaders of adolescent groups should exhibit:

1. Use responses that elaborate on feelings.
2. Clarify and summarize the participants' statements.
3. Use open-ended questions.
4. Facilitate both positive and negative feedback among group members.
5. Acknowledge the participants' statements.

6. Link members of the groups by the statements they make.

Adult Groups. In many ways adult groups will present the group leader with fewer challenges than child and adolescent groups, but in other ways they will be more difficult. Usually adult groups are self-selective. That is, each member has made the decision to participate. Occasionally however, group therapy is a requirement for receiving individual therapy. In situations such as these, clients may tolerate the group experience since it is the only way to have dyadic therapy. Even when initially reluctant to be involved in a group, adults tend to experience significantly more positive than negative interactions. The group becomes a supportive structure for clients and a place where they can experiment with new communicative behaviors. Although issues of control are usually not as problematic as with child and adolescent groups, task orientation can be more difficult. The group leader needs to be prepared to keep the group focused. Adult groups deal with adult issues, many of which the new clinician may not feel comfortable addressing in front of other people.

CULTURAL VARIABLES

Misunderstandings Between Cultures in Group Settings

A primary cultural identity in our country is ethnicity (Gollnick & Chinn, 1990). Many ethnic cultures express their identity through nonverbal behaviors and language. Within a group setting these nonverbal messages are especially prone to misunderstandings.

Nonverbal Behaviors. It is easy for the nonverbal behaviors of group members from different ethnic cultures to be misinterpreted. For example, the lack of eye contact, which is a sign of respect in one culture, may be misperceived as disrespectful in another (Cheng, 1987). Other behaviors, such as the physical distance between people may be misperceived as being sexually suggestive instead of civil and friendly (Saleh, 1986). The group leader needs to become the bridge between cultures. When it appears that group members are not relating to each other or are becoming segmented because of not understanding the nonverbal behaviors associated with a culture, it is the group leader's responsibility to discuss specific incidents and the way they are being misperceived. By understanding differences, strategies for avoiding future problems within the group can be developed.

Language Behaviors. Within a group setting, language can be used by members of one ethnic group as a form of identification and individuation from other group members. When this occurs, members of other ethnic groups may feel a sense of isolation or may form stereotypical impressions based on the language usage. A good example is contained in a study conducted with 13-year-old English-only speaking and 13-year-old Spanish bilingual students (McKirnan & Hamayan, 1984). The English-only students perceived the Spanish teenagers' style of speech as indicating a desire to remain isolated. Those English-only students with little or no contact with Spanish-speaking students also had negative perceptions of the Spanish-speaking students, based on their speech. Just as the group leader needed to address the consequences of ethnic-specific nonverbal behaviors, the consequences of linguistic-specific ethnic behaviors should also be discussed.

Groups and Ethnic Cultures

Group experiences are not perceived as identical in all ethnic cultures. Within certain cultures, the exhibition of disordered communicative ability and the discussion of personal problems is desirable, since it offers the individual the support of a community. Studies have shown that individuals from various Hispanic cultures may adapt to group work quite easily (Delgado & Humm-Delgado, 1984; McKinley, 1987). Similar results have been found for African-Americans (Higgins & Warner, 1975). For many Asian cultures though, group therapy may not be desirable for any of the stated group functions, because their cultures minimize the public display of emotions and disabilities (Cheng, 1987).

SUPPORT GROUPS

Support groups exist for individuals who stutter, are aphasic, or have had their larynx removed. Support groups have also been developed for parents of children who have communicative disorders. Many of the groups, such as the National Stuttering Project and many of the social aphasia and alaryngeal groups that can be found at senior centers, function without the leadership of a speech-language pathologist.

Functions of Support Groups

Support groups are different from therapy groups. They are homogeneous in nature and revolve around shared experiences. According to Rosenberg (1984), support groups can serve three useful functions. They can (a) increase the member's coping abilities, (b) stress interpersonal insight, and (c) operate as a feedback device. Additionally, reinforcement rather than reconstruction is emphasized.

View of the Profession

The leadership of support groups resides in the members. If a speech-language pathologist is present, it is usually as a participant. Discussions within these groups tend to focus on ways of adapting to the communicative disorder, discussion of personal problems resulting from the disorder, and presentation of examples of how individuals triumphed in spite of the disorder.

Some speech-language pathologists believe that support groups are antitherapeutic, because the focus of the group tends to be on the disorder rather than on the development of desirable behaviors. It has been suggested that much of the negative reaction towards self-help groups from professionals may be the result of an embarrassment that a need for self-help groups exists when trained professionals are available (Goldberg & Culatta, 1991). For example, if stutterers believed they were being adequately served by the profession, they would not find it necessary to form self-help groups. Faced with this rather negative indictment, some speech-language pathologists have chosen to ignore the reasons that self-help groups form and the many positive results they do achieve.

Other speech-language pathologists view support groups as basically positive, but ineffectual since they usually lack a trained leader and often are joined as a substitute for therapy. These professionals contend that although the individual may receive emotional support from the group interaction, the support is in the direction of reinforcing methods of coping with the disorder rather than developing new, more functional communicative behaviors.

A third and more objective position views support groups as a valuable adjunct to direct therapy by qualified individuals. For example, the San Francisco State University Center for Fluency Development has established a cooperative relationship with the local chapters of the National Stuttering Project. Clients at the center attend the chapter's meetings with specific speaking assignments. The cooperative relationship is one that has been beneficial to both the center and the National Stuttering Project. Similar relationships can be established with other types of support groups.

SUMMARY

Clinicians may be required to provide services in a group setting either because of the policies and economics of their place of employment or because of the experiences that are only possible through group therapy. Regardless of the reason, they need to understand that with each of the functions groups can serve, specific techniques are required. Although some techniques parallel those used in dyadic therapy, others are unique. Grouping clients appropriately, determining the functions that the group can serve, deciding on the techniques and activities to use, and implementing the activities in an effective and efficient manner, pose one of the greatest challenges for speech-language pathologists.

SUGGESTED READINGS

Corey, G. (1990). *Theory and practice of group counseling* (3rd ed.). Pacific Grove, CA: Brooks/Cole.

Delgado, M., & Humm-Delgado, D. (1984). Hispanics and group work: A review of the literature. *Social Work with Groups, 7* (3), 85–96.

Gladding, S. T. (1991). *Group work: A counseling specialty.* New York: Merrill/Macmillan.

Higgins, E., & Warner, R. (1975). Counseling blacks. *Personnel and Guidance Journal, 53,* 383–386.

Myrick, R. D. (1987). *Developmental guidance and counseling: A practical approach.* Minneapolis: Educational Media Corporation.

Rosenberg, P. P. (1984). Support groups: A special therapeutic entity. *Small Group Behavior, 15* (2), 173–186.

❏ **Activity 8.1**
Group Time Management

It is important to manage time effectively within a group. For this exercise observe a group session for 30 minutes. Assess the use of time for the following activities:

1. Time used by individual group members directly with leader (average)

    Member 1: _____

    Member 2: _____

    Member 3: _____

    Member 4: _____

    Member 5: _____

    Member n: _____

2. Time used by individual group members in general discussion (average)

    Member 1: _____

    Member 2: _____

    Member 3: _____

    Member 4: _____

    Member 5: _____

    Member n: _____

3. Time used by individual group members working/conversing with other group members (list approximate time).

            Member 1   Member 2   Member 3   Member 4   Member 5

    Member 1: _____

    Member 2: _____

    Member 3: _____

    Member 4: _____

    Member 5: _____

Activity 8.2
Group Control

It is important for the group leader to maintain control. This can be done in numerous ways. Observe a group for 15 minutes. Below are categories of control that can be exercised by the leader. Try to identify specific behaviors within each category. If there are behaviors that do not fit in any of the categories, place them in "Other."

Nonverbal

Direct Verbal

Indirect Verbal

Task Focus

Other

❑ **Activity 8.3**
Group Functions

Groups can serve four functions. Observe a group for 15 minutes. For each function observed, describe the methods the leader used for achieving the goal.

Changing Speech and Language Behaviors
Appropriate Groupings

Time Management

Competitiveness

Control

Orientation

Generalization of Behaviors
Formalized Clinician-Directed Activities

Simulations

Unstructured Communicative Activities

Discussion Groups
Focus of Topics

Orientation

Age of Groups

Baseline Data
Percentage of Correctly Produced Target Behaviors

Number of Target Behaviors Produced

Chapter 9
Clinical Strategies

STUDY GUIDE

- Describe the various types of implementation strategies.
- Given a client with a specific communicative disorder, design a competency-based clinical intervention program for the acquisition of one simple behavior.
- What are the advantages and disadvantages of computer-assisted instruction?
- What are the various strategies a client can be taught to use that will enhance memory and retention?

*C*lients with communicative disorders may lack not only basic skills but also the strategies for solving communicative problems. The purpose of therapy is to develop both communicative skills and communicative strategies. *Strategies* usually refer to mental steps that are undertaken in sequence to meet a specific goal (Mayer, 1983). They are sets of principles for solving problems for which the client has not been trained. Without the use of strategies the stutterer who is taught how to be fluent within a quiet therapy room will have difficulty remaining fluent in the presence of an aggressive employer. The child who is taught to produce "doggy run" only through modeling will have difficulty substituting "daddy" or "Billy" for the actor component in the Actor + Action construction. If therapy is to be effective and efficient, consideration must be given to strategies of implementation and strategies for learning.

Strategies of implementation deal with the sequencing and methodology of therapy. They are the structures that clinicians use to deliver therapy. Although strategies for learning may overlap with strategies of implementation, *strategies of learning* are primarily concerned with the teaching of abstract rules. These abstract rules enable clients to solve communicative problems that may be unique or never examined in therapy. Those solutions involve Gagné's sixth (rule-governed behavior) or seventh (problem-solving) learning level (Gagné, 1970).

❏ ❏ ❏ STRATEGIES OF IMPLEMENTATION

Strategies of implementation involve the methods of presenting clinical stimuli and their logical structuring. An analogy would be a carpenter's dovetail-joint template. The template, a steel plate that consists of a series of fingers, is placed on a piece of wood from which a cabinetry joint will be constructed. As a cutting tool is guided between the teeth of the template, the exposed wood is cut away. What remains is the joint. If therapy is to be effective and efficient, it requires a similar template, a structuring device that allows for the ordering of therapy elements. Speech-language pathologists can abstract implementation strategies from three disciplines in which extensive research on learning has been conducted: cognitive psychology, instructional technology, and computer-assisted instruction. In this section each area will be described and illustrated by an example applied to a communicative disorder.

Cognitive Psychology Scaffolding

Vygotsky (1978) developed a theory of learning for children that viewed adults as the mediating agents between environmental stimuli and the child. In this role, adults helped structure various learning situations that facilitated learning rather than merely providing it. This theory was developed into an educational application model by Wood, Bruner, & Ross (1976). They maintained that teachers should provide the means, or *scaffolding*, for individuals to go beyond their capabilities through the control of task components. Once the scaffolding has been provided, the learner eventually bridges the gap between present knowledge and new knowledge necessary for completing the task. They list six operations that the teacher should perform. These have been modified in the following descriptions to apply directly to speech-language pathologists.

Recruit the Client. Clients should have an initial desire to engage in the activity. It can be presented as something that either has immediate gratification or will provide long-term benefits. Wood et al. (1976) believe that unless a convincing argument can be made to a learner about why an activity should be engaged in, participation will be halfhearted, and although the task may be completed, the individual may not have learned what was intended.

Simplify the Task. A task may be so complex that its successful completion is beyond the cognitive capability of the client. Clinicians need to structure the activities so clients are not burdened with attending to elements that are not germane to mastery or are beyond the clients' current abilities.

Maintain Interest and Motivation. The activities necessary for the acquisition of a behavior should be reinforcing to the learner. Unless the client's interest in the activity is maintained, the likelihood of its successful completion is remote. Interest and motivation are maintained through reinforcement. Reinforcement can be intrinsic, extrinsic, or extraneous. Continued interest in an activity is more likely when the activity is intrinsically reinforcing.

Mark Relevant Features of the Task. In the mastery of any behavior, clients will produce responses that are not correct. An important function that clinicians serve is to identify the discrepancies between incorrect and correct productions. Then they determine the reasons for failures and, where necessary, provide scaffolding for learning.

Control the Level of Frustration. Learning can be a frustrating experience. Although a certain amount of frustration may be necessary in the acquisition of new behaviors, the clinician needs to limit it, especially when it no longer facilitates the development of problem-solving skills and begins to impede therapy.

Use Modeling When Necessary. The clinician should use modeling procedures when appropriate. This becomes especially important in the development of motor tasks that are difficult for the client to grasp without a visual model.

As clients gain greater competence, the scaffolding is gradually removed, allowing them to succeed with little or no assistance. According to Wood et al. (1976), the scaffolding model provides a way of reducing learner dependence and enhances cognitive development.

Competency-Based Clinical Intervention Format (CBCIF)

What appears to some as a very simple behavior may for the client constitute a complex behavior with many component parts. For example, the seemingly simple act of tying one's shoes involves over 100 specific movements. For a cognitively impaired child or an adult with a traumatic brain injury, this skill acquired by children in primary school may be viewed as more confusing than the complexity of microcircuits is to an intelligent adult with no knowledge of electronics. It is an appropriate clinical maxim to assume that any behavior the client is unable to perform is complex. Complexity is more a function of perception than actuality. The circuitry of a computer is basic for the doctoral student in computer science, but it is probably unfathomable to the music major who is computer illiterate. To provide clients with the greatest opportunity to master a complex behavior and experience more successes than failures, a logically structured, sequentially ordered intervention program can be used.

Educational technology has provided teachers and clinicians with a precise methodology for constructing intervention programs that can dissect complex behaviors into their component units. Competency-based instruction has been used in educational settings since the early 1970s. This mode of instruction begins by specifying what the end product of instruction or therapy is to be. An instructional program is then designed to take the students or clients from their current abilities and behaviors to the final goal of the intervention program. One of the first uses of this type of intervention model was by William and Diane Bricker (Bricker, 1972; Bricker & Bricker, 1970), who developed language lattice training models for cognitively impaired children. Throughout the years similar programs have been developed that use a successive approximation approach. Although competency-based instruction is based on the concept of successive approximations, its structure is somewhat more sophisticated. It not only uses successive approximations but provides precise formulations for implementing each of the approximations.

One model for this type of intervention program is the Competency Based Clinical Intervention Format (CBCIF). The model, which was developed by the author, is based on the sequential learning steps used in instructional technology and the training lattices developed by the Brickers.

The CBCIF incorporates successive approximations throughout the program and contains four structural levels: (a) terminal competency, (b) specific competencies, (c) instructional objectives, and (d) learning activities. In this section the definitions of each level are presented along with examples in Figures 9.1 through 9.5. Figure 9.1 shows a completed articulation program with each of the four levels completely delineated. Figures 9.2 through 9.5 illustrate partial programs for the treatment of other disorders, with only the first level under the first competency described. The examples in Figures 9.1 through 9.5 are provided to show the structure of competency-based instruction. They are not suggested intervention programs.

Terminal Competency. The *terminal competency* is an end product, the specific behavior the clinician would like the client to achieve. It can be as small as "the identification of car toys" or as large as "the correct usage of grammatical rules in all contexts." As a matter of practicality though, the smaller the terminal competency, the easier it will be for the clinician to construct a manageable

BEGIN

TERMINAL COMPETENCY
Production of /r/ in All Contexts

Specific Competency 1
Discrimination of /r/ in isolation

Specific Competency 2
Production of /r/ in nonsense words

Specific Competency 3
Production of /r/ in phonemic contexts

Specific Competency 4
Production of /r/ in words

Instructional Objective 1
Discrimination of /r/ juxtaposed to gross sounds

Learning Activity 1
Therapist vocalizes sounds, client raises fingers when she hears /r/

Instructional Objective 1
Production of /r/ with manual and auditory aids

Learning Activity 1
Peanut butter on palate, clinician produces /r/ first

Instructional Objective 1
/r/ within facilitating phonemes

Learning Activity 1
Nonsense words used within a game to advance position

Instructional Objective 1
/r/ in words surrounded by facilitating phonemes

Learning Activity 1
Words in structured settings

Learning Activity 2
Spontaneous production in play activity

Instructional Objective 2
Discrimination of /r/ from other consonants except /w/

Learning Activity 1
Therapist vocalizes sounds, client raises fingers when she hears /r/

Instructional Objective 2
Production of /r/ with auditory aid

Learning Activity 1
Clinician produces /r/ first

Instructional Objective 2
/r/ within non-facilitating phonemes

Learning Activity 1
Nonsense words used within a game to advance position

Instructional Objective 2
/r/ in words surrounded by non-facilitating phonemes

Learning Activity 1
Words in structured settings

Learning Activity 2
Spontaneous production in play activity

Instructional Objective 3
Discrimination of /r/ from /w/

Learning Activity 1
Therapist vocalizes sounds, client raises fingers when she hears /r/

Instructional Objective 3
Production of /r/ with no aids

Learning Activity 1
Client produces /r/ without any prompts or cues

Instructional Objective 3
Home program

Instructional Objective 3
Home program

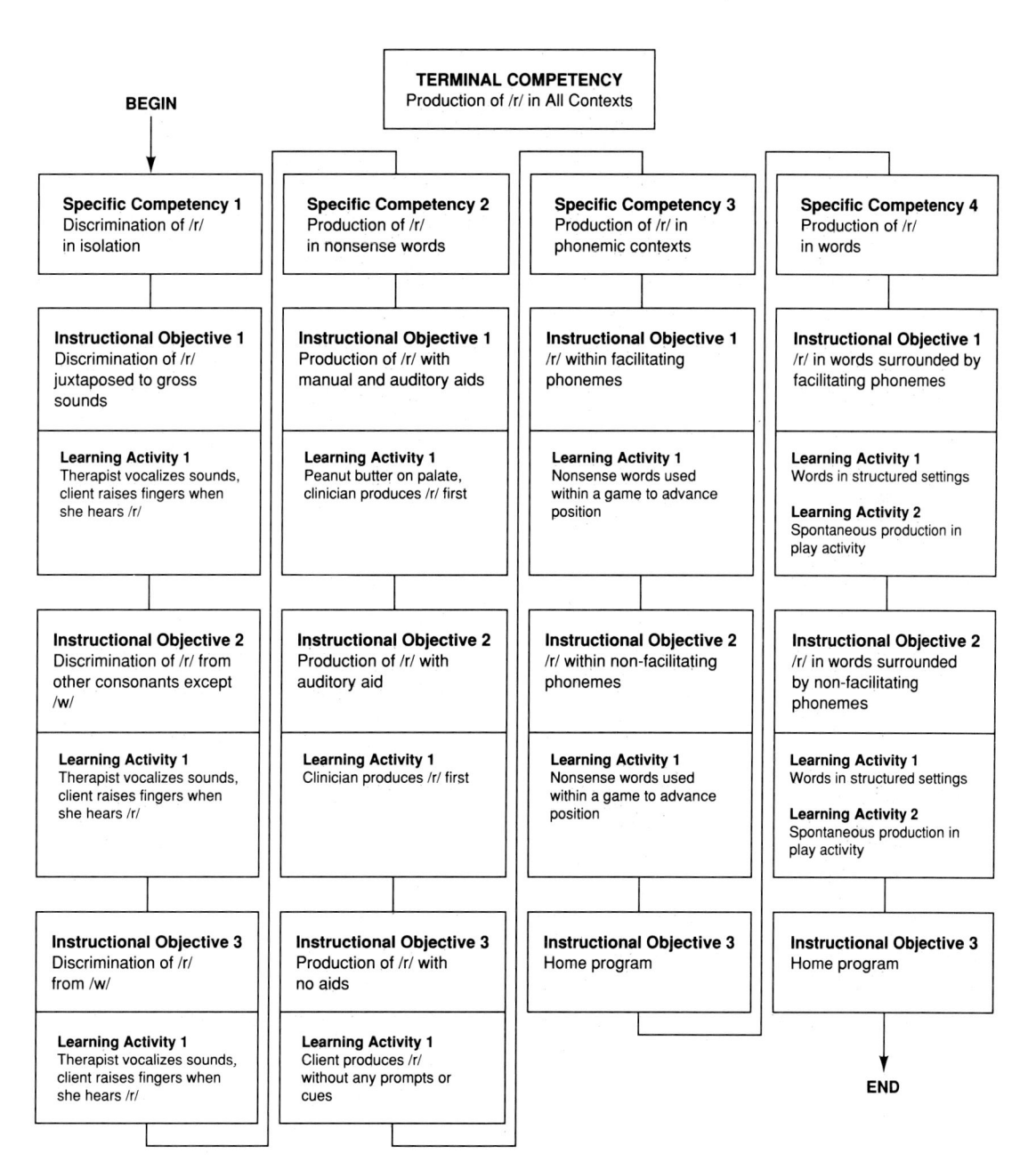

END

Figure 9.1
Articulation example

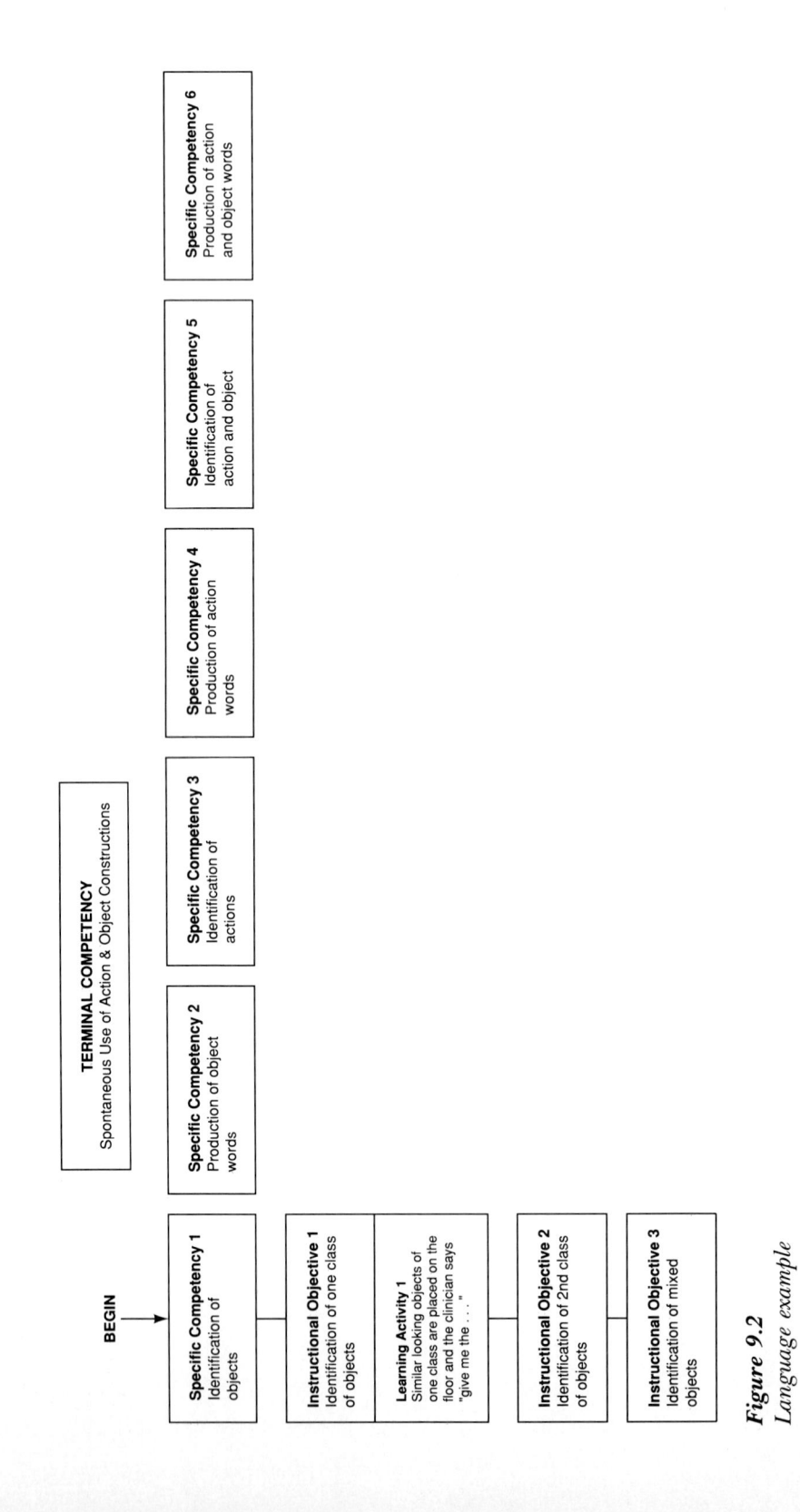

TERMINAL COMPETENCY
Spontaneous Use of Action & Object Constructions

Specific Competency 1
Identification of objects

Specific Competency 2
Production of object words

Specific Competency 3
Identification of actions

Specific Competency 4
Production of action words

Specific Competency 5
Identification of action and object

Specific Competency 6
Production of action and object words

BEGIN →

Instructional Objective 1
Identification of one class of objects

Learning Activity 1
Similar looking objects of one class are placed on the floor and the clinician says "give me the . . ."

Instructional Objective 2
Identification of 2nd class of objects

Instructional Objective 3
Identification of mixed objects

Figure 9.2
Language example

234

```
                    ┌─────────────────────────────────────┐
                    │         TERMINAL COMPETENCY         │
      BEGIN         │ Use of Appropriate Volume in All Situations │
                    └─────────────────────────────────────┘
        │
        ▼
```

Specific Competency 1	Specific Competency 2	Specific Competency 3	Specific Competency 4
Appropriate volume in quiet room	Appropriate volume in noisy setting	Appropriate volume with people talking	Appropriate volume with people talking in noisy setting

Instructional Objective 1
Monitoring level with use of a VU meter

Learning Activity 1
Select maximum volume level. Use quiet room and have client speak for a specified amount of time

Instructional Objective 2
Monitoring level by clinician

Instructional Objective 3
Monitoring level by client and clinician

Instructional Objective 4
Monitoring level by client

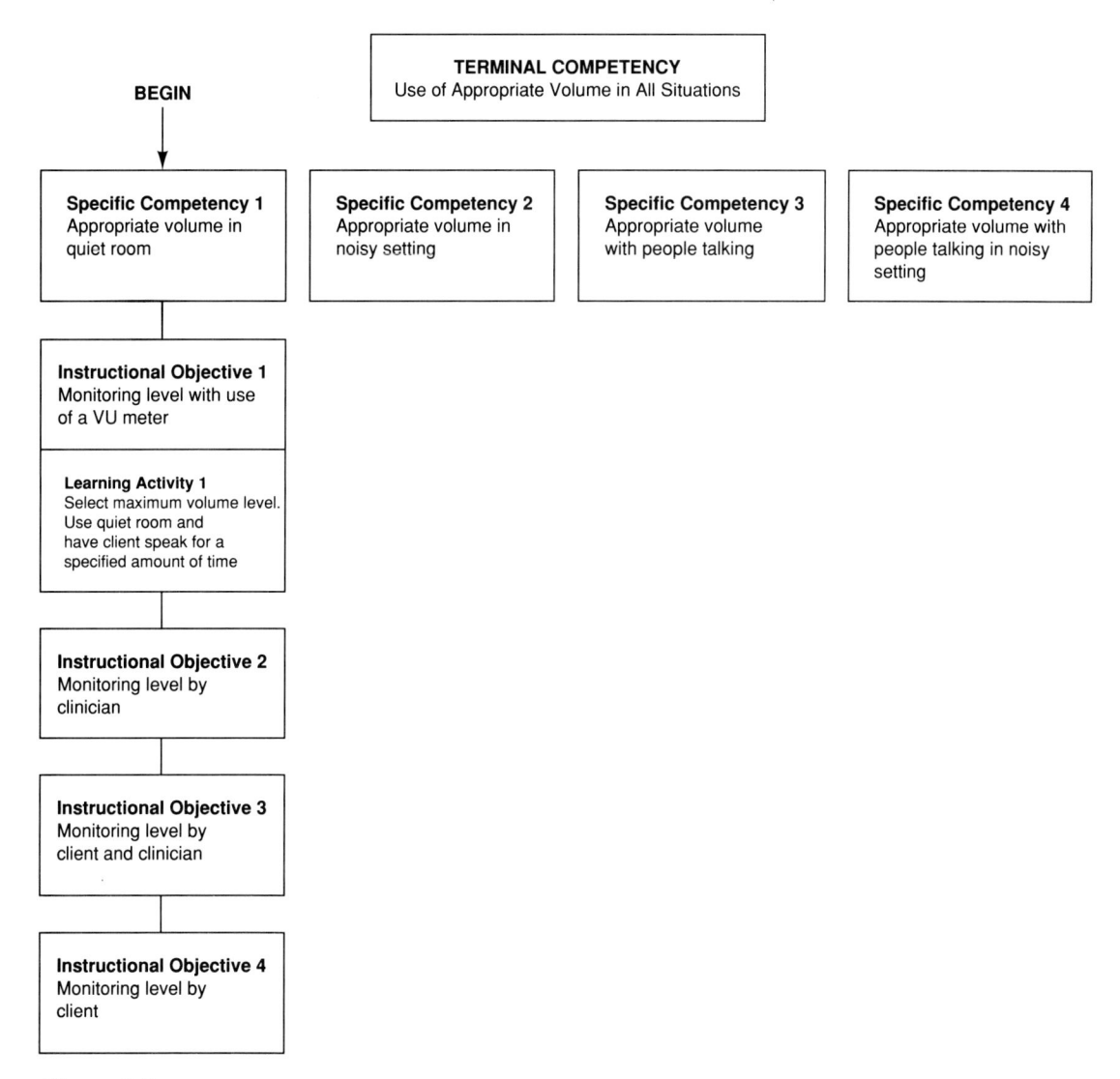

Figure 9.3
Voice example

intervention program. It is clinically a more viable approach to have a series of small interrelated intervention programs rather than one very complex and cumbersome one.

The designation of a behavior as a terminal competency is more a matter of ease than rigid guidelines. For example, "normal language usage" as the terminal competency for a nonverbal child would prove to be too complex a goal to develop, given the number of behaviors that would have to be traversed to achieve it.

In Figure 9.1 the terminal competency that is used as an example is "production of /r/ in all contexts." This constitutes a unit of behavior that has well-

```
                    ┌─────────────────────────┐
                    │  TERMINAL COMPETENCY    │
      BEGIN         │ Maintenance of Slow Rate│
                    └─────────────────────────┘
         │
         ▼
┌──────────────────┐  ┌──────────────────┐  ┌──────────────────┐  ┌──────────────────┐
│Specific Competency 1│ │Specific Competency 2│ │Specific Competency 3│ │Specific Competency 4│
│Use of 30 syllables per│ │Use of 60 syllables per│ │Use of 90 syllables per│ │Use of 120 syllables per│
│minute speech rate │  │minute speech rate │  │minute speech rate │  │minute speech rate │
└──────────────────┘  └──────────────────┘  └──────────────────┘  └──────────────────┘
         │
         ▼
┌──────────────────┐
│Instructional Objective 1│
│Use of instrument to│
│monitor speech rate│
└──────────────────┘

┌──────────────────┐
│Learning Activity 1│
│DAF set at feedback delay│
│resulting in 30 syllables per│
│minute speech rate│
└──────────────────┘

┌──────────────────┐
│Instructional Objective 2│
│Client maintains rate with-│
│out instrument, clinician│
│responsible for monitoring│
└──────────────────┘

┌──────────────────┐
│Instructional Objective 3│
│Client maintains rate with-│
│out instrument. Clinician│
│and client responsible for│
│monitoring│
└──────────────────┘

┌──────────────────┐
│Instructional Objective 4│
│Client responsible for│
│monitoring│
└──────────────────┘
```

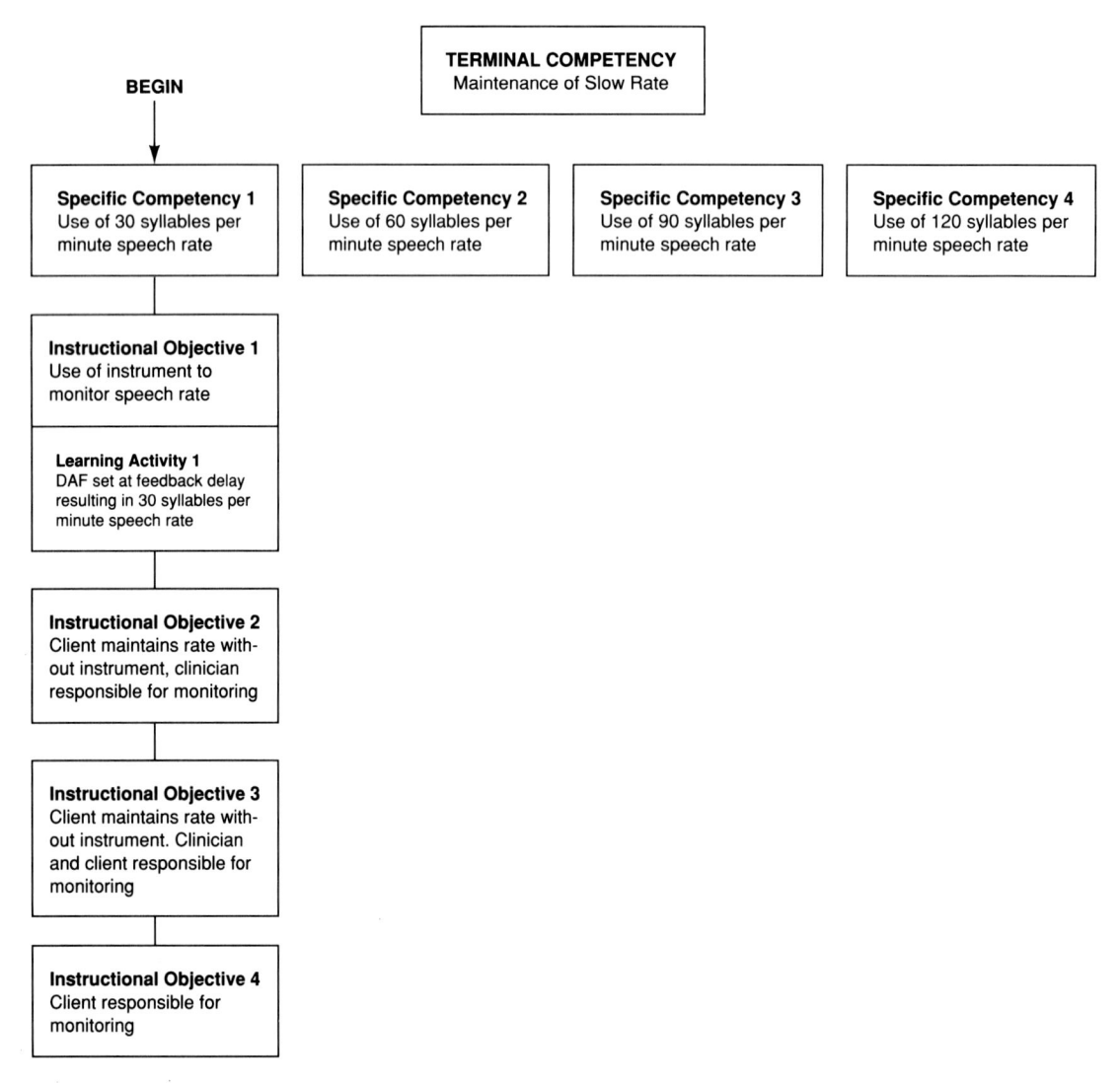

Figure 9.4
Stuttering example

defined limits and lends itself to being divided easily into basic component parts. Each component is designated as a specific competency.

Specific Competencies. Each terminal competency has two or more specific competencies. The *specific competencies* should be viewed as the major components of a terminal competency. The number of specific competencies that should be included under a terminal competency is determined by the scope of the terminal competency and the preferred method of acquiring it.

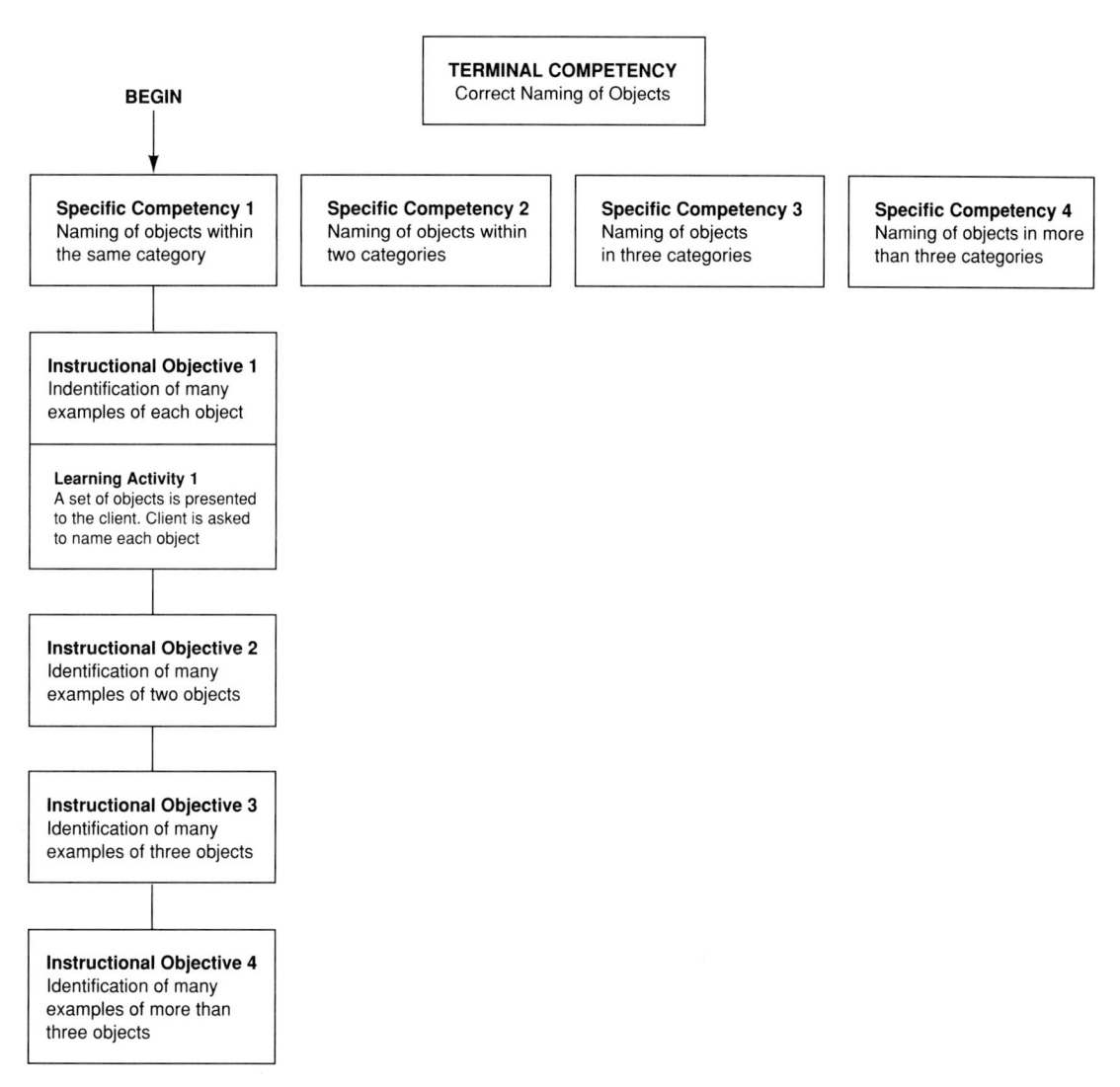

```
                        TERMINAL COMPETENCY
      BEGIN             Correct Naming of Objects
        │
        ▼
┌──────────────────┐  ┌──────────────────┐  ┌──────────────────┐  ┌──────────────────┐
│ Specific         │  │ Specific         │  │ Specific         │  │ Specific         │
│ Competency 1     │  │ Competency 2     │  │ Competency 3     │  │ Competency 4     │
│ Naming of objects│  │ Naming of objects│  │ Naming of objects│  │ Naming of objects│
│ within the same  │  │ within two       │  │ in three         │  │ in more than     │
│ category         │  │ categories       │  │ categories       │  │ three categories │
└──────────────────┘  └──────────────────┘  └──────────────────┘  └──────────────────┘
        │
┌──────────────────┐
│ Instructional    │
│ Objective 1      │
│ Identification of│
│ many examples of │
│ each object      │
└──────────────────┘

┌──────────────────┐
│ Learning         │
│ Activity 1       │
│ A set of objects │
│ is presented to  │
│ the client.      │
│ Client is asked  │
│ to name each     │
│ object           │
└──────────────────┘

┌──────────────────┐
│ Instructional    │
│ Objective 2      │
│ Identification of│
│ many examples of │
│ two objects      │
└──────────────────┘

┌──────────────────┐
│ Instructional    │
│ Objective 3      │
│ Identification of│
│ many examples of │
│ three objects    │
└──────────────────┘

┌──────────────────┐
│ Instructional    │
│ Objective 4      │
│ Identification of│
│ many examples of │
│ more than three  │
│ objects          │
└──────────────────┘
```

Figure 9.5
Aphasia example

The question of scope is illustrated in the following example. If "driving a car" is a terminal competency for a 16-year-old new driver, the specific competencies might be (a) knowing basic car controls, (b) understanding the rules of the road, and (c) being able to maneuver in traffic. The terminal competency for a new NASCAR racing driver might be (a) knowing controlled sliding techniques, (b) knowing the rules of slip streaming cars, and (c) being able to pass at very high speeds. In the area of speech-language pathology, similar differences exist. The specific competencies necessary for attaining the appropriate use of modifiers would look very different for the language-impaired child than for the adult aphasic who was a college professor before her stroke occurred.

Differences in methods of acquiring the terminal competency may be reflected in the choice of specific competencies. For example, a traditional method for training race car drivers involves the early placement of a driver in a low-powered car on a track. A more technologically based approach may use computerized simulations before actual track experience. In speech-language pathology, one's theoretical position is often reflected in the choice of specific competencies. For example, in stuttering therapy, someone who espoused a two-factor learning theory of stuttering may include the elimination of secondary behaviors in the terminal competency of increased fluency (Brutten & Shoemaker, 1967). For someone who views stuttering as purely an operant behavior (Shames & Florance, 1980), the elimination of secondary behaviors would not be a separate, specific competency.

Figure 9.1 lists four specific competencies. These involve discrimination, production of /r/ in isolation, production of /r/ within various phonemic contexts, and the production of /r/ within words. The selection of these four specific competencies reflects three theoretical positions. The first is that target sounds should be discriminated from error sounds before production begins (Winitz, 1969). The second position is that the easiest way to break the automaticity of error productions is to use unfamiliar contexts in which the target sound is produced (Holland, 1967). And the third is that the production of words should not be separated from their normal use within sentences (Elbert, 1989). Obviously, if one did not believe that these theories were relevant for the remediation of phonological disorders, a different set of specific competencies might be used.

Instructional Objectives. *Instructional objectives* are the means by which specific competencies are acquired. Often, the instructional objectives for more than one competency are identical or very similar. The criteria for selecting instructional objectives usually involve the principles of acquisition and retention. For example, we know that one of the problems of learning for individuals with cognitive deficits is the difficulty of learning new materials without concrete visual cues. Knowing this, an instructional objective could specify that easily discriminable visual cues be initially provided when learning any new task.

In Figure 9.1, under Specific Competency 1, three instructional objectives are listed. The goal for this competency is to teach the client to discriminate between the correct and his incorrect production of /r/. From educational research it has been determined that the most appropriate way to teach discrimination tasks is to do it with ever-increasing levels of fineness (Bandura, 1969). The instructional objectives are therefore designed to take the client from gross to fine phonetic discriminations.

Learning Activities. *Learning activities* refer to the materials or actual progression of events during an intervention program. Examples of materials are board games, puppets, or picture cards. An example of an event is "client raises hand before beginning fluency contract." It is a common mistake of new clinicians to focus more attention on this area than on the preceding three levels of construction. Learning activities should be constructed that (a) will facilitate the use of instructional objects, (b) will hold the client's interest, (c) are safe and inexpensive, and (d) facilitate the generalization of the behavior being developed.

The primary purpose of learning activities is to facilitate the completion of an instructional objective. Therefore, materials and activities should not be selected until the clinician has a clear idea of what is to be accomplished. It is a common mistake to select materials first and then determine how they can be effectively used in therapy. By reversing the order, the therapy becomes more organized and the parameters of what becomes a useful object or activity are also expanded. For example, if an instructional objective involved the use of visual cues to learn abstract concepts, the clinician could construct a number of excellent cues with merely a felt-tipped marker and blank cards.

Often materials for learning activities are selected for superficial reasons such as cost, availability, transportability, and assumed interest on the part of the client. To choose learning activities in this manner ignores a further dimension. Winnicott (1971) viewed play objects and activities as often simultaneously serving as toys, tools, and symbols. For him, activities and play objects were expressions of cultural values and elements of growth. Winnicott called these objects and activities "transitional," since they eased the child from the known to the uncertainties associated with aging. For example, the 6-year-old child who still carries a frayed piece of his baby blanket is not attached to the article, but rather to what it represents. The little girl who transforms the back seat of a car into a house and incessantly hits her doll for wetting herself is probably engaging in symbolic play rather than just creating a fanatasy on parenting. Understanding the relationship between objects and what they represent allows clinicians to identify objects and activities that are not only clinically useful but also intrinsically reinforcing and growth enhancing to clients. Approaching learning activities in this manner avoids having to outline each specific activity that is recommended for each age level. Rather, it provides a strategy for determining the most appropriate materials.

Researchers in the area of play have offered many ideas that speech-language pathologists can use in therapy. One very powerful concept is that of *discovery*, which involves encountering a new activity, object, or concept for the first time. Hodgkin (1985) believed that discovery was a critical element in the design of any play activity. For him it was the driving force for why some activities retain their fascination for children throughout the history of play.

Immersion is another element that has been mentioned extensively (Hodgkin, 1985). *Immersion* is the total involvement of the individual's senses. The best example of this was provided by Wickes (1982) in his analysis of the Suzuki method of teaching music. He describes a group of four children who share one violin. While one plays, the others sing or dance. By the end of the lesson each child has been involved with the music by playing it, singing it, dancing to it, and listening to it.

Another important, but controversial concept is competition. *Competition* is viewed by many as an expression of "achievement motivation," a motive thought by many to be a basic element of human behavior (Levy, 1978). Although pervasive throughout our culture, some researchers advise against using this as a teaching strategy for children and adolescents who are not motivated to strive for success at the cost of defeating a peer (Orlick & Botterill, 1975). Non-competitive activities or activities that involve self-competition are suggested for these clients.

Computer-Assisted Instruction

The purpose of computer-assisted instruction is to aid in the implementation of personalized therapy, not to replace it. Much of the commercially available application software, which dazzles clients with wonderful graphics and exciting games, still does not fully incorporate critical learning principles. Unfortunately even professionals often mistake technology for content. A client's interest in a game with complex graphics is no substitute for use of appropriate learning procedures. An additional problem results when an application designed for one purpose is used for another to which it is not applicable. Computer-assisted software can be divided into four different groups according to purpose: (a) tutorial, (b) drill and practice, (c) simulation, and (d) demonstration/information (Behrman, 1984). The features of each are shown in Table 9.1.

Tutorial Software. *Tutorial software* is designed to teach either skills or strategies to the learner. This form of software can serve the same functions as does competency-based instruction. Some programs are modeled after the competency-based format discussed in the previous section. Tutorial software advances in response to the client's input. When correct responses are given, it will advance to the next unit in the lesson. If incorrect responses are given, it will branch off to a remedial program (Lindsey, 1987).

Drill-and-Practice Software. Drill-and-practice software allows the client to master skills and concepts that will be needed for more difficult cognitive tasks. It should be used after a concept has been taught and at the point where practice is needed for the skill to become a part of the client's behavioral repertoire (Hofmeister, 1982). Well-designed software has the advantages of freeing the clinician to work with other clients and allowing for varied presentation of the material, eliminating the boredom that is usually associated with drill activities.

Although drill-and-practice activities could just as easily be conducted by the clinician, Silverman (1987) presents some convincing arguments why this task should be delegated to the computer. First, computer programs can present what may be repetitive and boring tasks in interesting, changing formats. Second, many people view the objectivity of the computer as being less threatening when mistakes are made. And third, the computer allows the client more opportunities to practice than might be possible if the clinician's presence was required.

Simulation Software. The importance of using simulations to facilitate generalization was discussed in Chapter 7. Although the simulations contained in

Table 9.1
Features of computer-assisted programs

Feature	Tutorial	Drill and Practice	Simulation	Demonstration/ Information
Assesses entry level knowledge and determines starting point in computer program	X			
Provides feedback	X	X		
Provides correct answers and questions	X	X		
Provides method for branching to more details, remedial programs, or practice	X	X	X	
Provides means for recording correct and incorrect answers	X	X		
Facilitates generalization			X	
Provides information	X	X	X	X

software programs may not have the reality that a person-to-person interaction has, one advantage is the vast number of simulations that the client can be engaged in effortlessly. Simulation software has the additional advantage of providing a bridge for the client from a controlled environment to one where few, if any, controls exist. Since simulations involve the greatest complexity in programming and knowledge of learning paradigms, they are the least available type of computer-assisted instruction (Behrmann, 1984).

Demonstration/Information. The purpose of this software is to provide basic information to the learner or to provide examples of the objectives being taught. For example, if *jumping* is a targeted word, the program could show graphics of people and animals jumping. Compact videodisk technology has now made it possible to display actual video images of the action. Unlike tutorial and drill-and-practice software, demonstration/information does not provide feedback to the learner.

STRATEGIES

It is not uncommon that the teaching of specific skills and the use of diagnostic activities are incorrectly identified as the teaching of strategies. The most common confusion exists between skills and strategies. According to Duffy and Roehler (1989), there is an important distinction between the two. A skill can be isolated and its component parts simply described. Its elements are usually memorized and become automatic. The cognitively impaired child who has been taught by memorization to introduce herself by saying, "Hello, my name is Sarah," is using a skill. A strategy, on the other hand, looks very different. It is distinguished from skills by three elements (Duffy & Roehler, 1989). Strategies are (a) idiosyncratic, (b) not always applied in the same way, and (c) usually applied in combinations.

The second confusion involves the use of diagnostic activities as if they were learning strategies. Many clinical manuals on aphasia therapy, for example, contain a series of hierarchically organized retrieval activities. In one book clients are asked to name as many fruits as they can (concrete concepts). After reaching a criterion of success, they then move on to the next activity, which involves naming things involved in transportation (abstract concepts). The mastery of each task involves little more than repetition and rote memorization with no specific concern for teaching learning strategies. With each repetition of the task, the clinician is determining if the client has learned the task; therefore, the activity is little more than an informal diagnostic assessment of a skill.

In Chapter 7 various methods for increasing attending, acquisition, and retention of new behaviors were discussed. All of these are important in teaching learning strategies. In the following section additional considerations will be presented.

Memory

Two basic types of strategies enhance memory: encoding strategies and organizational strategies. The effectiveness of each is increased if the task is understandable to the learner (Waters & Andreassen, 1983). For the clinician, this means that when teaching memory strategies to the client, the client should be cognizant of the task at hand. By not understanding the purpose of the activity, it is quite likely that attempts at learning memory strategies will fail.

Encoding Strategies. Encoding strategies are those that encourage attention to relevant aspects of the material and task and lead to more elaborate and meaningful representations in memory (Waters & Andreassen, 1983). Three types of encoding strategies have proven to be effective: rehearsal, associative learning, and saliency. In children, *rehearsal* can be seen when they are asked to remember certain things and appear, by their lip movements, to be silently identifying the components to themselves. In a classic study done by Keeney, Cannizzo, and Flavell (1967), children who rehearsed were found to perform significantly better than those who did not. Even more interesting was that when those children who did not rehearse were instructed to do so, they performed equally as well as the children who initially rehearsed. In a later article Flavell (1970) maintained that often a child's inability to remember information was probably related more to the child's failure to use the encoding strategy than to anything else. This would also apply to adults.

Associative learning is a process whereby two items are learned together and the memory of one triggers the memory of the second (Pressley, Levin, & Bryant, 1983). The most efficient form of this strategy is known as elaboration learning (Rohwer, 1973) and involves the development of either an interactive visual image or a verbal context like a phrase, sentence, or story involving the item to be remembered. For example, during a presentation, a professor tried to illustrate this point by unexpectedly throwing a hundred Styrofoam balls out into the audience. Four years following the presentation, a member of the audience approached him at a social gathering and said, "You know, there is little I remember of your presentation except for the balls being thrown at me to illustrate your point on associating things."

Saliency refers to the importance an item has to the learner. The importance of the item to be remembered will affect the extent of its retention (Brown & Smiley, 1978). Studies have shown that during experimental learning situations there is a greater probability that things deemed important by the learner will be retained better than those items deemed of lesser importance. The lesson for speech-language pathologists is that activities should be related to the client's priorities.

Organizational Strategies. Various studies have shown that if the materials to be remembered are organized into categories, memory and retention are significantly enhanced (Tulving & Donaldson, 1972). This memory strategy can be particularly effective with clients who have a cognitive deficit that impairs organizational abilities. By presenting the organizational structure before presenting the stimulus materials, memory can be enhanced. For example, in working with an adult aphasic on retrieval of names, the clinician might begin by stating, "Today we will be working on the names of vegetables and money." This seemingly simple statement acts as an organizing template for what will follow and will therefore enhance retention. The use of visible cues (i.e., symbols presenting vegetables and money) during the stimulus presentation also enhances memory.

Retrieval

To some extent, the ability to retrieve information is directly related to the method by which it was learned. Although the use of encoding and organizational strategies during learning will greatly facilitate the retrieval of learned material, the reaffirmation of the strategies prior to remembering the information increases the likelihood that the material will be retrieved (Brown, Smiley, & Lawton, 1978). For example if the aphasic client learned the names of objects by categorizing them into vegetables and money, he should be instructed, "First remember the two categories we used. Next, write the name of the category at the top of a column. Now, as you remember each object, write its name in the category."

The child who cannot use the rules of social interaction with anyone other than the clinician is unable to use a strategy for generalizing what was learned in a clinical setting. The methods used by clinicians to facilitate transfers of this type often parallel the methods of classroom instruction that have been criticized by McKeachie (1988):

> Students are directed to carry out learning activities, but grades and other feedback to the students are primarily directed to the correctness of the outcome, rather than to the strategy used to achieve the result. . . . (students) stumble upon effective strategies only when, by chance, they vary their approach and find that one method worked better than others. (p. 5)

If McKeachie's admonition is to be followed, then when clinicians observe communicative failures on the part of a client, they should not merely provide feedback on the behavior or model the appropriate behavior but rather determine what aspects of the client's cognitive processes are flawed.

An approach that is more positive than trying to identify flaws in cognition is one presented by Mayer (1988), whereby clinicians focus on teaching clients the components of three learning strategies: (a) selecting information, (b) building internal connections, and (c) building external connections.

Selecting Information. One type of learning strategy concentrates on teaching the client to focus only on those features of a situation that are salient to solving a problem. Methods of teaching how to attend selectively may involve structuring situations that will emphasize some aspects of a stimulus configuration while de-emphasizing others. In some stuttering approaches, the client is taught to concentrate only on the initial sound of words by emphasizing it through rate reduction and easy phonation (Webster, 1980). If this strategy for the production of fluent speech is effective, the client should be able to produce fluent speech in a variety of untrained situations.

Building Internal Connections. Strategies for building internal connections are designed to provide some sort of logical structuring for the items to be learned. For example, prior to beginning a classification task for an aphasic, the client is informed that he will be asked to learn and later identify the names of four fruits that are green. According to Mayer (1987), organizational strategies of this type are most effective when the person is unfamiliar with the material to be learned.

Building External Connections. These strategies are designed to build connections between new and existing information. The relationship between the two has been described as "mapping," where new information is related to what is already known (Resnick & Ford, 1981).

Generalization

If strategies are to be more than limited skills, they need to be generalizable. That is, the method of retrieval needs to be applicable to situations other than the one in which the client was trained. The greater the difference between the training situation and the situation in which the strategy is to be generalized, the more likely the ability to retrieve and use the strategy will be impaired (Borkowski & Buchel, 1981). For example, the child learning the two-word construction Actor + Action has been taught "daddy run" through a rule-governed intervention program. The program taught him not only the construction "daddy run" but also the strategy for combining Actor + Action words to form an acceptable communication. If the child has learned the rule, he will apply it when seeing his dog run and be able to say "doggie run."

Self-Instruction. Learning the strategy and applying it are not necessarily the same; this is especially true for individuals with cognitive impairments. In an interesting study on the teaching of mathematics to cognitively impaired children, it was found that self-instruction significantly helps the subjects to remember the strategy for adding numbers (Johnson, Whitman, & Johnson, 1980). Self-instruction merely involves teaching the individual to recite a set of instructions prior to attempting to solve a problem. The use of self-instruction was found to be effective in teaching both social and work skills to cognitively impaired adolescents and adults (Goetz et al., 1986).

Selection of Strategies

Individuals have differing cognitive aptitudes that they rely on to solve problems (Cronbach & Snow, 1977). Carroll (1981) has hypothesized that 10 fundamental cognitive processes are involved in learning and retrieving. Some gifted individuals are able to use these aptitudes to their fullest capacity. Others try to compensate for deficits by relying on strategies. Clients with communicative disorders may either have deficits in one or more areas or just not be able to use the cognitive processes as well as gifted individuals. Borkowski and Buchel (1981) maintain that if one can identify which of these cognitive processes is deficient, the appropriate strategy for enhancing it could be designed. In Table 9.2, Carroll's 10 cognitive processes are listed along with an explanation and an example. If known, a compensatory strategy is provided for each process.

SUMMARY

The time spent in therapy by clients is only a minute portion of the time spent communicating. The client who spends one hour a week in therapy but is in a communicating environment for 12 hours a day for 7 days a week receives direct help for only 1% of his or her communicating time. Although the teaching of specific behaviors is a necessary component of communicative structuring and restructuring, it should not be the primary focus. Given the limited amount of time available for therapy, the teaching of specific behaviors is less efficient than the teaching of strategies the client can use during the 99% of the time when direct help is not available.

Although teaching strategies is more complex than teaching discriminate behaviors, it can be accomplished if the clinician structures therapy using the methods described in this chapter. Constructing an effective intervention proto-

Table 9.2
Fundamental cognitive processes

Cognitive Process	Explanation	Example	Compensatory Strategy
Monitoring	Awareness of one's self in relation to environmental factors	Able to move around a room	
Attending	Directing attention to a given stimulus configuration	To teach discrimination of /r/, client must aurally attend to clinician's voice	Since most attending problems are really problems of encoding, see encoding for strategies
Apprehension	Ability to be aware of a particular stimulus configuration	To teach discrimination of /r/, client must aurally attend to sound pairs	
Perceptual Integration	Ability to identify critical attributes of a stimulus configuration	Distinctive features of /w/ and /r/ can be identified	
Encoding	Mental representation of stimulus and its attributes	Placement of articulator can be mentally visualized	Self-generated elaboration
Comparison	Ability to compare the critical attributes of two or more stimulus configurations	Distinctive features of /w/ and /r/ can be compared	
Corepresentation Formation	Finding in memory a representation associated with an older memory	Comparing two past memories of dog	Self-generated elaboration
Corepresentation Retrieval	Finding in memory a representation associated with another representation by a rule	Comparing a past memory of dog with the rule for what constitutes a dog	Self-generated elaboration
Transformation	Transforming retrieval into plan for execution	Deciding how to place the articulator in order to produce /r/	
Response Execution	Executing the response	Producing /r/	

col requires not only the specification of the next session's goals and procedures but also a vision of how the client should communicate at the end of the semester, in 1, 5, or maybe even 10 years. Therapy is not a finite event with consequences limited to immediate occurrences or the completion of an academic semester's requirements. It is a powerful stimulant in the lives of our clients and therefore should be viewed and constructed with long-term consequences in mind.

SUGGESTED READINGS

Duffy, G. G., & Roehler, L. R. (1989). Why strategy instruction is so difficult and what we need to do about it. In C. B. McCormick, G. Miller, and M. Pressley (Eds.), *Cognitive strategy research: From basic research to educational applications* (pp. 133-154). New York: Springer Verlag.
Gagné, R. M. (1970). *The conditions of learning.* New York: Holt, Rinehart & Winston.
Hodgkin, R. A. (1985). *Playing and exploring.* New York: Methuen.
Lindsey, J. D. (1987). *Computers and exceptional individuals.* Columbus, OH: Merrill/Macmillan.
Mayer, R. E. (1983). *Thinking, problem solving, cognition.* New York: W. H. Freeman.
McKeachie, W. J. (1988). The need for study strategy training. In C. E. Weinstein, E. T. Goetz, and P. A. Alexander (Eds.), *Learning and study strategies* (pp. 3–9). New York: Academic Press.
Winnicott, D. W. (1971). *Playing and reality.* London: Tavistock.

❑ ***Activity 9.1***
Skill and Strategy Observation

In this chapter, the distinction was drawn between diagnostic activities, skills, and strategies. Observe a client for a 30-minute period. Identify and describe those occurrences during the session where the clinician (a) utilized diagnostic activities, (b) attempted to teach the client specific skills, and (c) attempted to teach the client strategies.

Diagnostic Activities	Skill Activities	Strategy Activities

Chapter 10
The First Client

STUDY GUIDE

- What types of information should be noted when examining clinical records?
- Describe the purposes of the pre-clinical telephone interview.
- What are the goals of the first clinical session?
- Why are each of the goals of the first clinical session important?
- What behaviors of the client should be analyzed after the first clinical session?
- What behaviors of the clinician should be analyzed after the first clinical session?

The past nine chapters have introduced the component parts of clinical practice, beginning with the importance of accounting for cultural differences and ending with methods of teaching learning strategies. In this chapter, suggestions will be presented for how clinicians should prepare for the client's first session and the methods that can be used for analyzing the interaction.

❑ ❑ ❑ ## *PREPARING FOR THE FIRST SESSION*

The first step in preparing for clients is to examine all written records. Typically the student's first clinical experience occurs within a university clinic, where extensive diagnostic and intervention records exist if the client has been seen. Whether written records are or are not available, a telephone interview should also be conducted.

Clinical Records

Client reports within a university clinic are typically written by students and reviewed for accuracy by supervisors. Although all reports on the client should be reviewed, certain areas are of special value for the first meeting. Most diagnostic assessments have similar formats, regardless of the disorder or the clinical orientation of the clinician. Generally, the information is divided into four main headings: history, evaluation, results, and recommendations. As an example of this, Table 10.1 contains the diagnostic procedures that have been recommended for five different disorders. The information the authors suggest should be gathered for each of the disorders easily fits into these four categories. Although the contents of the reports usually reflect the clinical orientation of the diagnostician, the factual information contained within the report is relevant regardless of the clinician's theoretical orientation.

Overt Speech/Language Behaviors. The client's folder should contain detailed information regarding speech-language behaviors exhibited prior to, during, and after receiving therapy. Although the most useful information is data based, clinical impressions should also be noted since not all information can be conveyed in objective terminology.

Cognitive Ability. Since the design of the intervention program should account for the client's cognitive ability, information relative to Gagné's eight learning levels should be sought. Of particular interest are indications of where the client may be having problems either learning or using a communicative strategy.

Attitudes. The clinician should also examine the records for any information on client attitudes that may enhance or interfere with therapy. Of critical importance are indications that the client accepts responsibility for changing behaviors. The reports may contain information on how they believe their disorder has impacted their lives.

Table 10.1
Comparison of diagnostic procedures

	Stuttering[a]	**Voice**[b]	**Language**[c]	**Phonology**[d]	**Aphasia**[e]
History	1. Developmental history 2. Present speech-language problems 3. Health	1. Voice history 2. Psychological interview	1. Family interview	1. Etiology 2. Environment	1. Biography 2. Medical
Assessment	1. Feelings and attitudes 2. Speech-language behaviors 3. Interview	1. Laryngoscopy 2. Voice tests 3. Voice profile	1. Observing child in naturalistic setting 2. Transcription 3. Deep testing	1. Perception of problem 2. Oral cavity exam 3. Hearing 4. Phonological processes/rules	1. Behaviors 2. Speech 3. Language
Results	1. Determining developmental/treatment level	1. Interpretation of findings	1. Analyzing structures	1. Determining phonemes requiring treatment	1. Differential diagnosis
Recommendations	1. Stuttering therapy 2. Treatment plan	1. Voice therapy 2. Counseling and/or medical referral 3. Treatment plan	1. Need for therapy 2. Treatment plan	1. Articulation therapy 2. Treatment plan	1. Type of therapy

[a] Peters, T. J., & Guitar, B. (1991). *Stuttering: An integrated approach to its nature and treatment.* Baltimore, MD: Williams & Wilkins
[b] Aronson, A. E. (1990). *Clinical voice disorders.* New York: Thieme.
[c] Lund, N. J., & Duchan, J. F. (1988). *Assessing children's language in naturalistic contexts.* Englewood Cliffs, NJ: Prentice-Hall
[d] Bernthal, J. E., & Bankson, N. W. (1981). *Articulation disorders.* Englewood Cliffs, NJ: Prentice-Hall
[e] Rosenbek, J. C., LaPointe, L. L., & Wertz, R. T. (1989). *Aphasia: A clinical approach.* Austin, TX: Pro-Ed

Effective Reinforcers. For children and adolescents, the clinician should determine the effective intrinsic, extrinsic, and extraneous reinforcers used by previous clinicians. Additionally, the schedules of reinforcement should be noted. For adults, the only information recorded may be related to intrinsic reinforcement.

Effects of Specific Therapy Procedures and Techniques. Good clinical reports will indicate both what was done and how effective each procedure was. The reports should be written in such a manner as to allow someone unfamiliar with the client to replicate clinical procedures.

Cultural Values. Some information regarding the cultural values of the client can be derived from clinical records. Often basic information such as age, ethnic identity, and severity of disability can provide the clinician with a starting point for understanding the client's cultural values.

Non-Speech/Language Problems. Therapy should be a multidimensional process. Therefore, if the client has problems in motor, social, or self-help skills, these should be noted so that they can be addressed as secondary problems.

Pre-Clinical Telephone Interview

Types of Information to Be Gathered. The purposes of gathering information prior to the first meeting are to (a) prepare adequately for the session, (b) verify the information contained within the client's written file, and (c) determine changes in the client's communicative and general behaviors since the last therapy session was conducted. New students have found it helpful to use a telephone interview protocol to conduct this first interview. This form of "scripting" has proven to be effective in training individuals who have an adequate knowledge base but minimal experience with the area to be treated (Dreyfus & Dreyfus, 1986). Tables 10.2 and 10.3 show suggested protocols for children/adolescents and for adults. Obviously modifications are appropriate based on individual clinical situations. When written reports are unavailable, questions should be asked that will result in information similar to that gathered from an examination of the records.

Reducing Anxiety. The first meeting between a clinician and client may affect the entire course of therapy. New clients are entering what Scheuerle (1992) calls a "transition period," where familiar ways of interacting and viewing their problems may undergo changes.

Although clinical interactions have many of the same features as the client's everyday encounters, the uniqueness of the situation may result in feelings of anxiety that may interfere with the first session. Much of the anxiety can be eliminated through a simple phone call that is designed to make the client feel more comfortable during the first session and to gather important information that will be useful.

Changes in Behavior. The schedule of many university clinics follows that of their academic semesters. This can result in breaks in therapy lasting a few weeks to a few months. During this time, three things can occur that will affect therapy. Newly taught behaviors may (a) remain stable, (b) diminish or disappear, or (c) become the basis for the development of other behaviors.

It is always desirable that behaviors taught in therapy remain stable. However, this is not always the case. The stability of a behavior depends on various factors. Until the individual has had an adequate opportunity to practice a new behavior, it will remain fragile. New behaviors taught near the end of a semester may be forgotten or extinguished. Forgetting occurs when the individual has not

Table 10.2
Telephone protocol for children/adolescents

Making Contact

Contact your client's parent prior to the first scheduled session. The earlier the parent is called, the more time you will have to use the information provided.

Introduction

Introduce yourself to the parent as their child's clinician. First ask if this would be an appropriate time to ask some questions that may take from between 20 to 30 minutes to answer. If not, ask the parent what would be the most appropriate time.

Example:

Hello Mr./Ms. _____ . I am_____ and will be working with _____ during this semester. I would like to ask you some questions that will help me prepare for the first session. The questions will take between 20 and 30 minutes of your time. If it isn't convenient now, we can schedule a time that would be more convenient.

Dr. _____will be supervising the clinic this semester and will introduce herself to you during our first session.

I have examined _____'s file, but there still is some information I think would be helpful for me to plan for our first session.

Retained Behaviors

Before you start asking questions, have a clinical strategy in mind. In other words, do not use a shotgun approach. You should have a pragmatic purpose for each question you ask. Think about what you will be doing with the answer the parent will give you. If the answer to the question will not help you, do not ask it.

It's been _____weeks (months, years) since _____ has had therapy. I would like to know if she (he) has retained the behaviors that were worked on last semester. What I will do now is to ask you about each of the behaviors and then you can tell me if she (he) is still doing them.

Behaviors Listed in the File	Notes	Retained	Lost
1.			
2.			
3.			
4.			
5.			
6.			
7.			
8.			
9.			
10.			
11.			
12.			
13.			
14.			
15.			

continues

Table 10.2, continued

New Behaviors

In this section you will be inquiring about any new behaviors the parent has noticed. Since this is a generic form, some of the categories may not apply to your client.

I am also interested in knowing about any new behaviors you have seen _____ doing. I'll be asking about _____ groups of behaviors. The first is _____.

Articulation	Notes		Language	Notes

Voice	Notes		Fluency	Notes

Self-Help	Notes		Problem-Solving	Notes

SEPARATION *(Children to age 5 years)*

How easily does _____ separate from you and go with a new person?

1	2	3	4	5
Very Easily	Easily	Moderately Easily	With Difficulty	With Great Difficulty

What type of behavior does _____ exhibit when he/she has to separate from you?
How long does this behavior usually last? _____ minutes?

SAMPLING *(Speech/Language/Stuttering/Voice)*

During our first session I will be taking a _____ sample. Often we find that it is easier to get a good sample if we use toys and activities that the child likes. What are _____'s favorite toys. What are _____'s favorite activities?

If you do not have some of the more important toys or activities available in the clinic, ask the parent to bring a few of them in for the first session.

| Toys ||| Activities |||
Clinic	Home		Clinic	Home

REINFORCEMENT

I would like therapy to be a good and enjoyable experience for _____ . *Could you tell me what kinds of things or activities I can use to reward her/him for participating and doing well in therapy?*

Group the answers you receive into the following categories.

Intrinsic Reinforcers	Extrinsic Reinforcers	Extraneous Reinforcers

Other Information

Since I haven't worked with _____ *before, I would like to know if there is anything else you can tell me that would help my first meeting with her/him?*

Table 10.3
Telephone protocol for adults

Making Contact

Contact your client prior to the first scheduled session. The earlier the client is called, the more time you will have to use the information provided.

Introduction

Introduce yourself to the client. First ask if this would be an appropriate time to ask some questions that may take from between 20 to 30 minutes to answer. If not, ask the client what would be the most appropriate time.

Example:

> Hello Mr./Ms. _____ . I am _____ and will be working with you during this semester. I would like to ask you some questions that will help me prepare for our first session. The questions will take between 20 and 30 minutes of your time. If it isn't convenient now, we can schedule a time that would be more convenient.
>
> Dr. _____ will be supervising the clinic this semester and will introduce herself/himself to you during our first session.
>
> I have examined your file, but there still is some information I think would be helpful for me to know to plan for our first session.

Retained Behaviors

Before you start asking questions, have a clinical strategy in mind. In other words, do not use a shotgun approach. You should have a pragmatic purpose for each question you ask. Think about what you will be doing with the answer the client will give you. If the answer to the question will not help you, do not ask it.

It's been _____ weeks (months, years) since you have had therapy. I would like to know if you are still able to do the behaviors you learned in therapy. What I will do now is to ask you about each of the behaviors and then you can tell me if you are still able to do them.

Behaviors Listed in the File	Notes	Retained	Lost
1.			
2.			
3.			
4.			
5.			
6.			
7.			
8.			
9.			
10.			
11.			
12.			
13.			
14.			
15.			

Table 10.3, continued

New Behaviors

In this section you will be inquiring about any new behaviors the client has noticed. Since this is a generic form, some of the categories may not apply to your client.

I am also interested in knowing about any new behaviors you are able to do now that you couldn't do when you were in therapy. I'll be asking about _____ groups of behaviors. The first is _____.

Articulation	Notes	Language	Notes

Voice	Notes	Fluency	Notes

Self-Help	Notes	Problem-Solving	Notes

had the opportunity or desire to practice the behavior. Extinction occurs when the individual has produced the behavior but was not reinforced when it occurred. When the parent or client indicates that a previously taught behavior is no longer present, it is important to determine if it resulted either from forgetting or extinction, since the procedures used to prevent each are different.

New behaviors not taught in therapy can develop for two reasons: (a) developmental maturation and (b) generalization. Children mature with and without the help of clinicians. Even a break of three weeks with very young children can result in the development of behaviors due solely to maturation. Generalization occurs when the strategy for using a previously learned behavior is applied to another behavior.

Other Information. Experienced clinicians never fail to be amazed by the responses they get when asking parents and clients the simple question, "Is there anything else that you can tell me that would help me better prepare for our first session?" This allows the individual to focus on an important event or behavior that the clinician may have never thought of asking about.

GOALS FOR THE FIRST SESSION

The first session is important for setting goals and beginning diagnostic therapy. It should be used for more than just developing rapport, something that a well-known clinician described as "talking about the weather because you have no idea what to do." A better term for this much maligned word is *trust*, one of four specific goals clinicians should strive to achieve during the first session. The other goals are establishing the purpose of therapy, stating role relationships, and engaging in diagnostic therapy. Each goal is designed to structure the future interactions between the clinician and client.

Establishing the Purpose of Therapy

Children. Many children do not have the slightest idea why they are coming to therapy. Often, in an attempt not to frighten or stigmatize their children, parents try to conceal from their child the purpose of the clinic visit. The easiest way to determine what the child knows is simply to ask the question, "Do you know why you are here today?" To responses such as "to play" or "I don't know," clinicians should correct children's misperceptions by informing them that the purpose is to work on whatever communicative problem they are exhibiting. It is important that the explanation is presented in a positive manner, indicating that a new behavior will be taught which will help them be better understood. These are three examples of how to phrase the explanations:

- Yes, we will be playing games, but we will be doing other things as well, like showing you how to say the /r/ sound differently.
- We are going to show you how to use your voice so you won't have to go to the doctor again.
- We are going to show you how to say words smoothly, so children won't tease you anymore.

Of importance in each of these explanations is that the function of the session is clearly stated with an emphasis on the development of a new coping behavior rather than on the elimination of a deficient or disordered behavior.

Adolescents and Adults. Explanations for adolescents and adults should involve specifying the goals of therapy and the general procedures that will be used for achieving them. In an earlier chapter the importance of timing was discussed. Although clinicians should not go into detail concerning each aspect of their therapy program, the key points should be specified, and examples given of how the speech will change throughout the process. For example, in Goldberg's Behavioral Cognitive Stuttering Therapy (1981), audio-recorded examples of how the client will sound at each stage of fluency development are played. When audio- or videotapes are not available, clinicians should be prepared to simulate how the speech and language will sound.

Role Expectations

By establishing the role relationships in the first session, needless problems can be avoided. Clinicians should indicate that they are facilitators of change, and although they can provide information and techniques, the ultimate responsibility for change rests with the client. Shames and Rubin (1986) believe that the establishment of role relations within the first session is critical to the therapeutic process. Unless clients understand that the responsibility for behavioral changes rests with them, a symbiotic relationship may develop.

Trust

The therapeutic experience may require clients to reveal personal information that they may have never discussed with anyone or to engage in behaviors that may appear strange or embarrassing. It is unreasonable for clients to do any of these things without first trusting their clinician. According to Giffin and Patton (1971), trust is a complicated construct that involves both intellectual and emotional elements. Rogers (1965) conceived of it as a sense of psychological safety that allows an individual not to feel a need for defensive behaviors. To these, Goldberg (1981) added a third element, which is the feeling developed in clients as a result of clinical successes. Trust, therefore, is a complex feeling that involves the intellect, the emotions, and the experience of success.

Intellect. Unless clients can feel that clinicians are competent or being closely supervised by experienced individuals, there is little reason they should trust the clinicians' suggestions or judgments. It goes without saying that clinicians should be familiar with the characteristics of the disorder and with its variations. When a clinician does not know the answer to a question posed by a client, it is better to admit ignorance than to fabricate a response. An example of an acceptable response would be, "I'm sorry, I don't know the answer to that question. But I will ask my supervisor as soon as the session is over. We can discuss it at our next session."

Emotions. It is difficult for clients to place trust in a clinician whom they perceive as unfeeling, regardless of the clinician's level of competence. During the first session, impressions are created, some of which are indelibly etched in the memory of clients. It is important that clinicians are perceived as caring professionals whose primary concern is the welfare of clients. When clients begin discussing issues that are revealing, painful, or insightful, clinicians should acknowledge the legitimacy of the feelings and allow clients to remain on the topics until they feel that closure has been reached.

Successful Experiences. Nothing engenders a sense of trust and commitment to therapeutic activities more than a successful experience. If clients can successfully execute a simple behavior or use a technique suggested by the clinician, the clinician's ability to have the client engage in other, potentially more difficult behaviors is enhanced. If sufficient information has been gathered by examining the client's file and through the telephone interview, a simple therapeutic activity can be constructed that should result in an immediate successful experience for the client. It is important that clients leave the first session with a sense of accomplishment.

Diagnostic Therapy

Unless there have been no changes in the behaviors or attitudes of continuing clients, diagnostic therapy should begin during the first session. It should always occur with new clients. *Diagnostic therapy* is the implementation of specific techniques and procedures, rigorously documented and analyzed in terms of what may be appropriate and productive for the client. It is, in the very best sense, a scientific fishing trip. Diagnostic therapy may last only one session or span several sessions. It should be explained to clients who are old enough and capable of understanding that several different activities will be tried and that their purpose is to identify the most appropriate ones for inclusion within the intervention protocol.

Diagnostic therapy may involve both formal and informal tests or portions of tests in addition to the application of specific intervention procedures.

ANALYZING THE FIRST SESSION

The first session, as well as all subsequent sessions of new clinicians, should be audio-recorded to provide a precise analysis of the client's behaviors and to allow clinicians to assess their own performance. Analysis of the first session should involve both the client's behaviors and the clinician's performance.

Client Behaviors. Three basic areas should be part of the analysis: (a) formal test results, (b) informal test results, and (c) a behavioral analysis. Table 10.4 presents a summary form based on the information contained in Part II of this text, Clinical Behaviors.

Clinician Performance. The self-analysis of the clinician's performance is based on the information contained in Parts I and III of this text, Clinical Foundations and Clinical Intervention. A summary form appears in Table 10.5.

Table 10.4
Evaluation of client behaviors

CLINICAL RECORDS

Date of Last Audiological Examination_____

Information	Date	Description
Speech Behaviors		
Language Behaviors		
Cognitive Ability		
Attitudes		
Effective Reinforcers		
Effects of Specific Therapy Procedures		
Cultural Values		
Non-Speech/Language Problems		

CLINICAL OBSERVATION   Date_____

Information	Description	Confirmation*
Speech Behaviors		
Language Behaviors		
Cognitive Ability		
Attitudes		
Effective Reinforcers		
Effects of Specific Therapy Procedures		
Cultural Values		
Non-Speech/Language Problems		

*Under Confirmation   C = Confirms information in clinical records
X = Contradicts information in clinical records
— = No corroboration in clinical records

continues

Table 10.4 continued

FORMAL TEST RESULTS

	Assessment Instrument	Date	Results	Recommendation
Phonology				
Language				
Voice				
Stuttering				
Cognition				
Other				

INFORMAL TEST RESULTS

	Assessment Method	Date	Results	Recommendation
Phonology				
Language				
Voice				
Stuttering				
Cognition				
Other				

Table 10.5
Evaluation of clinician behaviors

Behavior	Yes/No	Description
CLINICAL FOUNDATIONS		
Sensitivity to cultural differences		
Established trust		
Used deductive reasoning		
Used inductive reasoning		
Used scientific method		
Displayed personality traits that facilitate positive change		
Displayed personality traits that do not facilitate positive change		
Clear expression of clinical values		
Self-image during session		
RECORDING OF CLINICAL BEHAVIORS		
Methods of permanent recording		
Units of measurement recorded		
Phonological behaviors		
Stuttering behaviors		
Vocal behaviors		
Language behaviors		
Metalinguistic behaviors		
Neurogenic behaviors		
Nonverbal behaviors		
Posture		
Vocalic		
Environmental factors		
Relationship between verbal and nonverbal		

continues

Table 10.5, *continued*

Behavior	Yes/No	Description
CLINICAL INTERVENTION		
Established purpose of therapy		
Explained roles		
Identified levels of learning		
Identified stages of learning and retrieval		
Used intrinsic reinforcement		
Used extrinsic reinforcement		
Used extraneous reinforcement		
Used negative reinforcement		
Used punishment		
Used reinforcement schedules		
Used response differentiation		
Started with behaviors client could perform		
Emphasized progress towards desired behaviors		
Eliminated maladaptive behaviors		
Developed problem-solving skills		
Incorporated decision-making activities into therapy		
Consistent		
Continuously assessed clinical progress		
Involved parents		
Reinforced behaviors in various settings		

Behavior	Yes/No	Description
Supplemented standardized test with analyses of conversational speech		
Established control of individual/group		
Formalized clinician-directed activities		
Used unstructured communicative activities		
Provided orientation for individual/group activity		
Implemented efficient therapy		
Used appropriate group activities		
Recruited client into activity		
Simplified tasks		
Maintained interest and motivation		
Marked relevant features of task		
Controlled level of frustration		
Used modeling when necessary		
Identified terminal competency of activity		
Identified specific competencies		
Used instructional objectives		
Used learning activities		
Used computer-assisted activities		
Used strategies for memory		
Used strategies for retrieval		
Applied generalization		

SUMMARY

In analyzing their own behavior, clinicians should try to view it as objectively as they would if they were performing a diagnostic evaluation on a client. The purpose of identifying inappropriate behaviors is not to impair the clinician's self-image but rather to determine what aspects of clinical behavior need more attention. Just as clients need to be taught how to use both skills and strategies, so do clinicians. The first step in the process is to identify as objectively as possible the problems and then develop a program for their remediation.

SUGGESTED READINGS

Dreyfus, H. L., & Dreyfus, S. E. (1986). *Mind over machine.* New York: The Free Press.

Scheuerle, J. (1992). *Counseling in speech-language pathology and audiology.* New York: Merrill/Macmillan.

Shames, G. H., & Rubin, H. (1986). The roles of the client and the clinician during therapy. In G. H. Shames and H. Rubin (Eds.), *Stuttering, then and now* (pp. 261–270). Columbus, OH: Merrill/Macmillan.

Appendix A
ASHA Observation Supplement

A requirement of the American Speech-Language-Hearing Association is that the first 25 hours of clinic practicum be directed clinical observation. Your training program may elect to use this form in conjunction with this text to fulfill the requirement. Be sure that an ASHA-certified supervisor signs off for each activity you have completed. Additional space is provided for other observations. This form should be placed in your file at the completion of the course.

(Name)

(Completion date)

(Observation site)

Observation Time in Minutes	Date	Supervisor	Activity
			1. Microcultural Values
			2. Clinical Experiment—ABA Design
			4. Simple Enumeration
			5. Type Token Ratio
			6. Rating Scales
			7. Articulation
			8. Fluency
			9. Voice
			10. Child/Adolescent Language
			11. Aphasia
			12a. Child Metalinguistics

Appendix A — ASHA Observation Supplement

Observation Time in Minutes	Date	Supervisor	Activity
			12b. Adult Metalinguistics
			13. Individual Behavioral Repertoires
			14. Linear-Temporal Behavioral Context
			15. Environmental Context
			16. Cognitive Learning Levels
			17. Intrinsic/Extrinsic/Extraneous Reinforcers
			18. Applications of Positive Reinforcers
			19. Applications of Aversive Stimuli
			20. Reinforcement Schedules
			21. Response Differentiation/Successive Approximations
			22. Individual Time Management
			23. Generalization Techniques
			24. Group Time Management
			25. Group Control
			26. Group Functions
			27. Application of Clinical Strategies
			CLASS VIDEO/AUDIOTAPES
			PROGRAMMED VIDEO/AUDIOTAPES
			OTHER OBSERVATIONS:

_____ TOTAL MINUTES
(25 hours = 1,500 minutes)

Appendix B
American Speech-Language-Hearing Association's Code of Ethics

Preamble*

The preservation of the highest standards of integrity and ethical principles is vital to the responsible discharge of obligations in the professions of speech-language pathology and audiology. This Code of Ethics sets forth the fundamental principles and rules considered essential to this purpose.

Every individual who is (a) a member of the American Speech-Language-Hearing Association, whether certified or not, (b) a nonmember holding the Certificate of Clinical Competence from the Association, (c) an applicant for membership or certification, or (d) a Clinical Fellow seeking to fulfill standards for certification shall abide by this Code of Ethics.

Any action that violates the spirit and purpose of this Code shall be considered unethical. Failure to specify any particular responsibility or practice in this Code of Ethics shall not be construed as denial of the existence of such responsibilities or practices.

The fundamentals of ethical conduct are described by Principles of Ethics and by Rules of Ethics as they relate to responsibility to persons served, to the public, and to the professions of speech-language pathology and audiology.

Principles of Ethics, aspirational and inspirational in nature, form the underlying moral basis for the Code of Ethics. Individuals shall observe these principles as affirmative obligations under all conditions of professional activity.

Rules of Ethics are specific statements of minimally acceptable professional conduct or of prohibitions and are applicable to all individuals.

Principle of Ethics I

Individuals shall honor their responsibility to hold paramount the welfare of persons they serve professionally.

Rules of Ethics

A. Individuals shall provide all services competently.
B. Individuals shall use every resource, including referral when appropriate, to ensure that high-quality service is provided.
C. Individuals shall not discriminate in the delivery of professional services on the basis of race, sex, age, religion, national origin, sexual orientation, or handicapping condition.
D. Individuals shall fully inform the persons they serve of the nature and possible effects of services rendered and products dispensed.
E. Individuals shall evaluate the effectiveness of services rendered and of products dispensed and shall provide services or dispense products only when benefit can reasonably be expected.
F. Individuals shall not guarantee the results of any treatment or procedure, directly or by implication; however, they may make a reasonable statement of prognosis.

---

* American Speech-Language-Hearing Association (1992). Code of Ethics. *Asha*, 34 (March, Suppl. 9), 1–2.

G. Individuals shall not evaluate or treat speech, language, or hearing disorders solely by correspondence.
H. Individuals shall maintain adequate records of professional services rendered and products dispensed and shall allow access to these records when appropriately authorized.
I. Individuals shall not reveal, without authorization, any professional or personal information about the person served professionally, unless required by law to do so, or unless doing so is necessary to protect the welfare of the person or of the community.
J. Individuals shall not charge for services not rendered, nor shall they misrepresent,[1] in any fashion, services rendered or products dispensed.
K. Individuals shall use persons in research or as subjects of teaching demonstrations only with their informed consent.
L. Individuals shall withdraw from professional practice when substance abuse or an emotional or mental disability may adversely affect the quality of services they render.

Principles of Ethics II

Individuals shall honor their responsibility to achieve and maintain the highest level of professional competence.

Rule of Ethics

A. Individuals shall engage in the provision of clinical services only when they hold the appropriate Certificate of Clinical Competence or when they are in the certification process and are supervised by an individual who holds the appropriate Certificate of Clinical Competence.

B. Individuals shall engage in only those aspects of the professions that are within the scope of their competence, considering their level of education, training, and experience.
C. Individuals shall continue their professional development throughout their careers.
D. Individuals shall delegate the provision of clinical services only to persons who are certified or to persons in the education or certification process who are appropriately supervised. The provision of support services may be delegated to persons who are neither certified nor in the certification process only when a certificate holder provides appropriate supervision.
E. Individuals shall prohibit any of their professional staff from providing services that exceed the staff member's competence, considering the staff member's level of education, training, and experience.
F. Individuals shall ensure that all equipment used in the provision of services is in proper working order and is properly calibrated.

Principle of Ethics III

Individuals shall honor their responsibility to the public by promoting public understanding of the professions, by supporting the development of services designed to fulfill the unmet needs of the public, and by providing accurate information in all communications involving any aspect of the professions.

Rules of Ethics

A. Individuals shall not misrepresent their credentials, competence, education, training, or experience.
B. Individuals shall not participate in professional activities that constitute a conflict of interest.
C. Individuals shall not misrepresent diagnostic information, services rendered, or products dispensed or engage in any scheme or artifice to defraud in connection with obtaining payment or reimbursement for such services or products.
D. Individuals' statements to the public shall provide accurate information about the nature

---

[1] For purposes of this Code of Ethics, misrepresentation includes any untrue statements or statements that are likely to mislead. Misrepresentation also includes the failure to state any information that is material and that ought, in fairness, to be considered.

and management of communication disorders, about the professions, and about professional services.

E. Individuals' statements to the public—advertising, announcing, and marketing their professional services, reporting research results, and promoting products—shall adhere to prevailing professional standards and shall not contain misrepresentations.

Principle of Ethics IV

Individuals shall honor their responsibilities to the professions and their relationships with colleagues, students, and members of allied professions. Individuals shall uphold the dignity and autonomy of the professions, maintain harmonious interprofessional and intraprofessional relationships, and accept the professions' self-imposed standards.

Rules of Ethics

A. Individuals shall prohibit anyone under their supervision from engaging in any practice that violates the Code of Ethics.

B. Individuals shall not engage in dishonesty, fraud, deceit, misrepresentation, or any form of conduct that adversely reflects on the professions or on the individual's fitness to serve persons professionally.

C. Individuals shall assign credit only to those who have contributed to a publication, presentation, or product. Credit shall be assigned in proportion to the contribution and only with the contributor's consent.

D. Individuals' statements to colleagues about professional services, research results, and products shall adhere to prevailing professional standards and shall contain no misrepresentations.

E. Individuals shall not provide professional services without exercising independent professional judgment, regardless of referral source or prescription.

F. Individuals who have reason to believe that the Code of Ethics has been violated shall inform the Ethical Practice Board.

G. Individuals shall cooperate fully with the Ethical Practice Board in its investigation and adjudication of matters related to this Code of Ethics.

Appendix C
Multicultural/Bilingual Assessment Materials

Articulation

Austin Spanish Articulation Test
Author: None listed
Publisher: Learning Concepts

Evaluating the English Articulation of Non-Native Speakers
Author: C. S. Wing
Publisher: ASHA-Language, Speech, and Hearing Services in Schools, 5, 3, 143–151, 1974.

Multiple-Choice Intelligibility Test for Spanish Discrimination in the Spanish Language
Author: C. A. Cancel
Publisher: ASHA, 5, 10, 1963

Southwestern Spanish Articulation Test (SSAT)
Author: A. S. Toronto
Publisher: Academic Tests, Inc.

Speech and Language Assessment for the Bilingual Handicapped
Authors: L. J. Mattes and D. R. Omark
Publisher: College-Hill Press

Test of Speech Intelligibility in the Spanish Language
Authors: L. Benitez and C. Speaks

Addresses for many of the publishers of these materials are listed in Appendix I.

Publisher: International Audiology, 7, 16–22, 1969

Language

Assessing Asian Language Performance
Author: L. L. Cheng
Publisher: Aspen Publishers

Bilingual Syntax Measure (BSM)
Authors: M. K. Burt, H. C. Dulay, and E. Hernandez Chavez
Publisher: The Psychological Corporation

Bilingualism and Language Disability: Assessment and Remediation
Author: N. Miller
Publisher: College-Hill Press

Del Rio Language Screening Test, English/Spanish (DRLST)
Authors: A. S. Toronto, D. Leverman, C. Hanna, P. Rosenzweig, and A. Maldonado
Publisher: National Educational Laboratory Publishers

Dos Amigos Verbal Language Scales (Dos Amigos)
Author: D. C. Critchlow
Publisher: United Educational Services

Hannah-Gardner Test of Verbal and Nonverbal Language Functioning—English/Spanish
Authors: E. P. Hannah and J. O. Gardner
Publisher: Lingua Press

James Language Dominance—English/Spanish
Author: P. James
Publisher: Learning Concepts

Language Assessment Instruments for Limited English-Speaking Students: A Needs Analysis
Authors: N. A. Locks, B. A. Pletcher, and D. F. Reynolds
Publisher: U.S. Department of Health, Education, and Welfare, National Institute of Education Report

Pre-School Language Scale-Spanish Version
Authors: I. L. Zimmerman, V. G. Steiner, and R. E. Pond
Publisher: The Psychological Corporation

Prueba Illinois de Habilidades Pscolinguisticas (Spanish adaptation of ITPA)
Authors: A. Von Isser and W. Kirk
Publisher: Department of Special Education, University of Arizona

Pruebas de Expresion Oral y Percepcion de la Lengua Espanola (PEOPLE)
Author: S. Mares
Publisher: Office of the Los Angeles County Superintendent of Schools

Screening Test of Spanish Grammar (STSG)
Author: A. S. Toronto
Publisher: Northwestern University Press

Speech and Language Assessment for the Bilingual Handicapped
Authors: L. J. Mattes and D. R. Omark
Publisher: College-Hill Press

Test de Vocabulario en Imagenes Peabody (TVIP)
Authors: L. M. Dunn, E. R. Padilla, D. E. Lugo, and L. M. Dunn
Publisher: American Guidance Service, Inc.

Test for Auditory Comprehension of Language, Revised—English/Spanish (TACL-R)
Author: E. Carrow-Woolfolk
Publisher: DLM Teaching Resources

Toronto Tests of Receptive Vocabulary (Spanish/English)
Author: A. S. Toronto
Publisher: National Education Laboratory

Woodcock Language Proficiency Battery—Spanish (WLPB-S)
Author: R. W. Woodcock
Publisher: DLM Teaching Resources

General

Assessment Instruments in Bilingual Education: A Descriptive Catalogue of 342 Oral and Written Tests
Author: None listed
Publisher: Center for Bilingual Education/National Dissemination and Assessment Center/Northwest Regional Educational Laboratory

Resource Guide to Multicultural Tests and Materials
Authors: L. Cole and T. Snope
Publisher: ASHA, 23, 639-649, 1981

Resource Guide to Multicultural Tests and Materials, Supplement II
Authors: V. R. Deal and M. A. Yan
Publisher: ASHA, 27, 6, 43-49, 1985

Resource Guide to Multicultural Tests and Materials in Communicative Disorders
Authors: V. R. Deal and V. L. Rodriguez
Publisher: American Speech-Language-Hearing Association

Appendix D
Phonological and Articulation Diagnostic Tests

Arizona Articulation Proficiency Scale (AAPS)
Author: J. B. Fudala
Publisher: Western Psychological Services

Assessment of Phonological Processes-Revised (APP-R)
Author: B. W. Hodson
Publisher: The Interstate Printers and Publishers

Austin Spanish Articulation Test
Author: None Listed
Publisher: Learning Concepts

Clinical Probes of Articulation Consistency—C-PAC
Author: W. Secord
Publisher: Psychological Corporation

Coarticulation Assessment in Meaningful Language Test
Authors: K. W. Kenney and E. M. Prather
Publisher: Communication Skill Builders

Compton-Hutton Phonological Assessment
Authors: A. J. Compton and J. S. Hutton
Publisher: Carousel House

Deep Test of Articulation
Author: E. McDonald
Publisher: Stanwix House

Deep Test of Articulation: Picture Form, Sentence Form, and Screening Deep Test of Articulation
Author: E. T. McDonald
Publisher: Stanwix House

Denver Articulation Screening Examination (DASE)
Author: A. F. Drumwright
Publisher: Ladoca Project and Publishing Foundation, Inc.

Developmental Articulation Test
Author: R. F. Hejna
Publisher: Speech Materials

Elicited Articulatory System Evaluation
Author: H. Steed
Publisher: Pro-Ed

Fisher-Logemann Test of Articulation Competence
Authors: H. B. Fisher and J. A. Logemann
Publisher: Riverside Publishing Company

Fluharty Preschool Speech and Language Screening Test
Author: N. Fluharty
Publisher: DLM Teaching Resources

Goldman Fristoe Test of Articulation (GFTA)
Authors: R. Goldman and M. Fristoe
Publisher: American Guidance Service, Inc.

Goldman-Fristoe-Woodcock Test of Auditory Discrimination
Authors: R. Goldman, M. Fristoe, and R. Woodcock
Publisher: American Guidance Service

Lindamood Auditory Conceptualization Test
Authors: C. H. Lindamood and P. C. Lindamood
Publisher: Teaching Resources

Multiple-Choice Intelligibility Test for Spanish Discrimination in the Spanish Language
Author: C. A. Cancel
Publisher: ASHA, 5, 10, 1963

Phonological Process Analysis
Author: F. F. Weiner
Publisher: University Park Press

Photo Articulation Test (PAT)
Authors: K. Pendergast, S. E. Dickey, J. W. Selmar, and A. L. Soder
Publisher: Interstate Printers and Publishers

Picture Articulation and Language Screening Test (PALST)
Author: W. C. Rodgers
Publisher: Word Making Productions

Predictive Screening Test of Articulation (PSTA)
Authors: C. Van Riper and R. L. Erickson
Publisher: Western Michigan University

Riley Articulation and Language Test (RALT)
Author: G. D. Riley
Publisher: Western Psychological Services

Screening Speech Articulation Test (SSAT)
Authors: M. J. Mecham, J. L. Jex, and J. D. Jones
Publisher: Communication Research Associates

Screening Test for Developmental Apraxia of Speech
Author: R. W. Blakeley
Publisher: Pro-Ed

Southwestern Spanish Articulation Test (SSAT)
Author: A. S. Toronto
Publisher: Academic Tests, Inc.

Speech and Language Assessment for the Bilingual Handicapped
Authors: L. J. Mattes and D. R. Omark
Publisher: College-Hill Press

Templin-Darley Tests of Articulation
Authors: M. C. Templin and F. L. Darley
Publisher: The University of Iowa

Test of Articulation Performance Diagnostic—TAP-D
Authors: B. Bryant and D. Bryant
Publisher: Pro-Ed

Test of Articulation Performance Screen—TAP-S
Authors: B. Bryant and D. Bryant
Publisher: Pro-Ed

Test of Minimal Articulation Competence—T-MAC
Author: W. Secord
Publisher: Psychological Corporation

Test of Speech Intelligibility in the Spanish Language
Authors: L. Benitez and C. Speaks
Publisher: International Audiology, 7, 16-22, 1969

Washington Speech Sound Discrimination Test
Authors: E. Prather, A. Miner, M. A. Addicott, and S. Sunderland
Publisher: Interstate Printers and Publishers

Weiss Comprehensive Articulation Test—WCAT
Author: C. Weis
Publisher: DLM Teaching Resources

Appendix E
Language Diagnostic Tests

Adolescent Language Screening Test (ALST)
Authors: D. Morgan and A. Guilford
Publisher: Pro-Ed

Advanced Communication Exercises
Author: K. Tomlin
Publisher: LinguiSystems

Assessing Asian Language Performance
Author: L. L. Cheng
Publisher: Aspen Publishers

Assessing Linguistic Behaviors (ALB)
Authors: Olswang, Stoel-Gammon, Cogins, & Carpenter
Publisher: University of Washington Press

Assessment of Children's Language Comprehension (ACLC)
Authors: R. Foster, J. J. Giddan, and J. Stark
Publisher: Consulting Psychologists Press

Auditory-Visual, Single Word Picture Vocabulary Test
Author: M. F. Gardiner
Publisher: Children's Hospital of San Francisco

Bankson Language Screening Test (BLST)
Author: N. W. Bankson
Publisher: University Park Press

Bankson Language Test—BLT-2
Author: N. W. Bankson
Publisher: Pro-Ed

Bilingual Syntax Measure (BSM)
Authors: M. K. Burt, H. C. Dulay, and E. Hernandez Chavez
Publisher: The Psychological Corporation

Boehm Test of Basic Concepts-Revised
Author: A. E. Boehm
Publisher: The Psychological Corporation

Carrow Elicited Language Inventory (CELI)
Author: E. Carrow
Publisher: Teaching Resources Corporation

CELF: Clinical Evaluation of Language Fundamentals—Revised
Authors: E. Semel-Mintz, E. Wiig, and W. Secord
Publisher: The Psychological Corporation

Communication Competence—A Functional Pragmatic Approach to Language Therapy
Author: C. Simon
Publisher: Communication Skill Builders

The Communication Screen—A Preschool Speech/Language Screening Tool
Authors: N. Striffler and S. Willig
Publisher: United Educational Services

Conversation-Language Intervention for Adolescents
Author: B. Hoskins
Publisher: DLM

Del Rio Language Screening Test, English/Spanish (DRLST)
Authors: A. S. Toronto, D. Leverman, C. Hanna, P. Rosenzweig, and A. Maldonado
Publisher: National Educational Laboratory Publishers

Developmental Sentence Scoring (DDS)
Authors: L. Lee and R. A. Koenigsknect
Publisher: Northwestern University Press

Dos Amigos Verbal Language Scales (Dos Amigos)
Author: D. C. Critchlow
Publisher: United Educational Services

Early Language Milestone Scale (ELM)
Author: Coplan
Publisher: Pro-Ed

Environmental Language Inventory (ELI)
Author: J. D. MacDonald
Publisher: The Psychological Corporation

Environmental Pre-Language Battery (EPB)
Authors: D. Horstmeier and J. D. MacDonald
Publisher: The Psychological Corporation

Evaluating Communicative Competence—A Functional Pragmatic Procedure
Author: C. Simon
Publisher: United Educational Services

Expressive One-Word Picture Vocabulary Test
Author: M. F. Gardiner
Publisher: Academic Therapy Publications

Expressive One-Word Picture Vocabulary Test—Upper Extension
Author: M. F. Gardiner
Publisher: Academic Therapy Publications

Fluharty Preschool Speeching and Language Screening Test
Author: N. Fluharty
Publisher: DLM Teaching Resources

Full-Range Picture Vocabulary Test
Authors: R. B. Ammons and H. S. Ammons
Publisher: Psychological Test Specialists

Fullerton Language Test for Adolescents
Author: A. Thorum
Publisher: Consulting Psychologists Press

Grammatical Analysis of Elicited Language (GAEL)
Authors: J. S. Moog, V. J. Kozak and A. E. Geers
Publisher: Central Institute for the Deaf

Hannah-Gardner Test of Verbal and Nonverbal Language Functioning—English/Spanish
Authors: E. P. Hannah and J. O. Gardner
Publisher: Lingua Press

The Houston Test for Language Development
Author: M. Crabtree
Publisher: The Houston Test Company

Interpersonal Language Skills Assessment—ILSA
Authors: C. Blagden and N. McConnell
Publisher: LinguiSystems

James Language Dominance—English/Spanish
Author: P. James
Publisher: Learning Concepts

Language Facility Test
Author: J. T. Dailey
Publisher: The Allington Corporation

Language Sampling, Analysis, and Training
Authors: D. Tyack and R. Gottsleben
Publisher: Consulting Psychologists Press

Let's Talk Inventory for Children
Authors: C. M. Bray and E. H. Wiig
Publisher: The Psychological Corporation

Michigan Picture Language Inventory
Authors: W. Wolski and L. Lerea
Publisher: University of Michigan, Department of Communication Disorders

Miller-Yoder Language Comprehension Test
Authors: J. F. Miller and D. E. Yoder
Publisher: University Park Press

Appendix E ❑ Language Diagnostic Tests

Multilevel Informal Language Inventory (MILI)
Author: C. Goldsworthy
Publisher: Psychological Corporation

Muma Assessment Program (MAP)
Authors: J. R. Muma and D. B. Muma
Publisher: Natural Child Publishing Company

Northwestern Syntax Screening Test (NSST)
Author: L. Lee
Publisher: Northwestern University Press

The Oral Language Sentence Imitation Diagnostic Inventory (OLSIDI)
Authors: L. Zachman, R. Huisingh, C. Jorgensen, and M. Barrett
Publisher: LinguiSystems, Inc.

The Oral Language Sentence Imitation Screening Test (OLSIST)
Authors: L. Zachman, R. Huisingh, C. Jorgensen, and M. Barrett
Publisher: LinguiSystems, Inc.

Peabody Picture Vocabulary Test-Revised (PPVT-R)
Authors: L. M. Dunn and L. M. Dunn
Publisher: American Guidance Service, Inc.

Picture Articulation and Language Screening Test (PALST)
Author: W. C. Rodgers
Publisher: Word Making Productions

Porch Index of Communicative Ability in Children (PICAC)
Author: B. E. Porch
Publisher: Consulting Psychologists Press

Preschool Language Scale
Authors: I. Zimmerman, V. Steiner, and R. Pond
Publisher: Psychological Corporation

Preschool Language Scale (PLS)
Authors: I. L. Zimmerman, V. G. Steiner, and R. E. Pond
Publisher: The Psychological Corporation

Preschool Language Scale—Spanish Version
Authors: I. L. Zimmerman, V. G. Steiner, and R. E. Pond
Publisher: The Psychological Corporation

Prueba Illinois de Habilidades Pscolinguisticas (Spanish Adaptation of ITPA)
Authors: A. Von Isser and W. Kirk
Publisher: Department of Special Education, University of Arizona

Pruebas de Expresion Oral y Percepcion de la Lengua Espanola (PEOPLE)
Author: S. Mares
Publisher: Office of the Los Angeles County Superintendent of Schools

Receptive-Expressive Emergent Language Scale (REEL Scale)
Authors: K. R. Bzoch and R. League
Publisher: The Tree of Life Press

Receptive-Expressive Emergent Language Test
Authors: K. R. Bzoch and R. League
Publisher: Pro-Ed

Receptive One-Word Picture Vocabulary Test
Author: M. F. Gardiner
Publisher: Academic Therapy Publications

Reynell Developmental Language Scales
Author: J. K. Reynell
Publisher: Western Psychological Services

Rhode Island Test of Language Structure
Authors: E. Engen and T. Engen
Publisher: Pro-Ed

Riley Articulation and Language Test (RALT)
Author: G. D. Riley
Publisher: Western Psychological Services

Rossetti-Infant-Toddler Language Scale
Author: L. Rossetti
Publisher: LinguiSystems

Screening Test of Spanish Grammar (STSG)
Author: A. S. Toronto
Publisher: Northwestern University Press

Appendix E — Language Diagnostic Tests

Screening Test of Adolescent Language (STAL)
Authors: E. Prather, S. Breecher, M. Stafford, and E. Wallace
Publisher: University of Washington Press

Sequenced Inventory of Communication Development—Revised (SICD-R)
Authors: D. Hedrick, E. Prather, and A. Tobin
Publisher: University of Washington Press

Slingerland Screening Tests for Identifying Children with Specific Language Disability, Revised
Author: B. H. Slingerland
Publisher: Educators Publishing Service

Synergistic Systems Clinical Model—Children's Language Battery I.
Author: G. H. Eggert
Publisher: Biolinguistic Clinical Institutes

Temple University Short Syntax Inventory
Authors: A. Gerber and H. Goehl
Publisher: University Park Press

Test de Vocabulario en Imagenes Peabody (TVIP)
Authors: L. M. Dunn, E. R. Padilla, D. E. Lugo, and L. M. Dunn
Publisher: American Guidance Service, Inc.

Test of Adolescent Language—2 (TOAL-2)
Authors: D. D. Hammill, V. L. Brown, S. C. Larsen, and J. L. Wiederholt
Publisher: Pro-Ed

Test for Auditory Comprehension of Language, Revised Edition—English/Spanish (TACL-R)
Author: E. Carrow-Woolfolk
Publisher: DLM Teaching Resources

Test for Examining Expressive Morphology
Authors: K. Shipley, T. A. Stone, and M. B. Sue
Publisher: Communication Skill Builders

Test of Language Competence
Authors: E. Wiig and P. L. Newcomer
Publisher: Psychological Corporation

Test of Language Development—2-Intermediate (TOLD-2-I)
Authors: P. L. Newcomer and D. D. Hammill
Publisher: Pro-Ed

Test of Language Development—2-Primary (TOLD-2-P)
Authors: P. L. Newcomer and D. D. Hammill
Publisher: Pro-Ed

Test of Pragmatic Skills
Author: B. Shulman
Publisher: Communication Skill Builders

Test of Syntactic Abilities
Authors: S. P. Quigley, M. Steinkamp, D. Power, and B. Jones
Publisher: Dormac, Inc.

Test of Word Finding (TWF)
Author: D. J. German
Publisher: DLM Teaching Resources

Test of Written Language—TOWL
Author: D. D. Hammill and S. C. Larsen
Publisher: Pro-Ed

Token Test for Children (TTC)
Author: F. DiSimoni
Publisher: DLM Teaching Resources

Toronto Tests of Receptive Vocabulary (Spanish/English)
Author: A. S. Toronto
Publisher: National Educational Laboratory

Utah Test of Language Development
Authors: M. J. Mecham, J. L. Jex, and J. D. Jones
Publisher: Communication Research Associates

Vane Evaluation of Language Scale (VANE-L)
Author: J. R. Vane
Publisher: Clinical Psychology Publishing Co. Inc.

Verbal Language Development Scale (VLDS)
Author: M. Mecham
Publisher: American Guidance Service, Inc.

Appendix E — Language Diagnostic Tests

Vocabulary Comprehension Scale
Author: T. E. Bangs
Publisher: Teaching Resources Corporation

Woodcock Language Proficiency Battery—Spanish (WLPB-S)
Author: R. W. Woodcock
Publisher: DLM Teaching Resources

The WORD Test
Authors: C. Jorgensen, M. Barrett, R. Huisingh, and L. Zachman
Publisher: LinguiSystems

Appendix F
Stuttering Tests

Behavioral Cognitive Stuttering Therapy

Author: S. A. Goldberg

Publisher: Quest Publishers

Checklist of Stuttering Behavior

Authors: D. E. Williams, F. L. Darley, & D. C. Spriestersbach. (1978).

Publisher: In F. L. Darley & D. C. Spriestersbach (Eds.). *Diagnostic methods in speech pathology.* New York: Harper & Row.

Cooper Personalized Fluency Control Therapy, Revised

Authors: E. B. Cooper & C. S. Cooper

Publisher: DLM Teaching Resources

Measures of Disfluency of Speaking and Oral Reading

Authors: D. E. Williams, F. L. Darley, & D. C. Spriestersbach. (1978).

Publisher: In F. L. Darley & D. C. Spriestersbach (Eds.). *Diagnostic methods in speech pathology.* New York: Harper & Row.

Scale for Rating Severity of Stuttering

Authors: D. E. Williams, F. L. Darley, & D. C. Spriestersbach. (1978).

Publisher: In F. L. Darley & D. C. Spriestersbach (Eds.). *Diagnostic methods in speech pathology.* New York: Harper & Row.

Stuttering Assessment Protocol

Authors: R. Culatta and S. A. Goldberg

Publisher: Merrill/Macmillan

Stuttering Intervention Program

Author: R. Pindzola

Publisher: Modern Education Corp.

Stuttering Severity Instrument

Author: G. Riley

Publisher: C.C. Publications

Systematic Fluency Training Assessment

Author: R. E. Shine

Publisher: Pro-Ed

Appendix G
Voice Tests

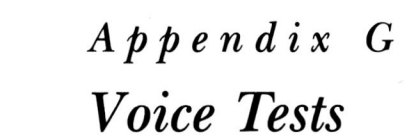

Boone Voice Evaluation in Boone Voice Program for Adults
Author: D. Boone
Publisher: Pro-Ed

Boone Voice Evaluation in Boone Voice Program for Children
Author: D. Boone
Publisher: Pro-Ed

Inventory for the Assessment of Laryngectomy Rehabilitation
Author: L. La Borwit
Publisher: C.C. Publications

Programmed Approach to Voice Therapy
Authors: F. B. Wilson and M. A. Rice
Publisher: Learning Concepts

Appendix H
Neurogenic/Cognitive Tests

Aphasia Language Performance Scales (ALPS)
Authors: J. S. Keenan and E. G. Brassel
Publisher: Pinnacle Press

Appraisal of Language Disturbance
Author: L. L. Emerick
Publisher: Northern Michigan University

Apraxia Battery for Adults
Author: B. L. Dabul
Publisher: Pro-Ed

The Assessment of Aphasia and Related Disorders
Authors: H. Goodglass and E. Kaplan
Publisher: Lea & Febiger

Assessment of Intelligibility of Dysarthric Speech
Authors: K. Yorkston, D. Beukelman, and C. Traynor
Publisher: Pro-Ed

Basic Concept Inventory
Author: S. Engelmann
Publisher: Follett Publishing Co.

Bedside Evaluation of Screening Test of Aphasia
Authors: J. Fitch-West and E. S. Sands
Publisher: Pro-Ed

Boehm Test of Basic Concepts—Revised
Author: A. E. Boehm
Publisher: The Psychological Corporation

Boston Assessment of Severe Aphasia
Authors: N. Helm-Estabrooks, G. Ramsberger, A. R. Moran, and M. Micholoas
Publisher: Pro-Ed

The Boston Diagnostic Aphasia Examination
Authors: H. Goodglass and E. Kaplan
Publisher: Lea & Febiger

Boston Naming Test
Authors: E. Kaplan, H. Goodglass, and S. Weintraub
Publisher: Lea & Febiger

Clinical Management of Right Hemisphere Dysfunction
Authors: M. S. Burns, A. S. Halper, and S. I. Mogil
Publisher: Aspen Systems Corporation

Cognitive Abilities Scale
Author: S. Bradley-Johnson
Publisher: Pro-Ed

Cognitive, Linguistic, and Social-Communicative Scales
Authors: D. Tanner and W. Lamb
Publisher: Modern Education Corporation

Communicative Abilities in Daily Living (CADL)
Author: A. L. Holland
Publisher: Pro-Ed

Computerized Assessment of Intelligibility of Dysarthric Speech
Authors: Yorkston, Beukelman, Traynor
Publisher: C.C. Publications, Inc.

Dysarthria Profile
Author: S. J. Robertson
Publisher: Communication Skill Builders, Inc.

Examining for Aphasia
Author: J. Eisenson
Publisher: The Psychological Corporation

Frenchay Dysarthria Assessment
Author: P. M. Enderby
Publisher: Pro-Ed

Functional Communication Profile
Author: M. T. Sarno
Publisher: Institute of Rehabilitation Medicine

Language Modalities Test for Aphasia
Authors: J. M. Wepman and L. V. Jones
Publisher: Education-Industry Service

Minnesota Test for Differential Diagnosis of Aphasia
Author: H. Schuell
Publisher: University of Minnesota Press

Multilingual Aphasia Examination
Author: A. Benton
Publisher: Benton Laboratory of Neuropsychology

Neurosensory Center Comprehensive Examination for Aphasia (NCCEA)
Authors: O. Spreen and A. Benton
Publisher: Neuropsychology Laboratory

The Porch Index of Communicative Ability
Author: B. Porch
Publisher: Consulting Psychologists Press

Proverbs Test
Author: D. Gorham
Publisher: Psychological Test Specialists

Raven's Progressive Matrices
Author: J. C. Raven
Publisher: The Psychological Corporation

Reading Comprehension Battery for Aphasia
Author: L. LaPointe and J. Horner
Publisher: C.C. Publications

The Revised Token Test
Authors: M. R. McNeil and T. Prescott
Publisher: University Park Press

RIC Evaluation of Communication Problems in Right Hemisphere Dysfunction (RICE)
Authors: M. S. Burns, A. S. Harper, and S. I. Mogil
Publisher: Aspens Systems Corp.

The Right Hemisphere Language Battery
Author: K. Bryan
Publisher: Far Communication

Screening Test for Developmental Apraxia of Speech
Author: R. Blakeley
Publisher: C.C. Publications

Short-Term Auditory Retrieval and Storage (STARS)
Author: A. Flowers
Publisher: Perceptual Learning Systems

Test of Listening Accuracy in Children
Authors: M. J. Mechan, J. L. Jex, and J. D. Jones
Publisher: DLM Teaching Resources

The Test of Nonverbal Intelligence (TONI)
Authors: L. Brown, R. J. Sherbenou, and S. J. Dollar
Publisher: Pro-Ed

Test of Practical Knowledge (TPK)
Authors: J. L. Wiederholt and S. Larsen
Publisher: Pro-Ed

Wachs Analysis of Cognitive Structures
Authors: H. Wachs and L. Vaughan
Publisher: DLM Teaching Resources

Weller-Strawser Scales of Adaptive Behavior for the Learning Disabled—WSSAB
Authors: C. Weller and S. Strawser
Publisher: Academic Therapy Publications

The Western Aphasia Battery (WAB)
Author: A. Kertesz
Publisher: The Psychological Corporation

Appendix I
Selected Publishers' Addresses for Listed Diagnostic Tests

Academic Tests, Inc.
PO Box 18613
Austin, TX 78760

Academic Therapy Publications
20 Commercial Blvd.
Novato, CA 94949-6191

The Allington Corporation
P.O. Box 125
Remington, VA 22734

American Guidance Service, Inc.
Publishers' Bldg.
Circle Pines, MN 55014

Aspen Publications
200 Orchard Ridge Road
Gaithersburg, MD 20878

Benton Laboratory of Neuropsychology
University of Iowa
Iowa City, IA

C.C. Publications
(Contact Pro-Ed concerning availability)

Carousel House
PO Box 4480
San Francisco, CA 94101

Center for Bilingual Education
Los Angeles, CA

Central Institute for the Deaf
818 South Euclid Avenue
St. Louis, MO 63110

Children's Hospital of San Francisco
Box 3805
San Francisco, CA 94119

Clinical Psychology Publishing Co., Inc.
4 Conant Square
Brandon, VT 05733

Communication Research Associates
PO Box 11012
Salt Lake City, UT 84147

Communication Skill Builders
3830 E. Bellvue
PO Box 42050
Tucson, AZ 85733

Consulting Psychologists Press, Inc.
3803 Bayshore Rd.
Palo Alto, CA 94303

DLM Teaching Resources
PO Box 4000
One DLM Park
Allen, TX 75002

Dormac, Inc.
PO Box 1699
Beaverton, OR 97075-1699

Education-Industry Service
1225 E. 60th St.
Chicago, IL

Educators Publishing Service, Inc.
75 Moulton St.
Cambridge, MA 02138-1104

Far Communication
5 Harcourt Estate
Kibworth
Leics LE8 ONE

Follett Publishing Co.
1000 W. Washington Blvd.
Chicago, IL 60607

Harper Collins
10 E. 53rd St.
New York, NY 10022

Institute of Rehabilitation Medicine
New York University Medical Center
400 East 34th St.
New York, NY 10016

The Interstate Printers and Publishers
19 N. Jackson
PO Box 50
Danville, IL 61834-0050

LADOCA Project and Publishing Foundation, Inc.
5100 Lincoln St.
Denver, CO 80216

Lea & Febiger
600 Washington Square
Philadelphia, PA 19106

Learning Concepts
2501 N. Lamar
Austin, TX 78705

Lingua Press
PO Box 293
Northridge, CA 91324

LinguiSystems
716 17th St.
Moline, IL 61265

National Educational Laboratory Publishers
813 Airport Blvd
Austin, TX 78702

Natural Child Publishing Co.
PO Box 3452
Lubbock, TX 79452

Northern Michigan University
Marquette, MI

Northwestern University Press
1735 Benson Ave.
Evanston, IL 60201

Office of the Los Angeles County Superintendent of Schools
9300 East Imperial Hwy.
Downey, CA 90241

Perceptual Learning Systems
PO Box 864
Dearborn, MI 48121

Pinnacle Press
PO Box 1122
Murfreesboro, TN 37130

Pro-Ed
8700 Shoal Creek Blvd.
Austin, TX 78758-6897

The Psychological Corporation
555 Academic Court
San Antonio, TX 78204

Psychological Test Specialists
Box 9229
Missoula, MT 59807

Quest Publishers
Suite 303
450 Taraval St.
San Francisco, CA 94116

Riverside Publishing Company
8420 West Bryn Mawr Road
Chicago, IL 60631

Slosson Educational Publications, Inc.
PO Box 280
East Aurora, NY 14052

Speech Materials
PO Box 1713
Ann Arbor, MI 48106

Stanwix House
Pittsburgh, PA

Teaching Resources Corporation
100 Boylston Street
Boston, MA 02116

The Tree of Life Press
1309 North East Second Street
Gainesville, FL 32601

Appendix I ❑ *Selected Publishers' Addresses for Listed Diagnostic Tests*

United Educational Services
Box 605
East Aurora, NY 14052

The University of Iowa
Iowa City, IA 52242

University of Michigan, Department of Communication Disorders
Ann Arbor, MI

University of Minnesota Press
2037 University Ave., S.E.
Minneapolis, MN 55414

University of Washington Press
PO Box 50096
Seattle, WA 98105-5096

Western Michigan University
Continuing Education Office
Kalamazoo, MI 49001

Western Psychological Services
12031 Wilshire Boulevard
Los Angeles, CA 90025

Word Making Productions
70 W. Louise Ave. S.
Salt Lake City, UT 84114

Appendix J
Language Therapy and Parent Involvement

Team Work

Understanding and using language may be difficult for your child. We can make it easier by doing certain things. The most important of these is to act as a team. *The clinician and the child's family should become co-therapists.* In this clinic your involvement in teaching your child language is important. We want you not only to do certain things at home, but also to **participate in therapy.**

Parent Involvement

The experience of therapy will be rewarding to you and your family and is very important for your child's progress. We see your child only 2 hours each week, but you are with him or her for the remaining 168 hours. We would like you to be present for each session. During that time you will either be meeting with the clinician or supervisor, observing your child, or directly working with your child.

Teaching a child something new is an enriching experience. Parents want to do all they can for their child. Unfortunately, many do not know the best techniques to use. The training that you will receive in this clinic will provide you with the knowledge necessary to help your child with language problems and other problems as well.

Therapy Approach

Most children with language disorders also have other problems. Some are related directly to the language problem; others are not. In this clinic we are concerned with treating the whole child, not just a specific language problem. Ten main areas of therapy will be emphasized:

Language. When teaching language to your child, we will be providing him or her with a strategy for learning new words and structures. In other words, your child will learn how to put words together, by him or herself.

Articulation. Some children with language problems also have difficulty in pronouncing certain sounds. Of greatest concern is when a child says only the first part of words and leaves off the endings. We will teach your child a strategy for remembering that a word has more than one sound.

Cognition. Some children with language problems also have problems with cognition, or abstract thinking. It may be difficult for them to think about (a) things that are not present; (b) time; (c) numbers; (d) relationships between things or people; and (e) solving problems. As we teach them certain parts of language, their cognitive ability should improve.

Decision-Making. Many times children who have a language or mental handicap are not given the opportunity to make decisions. Yet, having the opportunity to make decisions is important for children. It allows them to have some control over their life and learn that actions have consequences. Throughout therapy, we will constantly allow the children to make decisions.

Emotions. All children have feelings. Children who have a sufficient amount of language can express their feelings. Children who little language may be unable to. Often, the inability to express how they feel can result in behavior that is disruptive, hostile, or not understandable to you as a parent. We will help your child learn how to express verbally how he or she feels.

Normalization. It is important to your child that he or she "fits in" as much as possible with other children. There are some things we cannot change. The child who has Down syndrome will always be identified as a "different" child. But many things can be done to minimize that "differentness." These things can range from clothing to learning some slang expressions that are used by other children of the same age. Throughout therapy, we will emphasize "normalizing" your child.

Self-Help and Practical Skills. Language therapy must be useful. The words and structures used in therapy will be chosen with practicality in mind. We will teach only what the child can use. For example, if you are working on toileting at home, the word we teach your child could be *bathroom*.

Generalization. Whatever we teach your child in the clinic must be applicable in other settings. This can be achieved by designing therapy sessions that have much in common with what occurs at home, on the bus, on a playground, or any other place your child finds him or herself. Therefore, therapy will not be limited to the clinic room. We will be doing therapy in the hallway, outside on the campus, and in various buildings with different people throughout the university.

Reinforcement. Children learn best when they are reinforced for doing desired behaviors. It is important that we are consistent with reinforcement. There are three types of reinforcement that we will be using in therapy:

Intrinsic: This is when the activity itself is rewarding to the child (e.g., pushing a car on a floor for a child who loves this activity).
Extrinsic: The reward with this type of reinforcement is the completion of the activity (e.g., when a child finishes a puzzle and sees a picture).
Extraneous: This type of reward is not directly related to an activity or its completion. Examples would be candy or verbal praise.

In therapy, we will be using all three forms of reinforcement.

Shaping Behaviors. All children learn best when a complicated behavior is broken down into very small parts. This is even more important for children who have cognitive problems. We will identify a specific target behavior and then design a program for reaching it. The program will have many steps. The more steps we have in a program, the easier it will be for your child to be successful. Being successful is not only important for learning new behaviors, but it will also enhance your child's feelings of self-worth.

Having a child with a language or cognitive problem can be an immense strain on you and your family. We would like to reduce it in three ways:

1. Teach new behaviors that will allow your child to develop his or her maximum potential.
2. Involve you in therapy, providing the family an opportunity to have positive experiences with your child.
3. Provide you and your family with an opportunity to discuss specific problems or feelings you have about your child.

Appendix K
Articulation Therapy and Parent Involvement

Team Work

Using correct pronunciation may be difficult for your child. We can make it easier by doing certain things. The most important of these is to act as a team. *The clinician and the child's family should become co-therapists.* In this clinic your involvement in teaching your child the correct way to pronounce sounds is important. We want you not only to do certain things at home, but also to **participate in therapy.**

Parent Involvement

The experience of therapy will be rewarding to you and your family and is very important for your child's progress. We see your child only 2 hours each week, but you are with him or her for the remaining 168 hours. We would like you to be present for each session. During that time you will either be meeting with the clinician or supervisor, observing your child, or directly working with your child.

Teaching a child something new is an enriching experience. Parents want to do all they can for their child. Unfortunately, many do not know the best techniques to use. The training that you will receive in this clinic will provide you with the knowledge necessary to help your child with language problems and other problems as well.

Therapy Approach

Learning how to pronounce sounds correctly will involve much repetition. Like any new skill, it needs to be practiced before it can become automatic. Therapy will concentrate on making the practice natural and enjoyable.

Generalization. Whatever we teach your child in the clinic must be applicable in other settings. This can be achieved by designing therapy sessions that have much in common with what occurs at home, on the bus, on a playground, or any other place your child finds him or herself. Therefore, therapy will not be limited to the clinic room. We will be doing therapy in the hallway, outside on the campus, and in various buildings with different people throughout the university.

Reinforcement. Children learn best when they are reinforced for doing desired behaviors. It is important that we are consistent with reinforcement. There are three types of reinforcement that we will be using in therapy:

Intrinsic: This is when the activity itself is rewarding to the child (e.g., pushing a car on a floor for a child who loves this activity).
Extrinsic: The reward with this type of reinforcement is the completion of the activity (e.g., when a child finishes a puzzle and sees a picture).
Extraneous: This type of reward is not directly related to an activity or its completion. Examples would be candy or verbal praise.

In therapy, we will be using all three forms of reinforcement.

Shaping Behaviors. All children learn best when a complicated behavior is broken down into very small parts. We will identify a specific target behavior and then design a program for reaching it. The program will have many steps. The more steps we have in a program, the easier it will be for your child to be successful. Being successful is not only important for learning new behaviors, but it will also enhance your child's feelings of self-worth.

Having a child with a communicative problem can be stressful for you and your family. We would like to reduce it in three ways:

1. Teach new behaviors that will allow your child to develop his or her maximum potential.
2. Involve you in therapy, providing the family an opportunity to have positive experiences with your child.
3. Provide you and your family with an opportunity to discuss specific problems or feelings you have about your child.

Appendix L
Voice Therapy and Parent Involvement

Team Work

Using appropriate vocal volume or pitch may be difficult for your child. We can make it easier by doing certain things. The most important of these is to act as a team. *The clinician and the child's family should become co-therapists.* In this clinic your involvement in teaching your child the correct way to pronounce sounds is important. We want you not only to do certain things at home, but also to **participate in therapy.**

Parent Involvement

The experience of therapy will be rewarding to you and your family and is also very important for your child's progress. We see your child only 2 hours each week, but you are with him or her for the remaining 168 hours. We would like you to be present for each session. During that time you will either be meeting with the clinician or supervisor, observing your child, or directly working with your child.

Teaching a child something new is an enriching experience. Parents want to do all they can for their child. Unfortunately, many do not know the best techniques to use. The training that you will receive in this clinic will provide you with the knowledge necessary to help your child with language problems and other problems as well.

Therapy Approach

Learning how to correctly use vocal volume or pitch will require much practice on the part of your child. Like any new skill, it needs to be practiced frequently before it can become automatic. Therapy will concentrate on making the practice natural and enjoyable.

Generalization. Whatever we teach your child in the clinic must be applicable in other settings. This can be achieved by designing therapy sessions that have much in common with what occurs at home, on the bus, on a playground, or any other place your child finds him or herself. Therefore, therapy will not be limited to the clinic room. We will be doing therapy in the hallway, outside on the campus, and in various buildings with different people throughout the university.

Reinforcement. Children learn best when they are reinforced for doing desired behaviors. It is important that we are consistent with reinforcement. There are three types of reinforcement that we will be using in therapy:

Intrinsic: This is when the activity itself is rewarding to the child (e.g., pushing a car on a floor for a child who loves this activity).
Extrinsic: The reward with this type of reinforcement is the completion of the activity (e.g., when a child finishes a puzzle and sees a picture).
Extraneous: This type of reward is not directly related to an activity or its completion. Examples would be candy or verbal praise.

In therapy, we will be using all three forms of reinforcement.

Shaping Behaviors. All children learn best when a complicated behavior is broken down into very small parts. We will identify a specific target behavior and then design a program for reaching it. The program will have many steps. The more steps we have in a program, the easier it will be for your child to be successful. Being successful is not only important for learning new behaviors, but it will also enhance your child's feelings of self-worth.

Having a child with a communicative problem can be stressful for you and your family. We would like to reduce it in three ways:

1. Teach new behaviors that will allow your child to develop his or her maximum potential.
2. Involve you in therapy, providing the family an opportunity to have positive experiences with your child.
3. Provide you and your family with an opportunity to discuss specific problems or feelings you have about your child.

Appendix M
Stuttering Therapy and Parent Involvement

Team Work

The use of fluent speech may be difficult for your child. We can make it easier by doing certain things. The most important of these is to act as a team. *The clinician and the child's family should become co-therapists.* In this clinic your involvement in teaching your child the correct way to pronounce sounds is important. We want you not only to do certain things at home, but also to **participate in therapy.**

Parent Involvement

The experience of therapy will be rewarding to you and your family and is also very important for your child's progress. We see your child only 2 hours each week, but you are with him or her for the remaining 168 hours. We would like you to be present for each session. During that time you will either be meeting with the clinician or supervisor, observing your child, or directly working with your child.

Teaching a child something new is an enriching experience. Parents want to do all they can for their child. Unfortunately, many do not know the best techniques to use. The training that you will receive in this clinic will provide you with the knowledge to help your child with language problems and other problems as well.

Therapy Approach

Learning how to speak fluently will require much practice on the part of your child. Like any new skill, it needs to be practiced frequently before it can become automatic. Therapy will concentrate on making the practice natural and enjoyable.

Generalization. Whatever we teach your child in the clinic must be applicable in other settings. This can be achieved by designing therapy sessions that have much in common with what occurs at home, on the bus, on a playground, or any other place your child finds him or herself. Therefore, therapy will not be limited to the clinic room. We will be doing therapy in the hallway, outside on the campus, and in various buildings with different people throughout the university.

Reinforcement. Children learn best when they are reinforced for doing desired behaviors. It is important that we are consistent with reinforcement. There are three types of reinforcement that we will be using in therapy:

Intrinsic: This is when the activity itself is rewarding to the child (e.g., pushing a car on a floor for a child who loves this activity).

Extrinsic: The reward with this type of reinforcement is the completion of the activity (e.g., when a child finishes a puzzle and sees a picture).

Extraneous: This type of reward is not directly related to an activity or its completion. Examples would be candy or verbal praise.

In therapy, we will be using all three forms of reinforcement.

Shaping Behaviors. All children learn best when a complicated behavior is broken down into very small parts. We will identify a specific target behavior and then design a program for reaching it. The program will have many steps. The more steps we have in a program, the easier it will be for your child to be successful. Being successful is not only important for learning new behaviors, but it will also enhance your child's feelings of self-worth.

Having a child with a communicative problem can be stressful for you and your family. We would like to reduce it in three ways:

1. Teach new behaviors that will allow your child to develop his or her maximum potential.
2. Involve you in therapy, providing the family an opportunity to have positive experiences with your child.
3. Provide you and your family with an opportunity to discuss specific problems or feelings you have about your child.

References

Albertini, J. A., Smith, J. M., & Metz, D. E. (1983). Small-group versus individual speech therapy with hearing-impaired young adults. *Volta Review, 85,* 83–89.

American Speech-Language-Hearing Association (1992). Code of ethics. ASHA, 34: 3, pp. 1–2.

American Speech-Language-Hearing Association. (1992). *Demographic Data.*

Andrews, G., & Ingham, R. (1971). Stuttering: Considerations in the evaluation of treatment. *British Journal of Communication Disorders, 6,* 124–138.

Aronson, A. E. (1990). *Clinical voice disorders.* New York: Thieme.

Ausubel, D. P. (1968). *Educational psychology: A cognitive view.* New York: Holt, Rinehart & Winston.

Ayer, A. J. (1936). *Language, truth and logic.* London: Victor Gollancz, Ltd.

Ayer, A. J., & Winch, R. (1963). *British empirical philosophers.* London: Routledge & Kegan Paul Ltd.

Bales, R. F. (1950). *Interaction process analysis.* Cambridge: Addison-Wesley.

Bandura, A. (1969). *Principles of behavior modification.* New York: Holt, Rinehart & Winston.

Barfield, J. (1976). Biological influences on sex differences in behavior. In M. S. Teitelbaum (Ed.), *Sex differences: Social and biological perspectives* (pp. 62–121). Garden City, NY: Anchor Press.

Baxter, J. C., Winters, E. P., & Hammer, R. E. (1968). Gestural behavior during a brief interview as a function of cognitive variables. *Journal of Personality and Social Psychology, 8,* 303–307.

Beck, A. T. (1976). *Cognitive therapy and the emotional disorders.* New York: International Universities Press.

Behrmann, M. (1984). The computer and special education. In M. Behrmann (Ed.), *Handbook of microcomputers in special education* (pp. 29–46) San Diego: College-Hill Press.

Berlo, D. K. (1960). *The process of communication.* New York: Holt, Rinehart & Winston.

Berne, E. (1966). *Principles of group treatment.* New York: Oxford University Press.

Bernthal, J. E., & Bankson, N. W. (1981). *Articulation disorders.* Englewood Cliffs, NJ: Prentice-Hall, Inc.

Beukelman, D. R., & Yorkston, K. M. (1991). *Communication disorders following traumatic brain injury.* Austin, TX: Pro-Ed.

Binder, A. (1964). Statistical theory. In P. R. Farnsworth, O. McNemar, & Q. McNemar (Eds.), *Annual review of psychology, 15,* 277–310.

Birdwhistell, R. L. (1968). Certain considerations in the concepts of culture and communication. In C. E. Larson and F. X. Dance (Eds.), *Perspectives on communication* (pp. 144–165). Milwaukee: University of Wisconsin.

Bloodstein, O. (1960). The development of stuttering: I. Changes in nine basic features. *Journal of Speech and Hearing Disorders, 25,* 219–237.

―――― (1961). The development of stuttering: III. Theoretical and clinical implications. *Journal of Speech and Hearing Disorders, 26,* 67–82.

_____(1975). *A handbook on stuttering*. Chicago, IL: National Easter Seal Society for Crippled Children and Adults.

_____ (1979). *Speech pathology: An introduction*. Boston: Houghton Mifflin.

Bluemel, C. S. (1932). Primary and secondary stammering. *Quarterly Journal of Speech, 18*, 187–200.

Boone, D. R. (1988). *Voice and voice therapy*. Englewood Cliffs, NJ: Prentice-Hall.

Borkowski, J. G., & Buchel, F. P. (1981). Learning and memory strategies in the mentally retarded. In M. Pressley & J. R. Levin (Eds.), *Cognitive strategy research: Psychological foundations* (pp. 103–128). New York: Springer-Verlag.

Bosanquet, B. (1895). *The essentials of logic*. New York: Macmillan.

Bricker, W. A. (1972). A systematic approach to language training. In R. L. Schiefelbusch (Ed.), *Language of the mentally retarded*. Baltimore: University Park Press.

Bricker, W. A., & Bricker, D. D. (1970). A program of language training for the severely language handicapped child. *Exceptional Children, 37*, 101–111.

Brown, A. L., & Smiley, S. S. (1978). The development of strategies for studying text. *Child Development, 49*, 1076–1088.

Brown, A. L., Smiley, S. S., & Lawton, S. C. (1978). The effects of experience on the selection of suitable retrieval cues for studying text. *Child Development, 49*, 829–835.

Brown, R. (1970). *Psycholinguistics*. New York: Free Press.

_____ (1973). *A first language, the early stages*. Cambridge, MA: Harvard University Press.

Brutten, E. J., & Shoemaker, D. J. (1967). *The modification of stuttering*. Englewood Cliffs, NJ: Prentice-Hall.

Bull, P. E. (1987). *Posture and gesture*. New York: Pergamon Press.

Buscaglia, L. F. (1982). *Personhood*. New York: Fawcett Columbine.

California Department of Education. (1991). *Special education enrollment data: State totals, ages 0–22, enrollment and annual growth by disability*. Sacramento, CA: California Department of Education.

Campbell, J., with Bill Moyers. (1988). *The power of myth*. New York: Doubleday.

Carroll, J. B. (1981). Ability and task difficulty in cognitive psychology. *Educational Researcher, 10*, 11–19.

Case, J. L. (1991). *Clinical management of voice disorders*. Austin, TX: Pro-Ed.

Castaneda, C. (1968). *The teachings of Don Juan*. New York: Ballantine Books.

Cheng, L. R. I. (1987). Cross-cultural and linguistic considerations in working with Asian populations. *ASHA, 29*, 33–37.

Chomsky, N. (1972). *Language and mind*. New York: Harcourt Brace Jovanovich, Inc.

Chomsky, N., & Halle, M. (1968). *The sound patterns of English*. New York: Harper & Row.

Clark, E. V. (1973). What's in a word? On the child's acquisition of semantics in his first language. In T. E. Moore (Ed.), *Cognitive development and the acquisition of language*. New York: Academic Press.

Cole, G. D. H. (Trans.) (1950). *Rousseau: The social contract and Discourses*. New York: E. P. Dutton.

Cole, L., & Deal, V. R. (Eds.) (in press). *Communication disorders in multicultural populations*. Rockville, MD: American Speech-Language-Hearing Association.

Compton, C. (1990). *A guide to 85 tests for special education*. Belmont, CA: Fearon Education.

Cooper, E. B. (1979). Intervention procedures for the young stutterer. In H. H. Gregory (Ed.), *Controversies about stuttering therapy*. Baltimore: University Park Press.

Corey, G. (1990). *Theory and practice of group counseling* (3rd ed.). Pacific Grove, CA: Brooks/Cole.

Cornett, B. S., & Chabon, S. S. (1988). *The clinical practice of speech-language pathology*. Columbus, OH: Merrill/Macmillan.

Corsini, R. J. (1988). Adlerian groups. In S. Long (Ed.), *Six group therapies* (pp. 1–43). New York: Plenum Press.

Costello, J. (1982). Techniques of therapy based on operant conditioning. In W. Perkins (Ed.), *General Principles of Therapy*. New York: Thieme-Stratton.

Costello, J., & Ingham, R. J. (1984a). Stuttering as an operant disorder. In R. Curlee & W. Perkins (Eds.), *Nature and treatment of stuttering*. San Diego, CA: College-Hill Press.

_____ (1984b). Assessment strategies for stuttering. In R. Curlee & W. Perkins (Eds.), *Nature and Treatment of Stuttering*. San Diego: College-Hill Press.

Cronbach, L. J., & Snow, L. J. (1977). *Aptitudes and instructional methods*. New York: Irvington Publishers, Inc.

Culatta, R. (1984). Cognitive stuttering therapy. Lecture at San Francisco State University, San Francisco, CA.

Culatta, R., & Goldberg, S. A. (in press). *Stuttering therapy: An integration of theory and practice*. New York: Merrill/Macmillan.

Culatta, R., & Seltzer, H. (1976). Content and sequence analysis of the supervisory conference. *ASHA, 18*, 1.

Dale, P. S. (1976). *Language Development*. New York: Holt, Rinehart & Winston.

Darley, F. L., (Ed.) (1979). *Evaluation of appraisal techniques in speech and language pathology*. Reading, MA: Addison-Wesley.

Davis, I. P. (1938). The speech aspects of reading readiness: Newer practices in reading in the elementary school. *17th yearbook of the Dept. of Elementary School, NEA, 17*, 7, 282–289.

Deci, E. L. (1975). *Intrinsic motivation*. New York: Plenum Press.

Delgado, M., & Humm-Delgado, D. (1984). Hispanics and group work: A review of the literature. *Social Work with Groups, 7*(3), 85–96.

Deutsch, M. (1949). An experimental study of the effects of cooperation and competition upon group process. *Human Relations, 2*, 199–231.

De Charms, R. (1968). *Personal causation: The internal affective determinants of behavior*. New York: Academic Press.

Diedrich, W., & Bangert, J. (1980). *Articulation learning*. San Diego: College-Hill.

Dinkmeyer, D. C., Dinkmeyer, D. C., Jr., & Sperry, L. (1987). *Adlerian counseling and psychotherapy* (2nd ed.). New York: Merrill/Macmillan.

Dreyfus, H. L., & Dreyfus, S. E. (1986). *Mind over machine*. New York: The Free Press.

Duchan, J. F. (1984). Language assessment: The pragmatics revolution. In R. C. Naremore (Ed.), *Language science* (pp. 147–180). San Diego, CA: College-Hill Press.

Duffy, G. G., & Roehler, L. R. (1989). Why strategy instruction is so difficult and what we need to do about it. In C. B. McCormick, G. Miller, and M. Pressley (Eds.), *Cognitive strategy research: From basic research to educational applications* (pp. 133–154). New York: Springer-Verlag.

Dunn, L. (1965). *Peabody picture vocabulary test*. Circle Pines, MN: American Guidance Service.

Dunn, L., & Dunn, L. (1981). *Peabody picture vocabulary test—Revised*. Circle Pines, MN: American Guidance Service.

Dunn, R. (1990). Cross-cultural differences in learning styles of elementary-age students from four ethnic backgrounds. *Journal of Multicultural Counseling and Development, 18*(2), 68–93.

Dworkin, J. P. (1991). *Motor-speech disorders: A treatment guide*. St. Louis: Mosby.

Egolf, D. B., Shames, G. H., Johnson, P., & Kaspirison-Burelli, A. (1972). The use of parent-child interaction patterns in therapy for young stutterers. *Journal of Speech and Hearing Disorders, 37*, 222–232.

Egolf, D. B., Shames, G. H., & Seltzer, H. N. (1971). The effects of time-out on the fluency of stutterers in group therapy. *Journal of Communication Disorders, 4*, 111–118.

Eisenberg, A. M., & Smith, R. R., Jr. (1971). *Nonverbal communication*. New York: Bobbs-Merrill.

Ekman, P. (1964). Body position, facial expression, and verbal behavior during interviews. *Journal of Abnormal and Social Psychology, 68*, 3, 295–301.

_____ (1985). *Telling Lies*. New York: Norton.

Ekman, P., & Friesen, W. (1968). Nonverbal behavior in psychotherapy research. *Research in psychotherapy, 3*, 179–215.

_____ (1971). *Emotion in the human face*. New York: Bobbs-Merrill.

_____ (1974). Detecting deception from the body or face. *Journal of Personality and Social Psychology, 29*, 288–298.

Elbert, M. (1989). Generalization in the treatment of phonological disorders. In L. V. McReynolds and J. E. Spradlin (Eds.), *Generalization strategies in the treatment of communication disorders* (pp. 31–43). Philadelphia: B. C. Decker.

Ellis, A. (1962). *Reason and emotion in psychotherapy*. New York: Lyle Stuart.

Emmert, P., & Brooks, W. D. (Eds.) (1970). *Methods of research in communication.* Boston: Houghton Mifflin.

Fairbanks, G. (1954). A theory of the speech organism as a servosystem. *Journal of Speech and Hearing Disorders, 19,* 133–139.

Farver, J. A., & Howes, C. (1988). Cross-cultural differences in social interaction: A comparison of American and Indonesian children. *Journal of Cross-Cultural Psychology, 19*(2), 203–215.

Ferster, C. B. (1957). Withdrawal of positive reinforcement as punishment. *Science, 126,* 509.

Feyereisen, P., & de Lannoy, J. (1991). *Gestures and speech: Psychological investigations.* New York: Cambridge Press.

Fillmore, C. J. (1968). The case for case. In E. Bach and R. T. Harms (Eds.), *Universals in linguistic theory.* New York: Holt, Rinehart & Winston.

Fisher, H. B., & Logemann, J. A. (1971). *Fisher-Logemann test of articulation competence.* Boston: Houghton Mifflin.

Fishman, J. A., & Luders, E. (1972). What has the sociology of language to say to the teacher. In C. B. Cazden, V. P. John, and D. Hymes (Eds.), *The functions of language.* New York: Teachers College Press.

Flavell, J. H. (1970). Developmental studies of mediated memory. In H. W. Reese & L. P. Lipsett (Eds.), *Advances in child development and behavior* (Vol. 5). New York: Academic Press.

Flew, A. (1961). *Hume's philosophy of belief.* New York: The Humanities Press.

Flower, R. M. (1984). *Delivery of speech-language pathology and audiology services.* Baltimore, MD: Williams & Wilkins.

Frank, J. D. (1961). *Persuasion and healing.* Baltimore: Johns Hopkins Press.

Frankel, S. A., & Frankel, E. B. (1970). Nonverbal behavior in a selected group of negro and white males. *Psychosomatics, 11,* 2, 127–132.

Frazier, N., & Sadker, M. (1973). *Sexism in school and society.* New York: Harper & Row.

Freud, S. (1933). *A general introduction to psychoanalysis.* New York: Norton.

Fromm-Reichmann, F. (1963). Psychiatric aspects of anxiety. In M. R. Stein, A. J. Vidich, and D. M. White (Eds.), *Identity and anxiety* (pp. 129–144). New York: The Free Press.

Gagné, R. M. (1970). *The conditions of learning.* New York: Holt, Rinehart & Winston.

Gagné, R. M., Briggs, L. J., & Wager, W. W. (1988). *Principles of instructional design.* New York: Holt, Rinehart, & Winston.

Gardner, R. A. (1982). *Psychotherapeutic approaches to the resistant child.* New York: Aronson.

George, R. L., & Dustin, D. (1988). *Group counseling: Theory and practice.* Englewood Cliffs, NJ: Prentice-Hall.

Giffin, K., & Patton, B. R. (1971). *Fundamentals of interpersonal communication.* New York: Harper & Row.

Gladding, S. T. (1991). *Group work: A counseling specialty.* New York: Merrill/Macmillan.

Goldberg, S. A. (1981). *Behavioral cognitive stuttering therapy.* Tigard, OR: C.C. Publications.

_____ (1989). An analysis of children's case structure grammar. American Speech and Hearing Association, Annual Conference, St. Louis, MO.

_____ (1990). Identification of clinical skills and their relationship to clinical training. American Speech-Language-Hearing Association Annual Conference, Seattle.

_____ (1991). The demise of stuttering therapy. American Speech-Language-Hearing Association Annual Conference, Atlanta, GA.

Goldberg, S. A., & Culatta, R. (1991). The demise of stuttering therapy: An indictment. American Speech-Language-Hearing Association, Annual Conference, Atlanta, GA.

Goldiamond, I. (1965). Stuttering and fluency as manipulatable operant response classes. In L. Krasner and L. P. Ullman (Eds.), *Research in behavior modification.* New York: Holt, Rinehart & Winston.

Golffing, F. (Trans.). (1956). *Nietzsche: The birth of tragedy and The genealogy of morals.* Garden City, NY: Doubleday.

Gollnick, D., & Chinn, P. (1990). *Multicultural education in a pluralistic society* (3rd ed.). New York: Merrill/Macmillan.

Goodenough, W. (1987). Multi-culturalism as the normal human experience. In E. M. Effy & W. L. Partridge (Eds.), *Applied anthropology in America* (2nd ed.). New York: Columbia University Press.

Gotlib, I. H. (1982). Self-reinforcement and depression in interpersonal interaction: The role of performance level. *Journal of Abnormal Psychology, 91,* 3–13.

Grant, E. C. (1968). An ethological description of nonverbal behavior during interview. *British Journal of Medical Psychology, 41*, 2, 177–184.

Hall, E. T. (1959). *The silent language.* Garden City, NY: Doubleday.

Ham, R. E. (1990). *Therapy of stuttering.* Englewood Cliffs, NJ: Prentice-Hall.

Hammill, D., Brown, B. S., Larsen, S. C., & Wiederholt, J. (1980). *Test of adolescent language.* Austin, TX: Pro-Ed.

Hanson, M. J. (1990). *California early intervention personnel model, personnel standards and personnel preparation plan: Final report.* San Francisco, CA: San Francisco State University.

Hegde, M. N., & Davis, D. (1992). *Clinical methods and practicum in speech-language pathology.* San Diego: Singular Publishing Group.

Herbert, F. (1965). *Dune.* New York: Ace Books.

Hewes, G. W. (1957). World distribution of certain postural habits. *American Anthropologist, 57*, 231–244.

Higgins E., & Warner, R. (1975). Counseling blacks. *Personnel and Guidance Journal, 53*, 383–386.

Hill, J., & Carper, M. (1985). Group therapeutic approaches with the head injured. *Cognitive Rehabilitation, 3*, 18–29.

Hodge, R., & Kress, G. (1988). *Social semiotics.* Cambridge: Polity Press.

Hodgkin, R. A. (1985). *Playing and exploring.* New York: Methuen.

Hofmeister, A. (1982). Microcomputers in perspective. *Exceptional Children, 49*(2), 115–122.

Holland, A. (1977). Communicative ability in daily living: Its measurement and observation. Paper presented at *Academy of Aphasia*, Montreal, Canada.

Holland, A. L. (1967). Some applications of behavioral principles to clinical speech problems. *Journal of Speech and Hearing Disorders, 32*, 11–18.

Holland, A. L., & Matthews, J. (1963). Application of teaching machine concepts to speech pathology and audiology. *ASHA, 5*, 474–482.

Holland A. L., & Reinmuth, O. M. (1982). Aphasia in adults. In G. H. Shames and E. H. Wiig (Eds.), *Human communication disorders* (pp. 426–452). Columbus, OH: Merrill/Macmillan.

Hollander, M., & Kazaoka, K. (1988). Behavior therapy groups. In S. Long (Ed.), *Six group therapies* (pp. 257–326). New York: Plenum.

Hollingshead, A. B. (1958). Factors associated with prevalence of mental illness. In E. E. Maccoby, T. M. Newcomb, & E. L. Hartley (Eds.), *Readings in social psychology* (pp. 425–436). New York: Holt, Rinehart & Winston.

Holt, J. (1964). *How children fail.* New York: Dell.

Hunt, P., Goetz, L., Alwell, M., & Sailor, W. (1986). Teaching generalized communication responses through an interrupted behavior chain strategy. *Journal of the Association for Persons with Severe Handicaps, 11*, 196–204.

Husserl, E. (1964). *The idea of phenomenology.* The Hague: Maritnus Nijhoff.

Huxley, R., & Ingram, E. (Eds.). (1971). *Language acquisition: Models and methods.* New York: Academic Press.

Infield, L. (Ed.). (1963). *Kant: Lectures on ethics.* New York: Harper & Row.

Ingham, R. J. (1990). Commentary on Perkins (1990) and Moore and Perkins (1990): On the valid role of reliability in identifying "What is stuttering?" *Journal of Speech and Hearing Disorders, 55*(3), 394–397.

Ingram, D. (1989). *Phonological disability in children.* San Diego: Singular Press Group.

Johnson, M. B., Whitman, T. L., & Johnson, M. (1980). Teaching addition and subtraction to mentally retarded children: A self-instructional program. *Applied Research in Mental Retardation, 1*, 141–160.

Johnson, W. (1934). The influence of stuttering on the attitudes and adaptations of the stutterer. *Journal of Social Psychology, 5*, 410–420.

Johnson, W. & Associates. (1959). *The onset of stuttering.* Minneapolis: University of Minnesota Press.

Kalunger, G., & Kalunger, M. F. (1986). *Human development: The span of life* (3rd ed.). Columbus, OH: Merrill/Macmillan.

Kanfer, F. (1968). Issues and ethics in behavior manipulation. In H. N. Sloane Jr. and B. D. MacAulay (Eds.), *Operant procedures in remedial speech and language training* (pp. 411–423). New York: Houghton Mifflin.

Kausler, D. (1974). *Psychology of verbal learning and memory.* New York: Academic Press.

Keeney, T. J., Cannizzo, S. R., & Flavell, J. H. (1967). Spontaneous and induced verbal rehearsal in a recall task. *Child Development, 38,* 953–966.

Kent, R. (1981). Normal aspects of articulation. In J. E. Bernthal and N. W. Bankson, *Articulation disorders* (pp. 5–60). Englewood Cliffs, NJ: Prentice-Hall.

Kockelmans, J. (1965). *Martin Heidegger: A first introduction to his philosophy.* Pittsburgh: Duquesne University Press.

Korzybski, A. (1958). *Science and sanity.* Lakeville, CN: The International Non-Aristotelian Library.

Krishnamurti, J. (1970). *Think on these things.* New York: Harper & Row.

——— (1976). *The awakening of intelligence.* New York: Avon Books.

Kupfer, D. J., Maser, J. D., Blehar, M. C., & Miller, R. (1987). Behavioral assessment in depression. In J. D. Maser (Ed.), *Depression and expressive behavior* (pp. 1–15). Hillsdale, NJ: Lawrence Erlbaum.

Kwant, R. C. (1963). *The phenomenological philosophy of Merleau-Ponty.* Pittsburgh, PA: Duquesne University Press.

Kyrios, M., Prior, M., Oberklaid, R., Demetriou, A., La Trobe, U., and Bundoora, V. (1989). Cross-cultural studies of temperament: Temperament in Greek infants. *International Journal of Psychology, 24*(5), 585–603.

Lambert, M. C., Weisz, J. R., & Knight, F. (1989). Over- and undercontrolled clinic referral problems of Jamaican and American children and adolescents: The culture general and the culture specific. *Journal of Consulting and Clinical Psychology, 57,* 4, 467–472.

Lahey, M. (1988). *Language disorders & language development.* New York: Macmillan.

Lafleur, L. J. (1960). (Trans.) *Descartes: Discourse on method and meditations.* New York: Bobbs-Merrill.

Larson, G. W., & Summers, P. A. (1976). Response patterns of preschool-age children to the Northwestern Syntax Screening Test. *Journal of Speech and Hearing Disorders, 41,* 486–497.

Latner, J. (1973). *The gestalt therapy book.* New York: Julian Press.

Le Croy, C. W. (1986). An analysis of the effects of gender on outcome in group treatment with young adolescents. *Journal of Youth and Adolescence, 15,* 497–508.

Lee, L. (1971). *Northwestern syntax screening test (NSST).* Evanston, IL: Northwestern University Press.

Leonard, L. B. (1984). Normal language acquisition: Some recent findings and clinical implications. In A. L. Holland (Ed.), *Language disorders in children* (pp. 1–36). San Diego, CA: College-Hill Press.

Lindsey, J. D. (1987). *Computers and exceptional individuals.* Columbus, OH: Merrill/Macmillan.

Long, S. (1988). The six group therapies compared. In S. Long (Ed.), *Six group therapies* (pp. 327–338). New York: Plenum.

Lovaas, O. I. (1966). A program for the establishment of speech in psychotic children. In J. K. Wing (Ed.), *Early childhood autism.* New York: Pergamon.

Lovaas, O. I., Freitag, G., Gold, V. J., & Kassorla, I. C. (1965). Experimental studies in childhood schizophrenia: Analysis of self-destructive behavior. *Journal of Experimental Child Psychology, 2,* 67–84.

Lund, N. J., & Duchan, J. F. (1988). *Assessing children's language in naturalistic contexts.* Englewood Cliffs, NJ: Prentice-Hall.

Martin, R., Haroldson, S. K., & Friden, K. A. (1984). Stuttering and speech naturalness. *Journal of Speech and Hearing Research, 49,* 53–58.

Maslow, A. H. (1968). *Towards a psychology of being.* New York: Van Nostrand Reinhold.

Matthews, J. (1990). The professions of speech-language pathology and audiology. In G. H. Shames and E. H. Wiig (Eds.), *Human communication disorders: An introduction* (3rd ed.). New York: Merrill/Macmillan.

——— (1986). Historical prologue. In G. H. Shames and H. Rubin (Eds.), *Stuttering, then and now* (pp. 5–18). Columbus, OH: Merrill/Macmillan.

May, R. (1961). The emergence of existential psychology. In R. May (Ed.), *Existential psychology* (pp. 11–51). New York: Random House.

Mayer, R. E. (1983). *Thinking, problem solving, cognition.* New York: W. H. Freeman.

——— (1987). Instructional variables that influence cognitive processes during reading. In

B. K. Britton & S. M. Glynn (Eds.), *Historical foundations of educational psychology* (pp. 327–347). New York: Plenum Press.

——— (1988). Learning strategies: An overview. In C. E. Weinstein, E. T. Goetz, & P. A. Alexander (Eds.), *Learning and study strategies* (pp. 11–12). New York: Academic Press.

McDonald, F. I. (1964). *Screening deep test of articulation.* Pittsburgh: Stanwix House.

McKeachie, W. J. (1988). The need for study strategy training. In C. E. Weinstein, E. T. Goetz, & P. A. Alexander (Eds.), *Learning and study strategies* (pp. 3–9). New York: Academic Press.

McKinley, V. (1987). Group therapy as a treatment modality of special value for Hispanic patients. *International Journal of Group Psychotherapy, 37*(2), 255–268.

McKirnan, D. J., & Hamayan, E. V. (1984). Speech norms and attitudes toward outgroup members: A test of a model in a bicultural context. *Journal of Language and Social Psychology, 3,* 21–38.

McReynolds, L. V., & Kearns, K. P. (1983). *Single-subject experimental designs in communicative disorders.* Baltimore: University Park Press.

McShane, J. (1980). *Learning to talk.* Cambridge, England: Cambridge University Press.

Mead, M. (1930). Adolescence in primitive and modern society. In V. F. Calverton and S. D. Schmalhausen (Eds.), *The new generation.* New York: Macauley.

Meichenbaum, D. (1977). *Cognitive-behavior modification.* New York: Plenum Press.

Merleau-Ponty, M. (1962). *Phenomenology of perception.* (C. Smith, Trans.). New York: Humanities Press.

Miller, E. S. (1979). *Introduction to cultural anthropology.* Englewood Cliffs, NJ: Prentice-Hall.

Miller, G. A., & Nicely, P. E. (1955). An analysis of perceptual confusions among some English consonants. *Journal of the Acoustical Society of America, 27,* 347.

Molyneaux, D., & Lane, V. W. (1982). *Effective interviewing.* New York: Allyn & Bacon.

——— (1992). *Dynamics of Communication Development.* Englewood Cliffs, NJ: Prentice-Hall.

Montagu, A. (1972). *Statement on race: An annotated elaboration and exposition of the four statements on race issues by the United Nations Educational, Scientific, and Cultural Organization.* New York: Oxford University Press.

Montes, J., & Erickson, J. G. (1990). Bilingual stuttering: Exploring a diagnostic dilemma. *Ethnotes, 1,* 14–15.

Morgenstern, J. (1956). Socioeconomic factors in stuttering. *Journal of Speech and Hearing Disorders, 21,* 25–33.

Mowrer, D. E. (1982). *Methods of modifying speech behaviors.* (2nd ed.). Columbus, OH: Merrill/Macmillan.

Murphy, A. T. (1982). The clinical process and the speech-language pathologist. In G. H. Shames and E. H. Wiig, *Human communication disorders* (pp. 453–474). Columbus, OH: Merrill.

Myrick, R. D. (1987). *Developmental guidance and counseling: A practical approach.* Minneapolis: Educational Media Corporation.

Nagel, E. (1961). *The structure of science.* New York: Harcourt, Brace & World.

Naremore, R. C. (Ed.). (1984). *Language science.* San Diego, CA: College-Hill Press.

Naroll, R., & Naroll, F. (1963). On the basis of exotic data. *Man, 25,* 24–26.

Nicolosi, L., Harryman, E., & Kresheck, J. (1978). *Terminology of communication disorders: Speech, language, hearing.* Baltimore: Williams & Wilkins.

Orlick, T., & Botterill, C. (1975). *Every kid can win.* Chicago: Nelson-Hall.

Ostwald, M. (Trans.) (1962). *Aristotle: Nicomachean ethics.* New York: Bobbs-Merrill.

Pachalska, M. K. (1982). Presentation of the state of social dependence of patients afflicted with aphasia. *American Journal of Social Psychiatry, 2,* 51–53.

Paden, E. P. (1970). *A history of the American speech and hearing association, 1925–1958.* Washington, DC: American Speech and Hearing Association.

Pap, A. (1962). *An introduction to the philosophy of science.* New York: The Free Press of Glencoe.

Parsons, T. (Ed.) (1947). *Max Weber: The theory of social and economic organization.* New York: Oxford University Press.

Perkins, W. H. (1986). Functions and malfunctions of theories in therapies. *ASHA, 28,* 2, 31–33.

——— (1990). What is stuttering? *Journal of Speech and Hearing Disorders, 55*(3), 370–382.

Perls, F. S. (1965). *Three approaches to psychotherapy I: Frederick Perls.* Psychological Films, Inc.

────── (1969). *Gestalt therapy verbatim.* Lafayette, CA: Real People Press.

Perls, F. S., Hefferline, R. E., & Goodman, P. (1951). *Gestalt therapy.* New York: Dell Publishing.

Peters, T. J., & Guitar, B. (1991). *Stuttering: An integrated approach to its nature and treatment.* Baltimore: Williams & Wilkins.

Piaget, J. (1954). *The construction of reality in the child.* New York: Basic Books.

Piercy, F., & Sprenkle, D. (1986). *Family therapy sourcebook.* New York: Guilford.

Poole, E. (1934). Genetic development of articulation of consonant sounds in speech. *Elementary English Review, 11,* 159–161.

Pressley, M., Levin, J. R., & Bryant, S. L. (1983). Memory strategy instruction during adolescence: When is explicit instruction needed? In M. Pressley and J. R. Levin (Eds.), *Cognitive strategy research: Psychological foundations* (pp. 25–49). New York: Springer-Verlag.

Ramirez, M., & Castaneda, A. (1974). *Cultural democracy, bicognitive development, and education.* New York: Academic Press.

Reichenbach, H. (1961). *The rise of scientific philosophy.* Berkeley, CA: University of California Press.

Resendiz, P. S., & Fox, R. A. (1985). Reflection-impulsivity in Mexican children: Cross-cultural relationships. *Journal of General Psychology, 112*(3), 285–290.

Resnick, L., & Ford, W. (1981). *The psychology of mathematics for instruction.* Hillsdale, NJ: Erlbaum.

Rogers, C. R. (1965). *Client-centered therapy.* Boston: Houghton Mifflin.

────── (1970). *On becoming a person.* Boston: Houghton Mifflin.

Rohwer, W. D., Jr. (1973). Elaboration and learning in childhood and adolescence. In H. W. Reese (Ed.), *Advances in child development and behavior* (pp. 2–57). (Vol. 8). New York: Academic Press.

Rollin, W. J. (1987). *The psychology of communication disorders in individuals and their families.* Englewood Cliffs, NJ: Prentice-Hall.

Rosenbek, J. C., LaPointe, L. L., & Wertz, R. T. (1989). *Aphasia: A clinical approach.* Austin, TX: Pro-Ed.

Rosenberg, P. P. (1984). Support groups: A special therapeutic entity. *Small Group Behavior, 15* (2), 173–186.

Rubin, H. (1986). Cognitive therapy. In G. Shames & H. Rubin (Eds.), *Stuttering then and now.* Columbus, OH: Merrill/Macmillan.

Rubin H., & Culatta, R. A. (1971). A point of view about fluency. *ASHA, 13,* 380–384.

────── (1974). Stuttering as an after effect of normal developmental disfluency. *Clinical Pediatrics, 13,* 172–176.

Russell, B. (1961). *The basic writings of Bertrand Russell.* R. E. Egner and L. E. Denonn (Eds.). New York: Simon & Schuster, p. 345.

Sadker, M., Sadker, D., & Steindam, S. (1989). Gender equity and educational reform. *Educational Leadership, 46,* 6, 44–47.

Sailor, W., Gee, K., & Karasoff, P. (1991). Restructuring schools to enable full inclusion. In M. Snell (Ed.), *Systematic instruction of persons with severe disabilities* (4th ed.). New York: Merrill/Macmillan.

Saleh, M. A. (1986). Cultural perspectives: Implications for counseling in the Arab world. *School Psychology International, 7*(2), 71–75.

Sapir, E. (1921). *Language.* New York: Harcourt, Brace & World.

Satir, V. (1967). *Conjoint family therapy* (Rev. Ed.). Palo Alto, CA: Science and Behavior Books.

Scheflen, A. E. (1967). On the structuring of human communication. *American Behavioral Scientist, 10,* 8, 8–12.

Scheuerle, J. (1992). *Counseling in speech-language pathology and audiology.* New York: Merrill/Macmillan.

Schneewind, J. B. (Ed.) (1965). *Mill's ethical writings.* New York: Collier Books.

Shames, G. H. (1989). Stuttering: An RFP for a cultural perspective. *Journal of Fluency Disorders, 14,* 67–77.

Shames, G. H., & Egolf, D. B. (1976). *Operant conditioning and the management of stuttering: A book for clinicians.* Englewood Cliffs, NJ: Prentice-Hall.

Shames, G. H., & Florance, C. L. (1980). *Stutter-free speech: A goal for therapy.* Columbus, OH: Merrill/Macmillan.

Shames, G. H., & Rubin, H. (1986). The roles of the client and the clinician during therapy. In G. H. Shames and H. Rubin (Eds.), *Stuttering,* *then and now* (pp. 261–270). Columbus, OH: Merrill/Macmillan.

Shames, G. H., & Sherrick, C. E., Jr. (1963). A discussion of nonfluency and stuttering as operant behavior. *Journal of Speech and Hearing Disorders, 28,* 13–18.

Shine, R. E. (1980). *Systematic fluency training for children.* Tigard, OR: C.C. Publications.

Shipley, K. G. (1992). *Interviewing and counseling in communicative disorders.* New York: Merrill/Macmillan.

Silverman, F. H. (1983). *Legal aspects of speech-language pathology and audiology.* Englewood Cliffs, NJ: Prentice-Hall.

_____ (1987). *Microcomputers in speech-language pathology and audiology: A primer.* Englewood Cliffs, NJ: Prentice-Hall.

Skinner, B. F. (1948). *Walden two.* New York: Macmillan.

_____ (1953). *Science and human behavior.* New York: Macmillan.

_____ (1957). *Verbal behavior.* New York: Appleton-Century-Crofts.

Sloane, H. N., Jr., & MacAulay, B. D. (Eds.). (1968). *Operant procedures in remedial speech and language training.* New York: Houghton Mifflin.

Snidecor, J. C. (1947). Why the Indian does not stutter. *Quarterly Journal of Speech, 33,* 493–495.

Spolsky, B. (1972). The language education of minority children. In B. Spolsky (Ed.), *The language education of minority children* (pp. 1–10). Rowley, MA: Newbury House.

Stockard, J., & Johnson, M. M. (1980). *Sex roles: Sex inequality and sex role development.* Englewood Cliffs, NJ: Prentice-Hall.

Suzuki, D. T. (1955). *Studies in Zen.* New York: Dell Publishing.

Taylor, O. (1989). Old wine and new bottles: Some things change yet remain the same. *ASHA, 31,* 9, 72–73.

Taylor, O. L. (1992). In L. Cole & V. R. Deal (Eds.), *Communication disorders in multicultural populations.* Rockville, MD: American Speech-Language-Hearing Association.

Teasdale, G., & Jennett, B. (1974). Assessment of coma and impaired consciousness. *Lancet, 2,* 81.

Templin, M. C. (1957). *Certain language skills in children, their development and interrelationships. Institute of child welfare, monograph series, No. 26, 54.* Minneapolis: University of Minnesota Press.

Tulving, E., & Donaldson, W. (Eds.). (1972). *Organization of memory.* New York: Academic Press.

Turkel, S. (1972). *Working.* New York: Avon Books.

Tyack, D., & Gottsleben, R. (1974). *Language sampling, analysis, and training: A handbook for teachers and clinicians.* Palo Alto, CA: Consulting Psychologists Press.

Van Riper, C. (1971). *The nature of stuttering.* Englewood Cliffs, NJ: Prentice-Hall.

_____ (1978). *Speech correction principles and methods.* Englewood Cliffs, NJ: Prentice-Hall.

Vygotsky, L. S. (1978). *Mind in society: The development of higher psychological processes.* M. Cole, V. John-Steiner, S. Scribner & E. Souberman (Eds.). Cambridge, MA: Harvard University Press.

Walker, H. M. (1979). *The acting-out child.* Boston: Allyn & Bacon.

Waters, H. S., & Andreassen, C. (1983). Children's use of memory strategies under instruction. In M. Pressley & J. R. Levin (Eds.), *Cognitive Strategy Research: Psychological Foundations* (pp. 3–24). New York: Springer-Verlag.

Watts, A. W. (1957). *The way of Zen.* New York: New American Library.

Webb, E. J., Campbell, D. T., Schwartz, R. D., & Sechrest, L. (1966). *Unobtrusive measures.* Chicago: Rand McNally & Co.

Webster, R. (1980). Evolution of a target-based therapy for stuttering. *Journal of Fluency Disorders, 5,* 303–320.

Wellman, B. I., Case, I., Mengurt, I., and Bradbury, D. (1931). Speech sounds of young children. *University of Iowa Studies in Child Welfare, 5.*

Wepman, J., Jones, L. V., Bock, R. D., & Van Pelt, D. (1960). Studies in aphasia: Background and theoretical formulations. *Journal of Speech and Hearing Disorders, 25,* 323–332.

Wessler, R. L. (1986). Rational-emotive therapy in groups. In A. Ellis & R. Grieger (Eds.), *Handbook of Rational-Emotive Therapy* (Vol. 2), (pp. 295–314). New York: Springer.

West, R. W., & Ansberry, M. (1968). *The rehabilitation of speech* (4th ed.). New York: Harper & Row.

Whitaker, C. A., & Malone, T. P. (1953). *The roots of psychotherapy.* New York: McGraw-Hill.

Whorf, B. (1956). Science and Linguistics. In J. Carrol (Ed.), *Language, thought and reality* (pp. 207–219). New York: John Wiley & Sons.

Williams, D. E., Darley, F. L., & Spriesterbach, D. C. (1978). *Diagnostic methods in speech pathology*. New York: Harper & Row.

Wilson, G. T. (1989). Behavior therapy. In R. J. Corsini & D. Wedding (Eds.), *Current psychotherapies* (4th ed.) (pp. 241–282). Itasca, IL: Peacock.

Winitz, H. (1969). *Articulatory acquisition and behavior*. Englewood Cliffs, NJ: Prentice-Hall.

Winnicott, D. W. (1971). *Playing and reality*. London: Tavistock.

Wolf, A. (1963). The psychoanalysis of groups. In M. Rosenbaum & M. Berger (Eds.), *Group psychotherapy and group function*. New York: Hawthorn.

Wood, D., Bruner, J. S., & Ross, G. (1976). The role of tutoring in problem-solving. *Journal of Child Psychology and Psychiatry, 17,* 89–100.

Woolf, G. (1967). Perceptions of stuttering inventory. *British Journal of Disorders of Communication, 2,* 158–177.

Wulf, H. H. (1973). *Aphasia: My world alone*. Detroit: Wayne State University Press.

Yetman, N. R. (Ed.) (1985). *Majority and minority: The dynamics of race and ethnicity in American life* (4th ed.). Boston: Allyn & Bacon.

Zeskind, P. S. (1983). Cross-cultural differences in maternal perceptions of cries of low- and high-risk infants. *Child Development, 54,* 5, 1119–1128.

Index

Activities. *See* Client activities; Student learning activities
Adolescents. *See individual topics*
Adults. *See individual topics*
African American. *See* Culture
Age. *See* Culture
Albertini, J. A., 210
Alexander, P. A., 247
American Speech-Language-Hearing Association, 47–48, 208
　observation supplement, 267–268
　code of ethics, 269–271
Amplitude of response, 76
Andreassen, C., 242
Andrews, G., 186
Ansberry, M., 109
Anxiety, 210, 252
Aphasia, 130–133
　apraxia, 9
　auditory agnosia, 9
　changing behaviors, 214
　communicative behavior, 132, 133
　diagnostic procedures, 251
　dysarthria, 10
　intervention, 42–43, 209, 210, 237
　labels, 4–5
　motor behavior, 132
　sensory behavior, 132
　support groups, 222
　unstructured activities, 216
　Wepman's operational levels of CNS, 6–10
Aristotle, 44
Aronson, A. E., 67, 251
Articulation disorders. *See* Phonological and articulation disorders
Asian. *See* Culture
Assessment, *See* Diagnostic Tests
Audiological screening, 196–197
Audiotapes. *See* Data collection, audiotapes

Aversive stimuli, 185–186, 189–191
Ayer, A. J., 27, 45

Bales, R. F., 65
Bandura, A., 185, 203, 238
Bangert, J., 70, 195
Bankson, N. W., 87, 92, 95, 112, 249
Barfield, J., 16
Beck, A. T., 214
Behaviors. *See also* Nonverbal behaviors
　consequences for actions, 213–214
　setting limits, 213
Behavior modification. *See* Operant conditioning
Behrmann, M., 239
Berkeley, G., 27
Berlo, D. K., 159
Berne, E., 217
Bernthal, J. E., 87, 92, 95, 112, 251
Beukelman, D. R., 140
Birdwhistell, R. L., 154, 160
Blehar, M. C., 159
Block, R. D., 6
Bloodstein, O., 98, 99, 110, 112
Bluemel, C. S., 99
Boone, D. R., 35, 112, 184
Borkowski, J. G., 245
Bosanquet, B., 32
Botterill, C., 240
Bricker, D. D., 232
Bricker, W. A., 232
Briggs, L. J., 203
Brooks, W. D., 69
Brown, A. L., 243
Brown, B. S., 17
Brown, R., 64, 122, 126, 140
Bruner, J. S., 230
Brutten, E. J., 184, 238
Bryant, S. L., 243
Buchel, F. P., 245

INDEX

Bull, P. E., 163
Buscaglia, L. F., 49

California Department of Education, 209
Campbell, D. T., 77
Campbell, J., 21, 45
Cannizzo, S. R., 242
Carper, M., 211, 216
Carroll, J. B., 243
Case, J. L., 112
Castaneda, A., 15
Castaneda, C., 51
Center for Fluency Development, 223
Chabon, S. S., 208, 210
Chaining, 175
Cheng, L.R.I., 15, 29, 221, 222
Child Development, 20–21
Children. *See individual topics*
Chinn, P., 12, 16, 18, 29, 209, 221
Clark, F. V., 26
Cleft palate speech, 110–111
   articulation, 111
   hypernasality, 110–111
   nasal fricative, 111
Client activities, elements of
   clinician directed, 214–215
   competition, 237
   discovery, 237
   group settings, 212
   immersion, 237
   instructional objectives, 238
   learning activities, 238–240
   simulations, 215
   specific competencies, 236–238
   terminal competencies, 232–236
   transitional, 237
   unstructured, 215
Client behavioral analysis, 260–262
Clinical goals
   diagnostic therapy, 258
   purpose of therapy, 256–257
   role expectations, 259
   trust, 257–258
Clinical intuition, 35–37
Clinical preparation
   goals, 258–260
   reviewing clincal records, 250–252
   telephone interview, 250–256
Clinical records, 250–252
Clinical strategies
   cognitive psychology scaffolding, 228–229
   competency based clinical intervention, 229–238
   computer-assisted instruction, 240–241
   memory, 242–243
   retrieval, 243–245

Clinician behavioral analysis, 260, 263–266
Clinician personality traits
   charisma, 39
   empathy, 39, 219
   group leadership, 219–220
   negative traits, 41–44
   positive traits, 40–41
   self-image, 50
Chomsky, N., 91, 94–97, 175
Cognition
   accommodation, 25
   adaptive behavior, 25
   assimilation, 25
   associative learning, 241
   cognitive psychology scaffolding, 230–231
   concrete operations, 25
   fundamental processes, 246
   learning styles, 22–23, 177
   levels of learning, 26
   memory, 242–243
   processes, 246
   retrieval, 241–244
   saliency, 241
   sensorimotor period, 25
   strategies, 240–243
Cole, G. D. H., 44
Cole, L., 12, 29
Coma, 134
Compton, C., 140
Cooper, E. B., 20
Communication models
   cultural communication model, 10–11
   general communication system, 5–6
   Wepman's operational levels of CNS, 6–9
Community centers, 209–210
Computer-assisted instruction
   demonstration/information, 239
   drill-and-practice software, 238, 241
   simulation software, 240–241
   tutorial software, 240, 241
Consistency, 200
Consultative model, 209
Corey, G., 211, 214, 223
Cornett, B. S., 208, 210
Corsini, R. J., 217, 219
Costello, J., 20, 67, 70, 104
Counseling
   Adlerian, 217
   counselor traits, 39–44
   gestalt, 217
   group settings, 216–218
   Jungian, 217
   nondirective, 216
   psychoanalysis, 217
   role of nonverbal behaviors, 155–158

INDEX

rational-emotive, 217
transactional analysis, 217
Counters. *See* Data collection, counters
Criteria for advancement, 70, 194–195
Cronbach, L. J., 22, 29, 178, 203, 245
Culatta, R., 12, 15, 22, 44, 51, 98, 112, 135, 217, 223
Cultural communication model, 10–11
Culture
   African American, 12, 13, 15, 222
   age, 17, 220–221, 252
   Asian, 14, 15, 20, 21, 222
   class, 18–19, 24
   differences and disorders, 24, 252
   ethnicity, 14, 221–222, 252
   exceptionality, 17–18
   gender/sex, 16–17
   group variables, 221–222
   Hispanic, 15, 221–222
   interaction rules and behaviors, 21
   language, 23–25, 221–222
   learning styles, 22
   macroculture, 3, 12, 19
   microculture, 3, 12–19
   Native American, 15, 21
   nonverbal behaviors, 160
   regional, 18
   religion, 16, 22
   societal reactions, 21–22

Darley, F. L., 99, 120, 140
Data collection
   amplitude of response, 76
   audiotapes, 66
   counters, 66–67
   group settings, 218–219
   latency of response, 73–76
   learning curve, 72–73
   number of correct responses, 69, 218
   percentage of correct repsonses, 69, 218
   rating scales, 76
   reasons for, 60–61
   simple enumeration, 69
   type token ratio, 73
   units of measurement, 68–77
   videotapes, 65–66
   written forms, 67
Davis, D., 70
Deal, V. R., 15, 29
Deci, E. L., 61, 77
De Charms, R., 61, 77
De Lannoy, J., 163
Delgado, M., 222, 223
Dependent variable, 38
Descartes, R., 27

Descrimination learning, 175
Deutsch, M., 65
Diagnostic tests
   Communicative Ability in Daily Living (CADL), 4
   language sampling, 64
   Northwestern Syntax Screening Test, 19
   Peabody Picture Vocabulary Test, 23
Diagnostic therapy, 260
Diedrich, W., 70, 195
Dinkmeyer, D. C., 219
Dinkmeyer, D. C., Jr., 219
Disabled. *See* Culture, exceptionality
Donaldson, W., 243
Dreyfus, H. L., 35, 51, 252, 266
Dreyfus, S. E., 35, 51, 252, 266
Duchan, J. F., 125, 140, 159, 251
Duffy, G. G., 242, 247
Dunn, R., 22
Dustin, D., 220
Dworkin, J. P., 67

Egolf, D. B., 20, 22, 211, 214
Eisenberg, A. M., 154
Ekman, P., 158, 159, 160, 162, 163
Elbert, M., 238
Ellis, A., 44, 217
Emblems, 155
Emmert, P., 69
Empathy. *See* Clinician personality traits
Encoding, 242–243
Erickson, J., 16
Ethics, ASHA code of, 47–48, 269–270
Experience
   perceptions, 28
   private meanings, 27

Fairbanks, G., 5
Farver, J. A., 21
Ferster, C. B., 190
Feyereisen, P., 163
Filmore, C. J., 123
Fisher, H. B., 64
Flavell, J. H., 242, 243
Flew, A., 195
Florence, C. L., 98, 215, 238
Flower, R. M., 208
Fluency. *See* Stuttering
Ford, W., 244
Fox, R. A., 23
Frank, J. D., 216
Frankel, E. B., 159
Frankel, S. A., 159
Frazier, N., 16
Freud, S., 44
Friesen, W., 158, 160, 162, 163

Gagné, R. M., 26, 29, 35, 172, 173, 203, 230, 245, 250
Gardner, R. A., 212
Gee, K., 209
Generalization
 new behaviors, 202
 group settings, 214–216
 strategies, 242–245
George, R. L., 20
Giffin, K., 50, 259
Gladding, S. T., 210, 211, 220, 223
Goals. *See* clinical goals
Goetz, L., 243
Goldberg, S. A., 12, 15, 17, 36, 44, 49, 51, 64, 99, 100–101, 112, 123, 209, 215, 223, 259
Goldiamond, I., 189
Golffing, F., 45
Gollnick, D., 12, 16, 18, 29, 209, 221
Goodenough, W., 12
Goodman, P., 48
Gotlib, I. H., 159
Gottsleben, R., 64
Group therapy, 207–223
 adolescents, 217, 220
 adults, 218, 221
 children, 217, 220
 competitiveness, 212
 control, 212–214
 cultural variables, 221–222
 functions, 210–219
 generalization, 214–216
 membership, 211, 212
 orientation, 214, 217
 qualities of group leader, 219–221
 setting, 208–210
 simulations, 215
 support groups, 222–223
 time management, 211–212
Guitar, B., 67, 251

Hall, E. T., 14, 29, 160, 163
Halle, N., 91, 94–97
Ham, R. E., 38
Hamayan, E. V., 221
Hammill, D., 17
Hanson, M. J., 208
Haroldson, S. K., 105
Harryman, E., 107, 112, 120
Hearing impaired, 209
Hedge, M N., 70
Hefferline, R. E., 48
Herbert, F., 36
Higgins, E., 222, 223
Hill, J., 211, 216
Hispanic. *See* Culture
Hodge, R., 160

Hodgkin, R. A., 237, 245
Holland, A. L., 4, 132, 133, 140, 179, 238
Hollander, M., 217
Hollingshead, A. B., 18
Holt, J., 177
Homosexuality, 16–17
Hume, D., 27, 195
Humm-Delgado, D., 222, 223
Hunt, P., 247
Husserl, E., 63
Huxley, R., 175

Illustrators, 156
Independent variable, 38
Infield, L., 44
Ingham, R. J., 20, 37, 64, 67, 104, 186
Ingram, D., 175

Johnson, B., 245
Johnson, M. B., 245
Johnson, M. M., 16
Johnson, W., 98
Jones, L. V., 6, 8

Kalunger, G., 17
Kalunger, M. F., 17
Kant, E., 44
Kausler, D., 175
Kazaoka, K., 217
Kearns, K. P., 37, 51
Keeney, T. J., 242
Kockelmans, J., 45
Korzybski, A., 4, 29
Kresheck, J., 107, 112, 120
Kress, G., 160
Krishnamurti, J., 49
Kupfer, D. J., 159
Kwant, R. C., 27
Kyrios, M., 20

Labels, 4
Lafleur, L. J., 27
Lahey, M., 64
Lambert, M. C., 16
Lane, V. W., 137, 138–139, 140, 215
Language and language disorders, child and adolescent
 diagnostic procedures, 251
 dialect, 24, 221–222
 English as a second language, 24, 209
 generalization, 242–243
 group setting, 210–211
 intervention, 73, 230, 232–235, 243
 labels, 4–5
 lexicon, 120, 121

INDEX

limited English proficiency, 24
metalinguistics, 134–140
morphology, 120, 121
parent information handout, 295–296
pragmatics, 123–128
retrieval strategies, 243–244
semantics, 26, 123
syntax, 122, 124–125, 127
LaPointe, C., 251
Larson, G. W., 19
Larson, S. C., 17
Latency of response, 73–74
Latino. *See* Culture
Latner, J., 217
Lawton, S. C., 243
Learning and retrieval
  levels, 173–177
  learning curve, 72
  stages, 172–173
LeCroy, C. W., 217
Lee, L., 19
Leonard, L. B., 127
Levin, J. R., 243
Lindsey, J. D., 240, 247
Locke, J., 27
Logemann, J. A., 64
Long, S., 220
Lovaas, O. I., 179, 189, 190
Lund, N. J., 159, 251

MacAulay, B. D., 179
McCormick, C. B., 247
McDonald, F. I., 64
McKeachie, W. J., 244, 247
McKinley, V., 222
McKirnan, D. J., 221
McReynolds, L. V., 37, 51
McShane, J., 135, 136–137, 140
Maladaptive behaviors, 198–199
Martin, R., 105
Maser, J. D., 159
Maslow, A. H., 49
Matthews, J., 47, 49, 51, 179
Maturation, 48–49
May, R., 45
Mayer, R. E., 230, 244, 247
Mead, M., 14
Mediation, 183
Memory
  encoding strategies, 240–241
  organizational strategies, 241
Meichenbaum, D., 183, 203, 214
Merleau-Ponty, M., 27
Metalinguistics, 134–139
Mill, J., 27, 44
Miller, E. S., 29

Miller, G., 247
Miller G. A., 97
Miller, R., 159
Molyneaux, D., 137, 138–139, 140, 215
Monitoring groups, 211, 217
Montagu, A., 15
Montes, J., 16
Morgenstern, J., 18
Motivation, 61
Mowrer, D. E., 69, 77
Multicultural. *See* Cultural
Murphy, A. T., 32, 40, 41, 220
Myrick, R. D., 212, 220, 223

Nagel, E., 37, 57
Naremore, R. C., 175
Naroll, F., 65
Naroll, R., 65
National Stuttering Project, 222, 223
Nicely, P. E., 97
Nicolosi, L., 107, 112, 120
Nietzsche, F. W., 44
Nonverbal behaviors
  arms/hands, 155–157
  clinical implications, 161–162, 221
  context, 158–160
  cultural variables, 221
  facial behaviors, 155
  feet/legs, 157
  functions of, 160–161
  microkinesics, 154
  posture, 157
  prekinesics, 154
  sending abilities, 162
  social kinesics, 158
  vocalic behaviors, 157–158

Observation, 61–65
  contexts, 63–64
  number and length, 64
  observation form, 267–268
  observer roles, 64–65
Open head injuries, 134
Operant conditioning, 178–203
  basic concepts, 183–191
  consequences for behaviors, 213
  criteria for advancement, 194–195
  ethics of, 180–183
  extinction, 252–257
  forgetting, 252–257
  group settings, 214, 217
  history, 178–180
  mediation, 183
  principles of therapeutic intervention,
    195–203
  reinforcement and reinforcers, 251

Operant conditioning, *continued*
   reinforcement schedules, 191–192
   response differentiation, 192–195
Orlick, T., 240
Ostwald, M., 44
Overt behaviors, 99–105

Pachalska, M. K., 210
Paden, E. P., 47
Pap, A., 37
Parents
   language therapy information handout, 295–296
   phonological and articulation therapy information handout, 297–298
   stuttering therapy information handout, 301–302
   voice therapy information handout, 299–300
Parsons, T., 18
Patton, B. R., 50, 259
Perkins, W., 4, 5, 29, 37
Perls, F. S., 44, 48, 161, 169
Peters T. J., 67, 249
Phenomenology, 27
Phonological and articulation disorders
   additions, 87
   diagnostic procedures, 251
   distortions, 87–89
   group settings, 210–211, 212, 217
   intervention, 38, 50, 72–73, 215–216, 232–238
   labels, 4–5
   misarticulations, 86
   omissions, 89
   substitutions, 89
   unstructured activities, 215–216
Phonology
   consonants, 93
   diagnostic procedures, 251
   dipthongs, 91
   distinctive feature analysis, 91–93, 94–97
   parent information handout, 297–298
   phonemes, 86
   traditional analysis, 90–91, 93–94
   vowels, 89–91
Piaget, J., 25
Piercy, F., 214, 243
Posttraumatic amnesia, 134
Prenatal exposure to drugs and alcohol, 209
Preschools, 209
Pressley, M., 247
Prosody, 157. *See also* Voice.
Public laws, 208–209
Public schools, 208–209
Punishment. *See* Aversive stimuli

Radical empiricism, 27
Ramirez, M., 15
Rating scales, 76–77

Reductionism, 57
Reflexive conditioning, 173–174, 184–185
Reichenbach, H., 33–34, 51
Reid, T., 27
Reinforcement
   ethics of, 180–183
   generalized reinforcer, 187
   group setting, 211
   intrinsic/extrinsic/extraneous, 187–188
   negative, 188–189
   reinforcers, 249
   schedules, 191–192, 198
   unconditioned and conditioned reinforcers, 186–187
   various settings, 202
Reinmuth, O. M., 132, 133, 140
Resendiz, P. S., 23
Resnick, L., 244
Response differentiation
   multiple cuing, 194
   successive approximation, 192–194
Responses. *See* Data collection
Retrieval, 241–242
Roehler, L. R., 242, 247
Rogers, C. R., 40, 44, 49, 51, 183, 216, 217, 259
Rohwer, W. D., Jr., 243
Role expectations, 1, 13, 259
Rollin, W. J., 41, 48, 51, 217
Rosenbek, J. C., 251
Rosenberg, P. P., 222, 223
Ross, G., 230
Rousseau, J. J., 44
Rubin, H., 1, 22, 98, 216, 217, 259, 266
Russell, B., 41, 45, 51

Sadker, D., 16
Sadker, M., 16
Sailor, W., 209
Saleh, M. A., 20, 221
Saliency, 243
Sampling procedures, 67–68
Satir, V., 40, 51
Scheflen, A. E., 163
Scheuerle, J., 220, 252, 266
Schneewind, J. B., 44
Schwartz, R. D., 77
Scientific method
   ABA design, 64
   academic contexts, 35
   clinical contexts, 35–37
   clinical experimentation, 37–39
   control, 38
   criteria, 69
   deductive knowledge, 32–33
   dependent variables, 38
   independent variables, 38

INDEX

inductive knowledge, 33–34
operational definitions, 37–38
reliability, 38–39
sampling procedures, 67–68
Sechrest, L., 77
Self-instruction, 243
Seltzer, H., 135, 214
Senior centers, 209
Shames, G., 1, 12, 22, 98, 140, 179, 211, 214, 215, 238, 259, 266
Sherrick, E. E., Jr., 98, 179
Shine, R. E., 17
Shoemaker, D. J., 184, 238
Silverman, F. H., 77, 240
Simple enumeration, 69
Simulations, 215
Skinner, B. F., 175, 178, 180, 189, 203
Sloane, H. N., Jr., 179
Smiley, S. S., 241
Smith, R. R., Jr., 154
Snidecor, J. C., 21
Snow, R. E., 22, 29, 178, 203, 245
Speech disorders. *See individual disorders*
Sperry, L., 219
Spolsky, B., 24
Sprenkle, D., 214
Spriestersbach, D. C., 99
Steindam, S., 16
Stimulus-response learning, 174
Stockard, J., 16
Student learning activites
 aphasia observation, 145
 articulation, 113–114
 clinical experiment-ABA design, 52
 environmental context, 167
 fluency, 115–116
 group control, 225
 group functions, 226–227
 group time management, 224
 individual behavior repertoires, 164–165
 language observation, 141–144
 learning continua, 204
 linear temporal context, 166
 metalinguistic analysis, 146–151
 microcultural values, 30
 operant procedures, 205
 rating scales, 84
 self-evaluation of values and ethics, 53
 simple enumeration, 78–79
 skill and strategy observation, 248
 type token ratio, 80–83
 voice, 117
Stuttering
 anxiety, 99
 associated behaviors, 103
 Center for Fluency Development, 223
 changing behaviors, 214
 covert behaviors, 98–99
 definition, 37–38
 diagnostic procedures, 251
 disfluency types, 99
 expectations of fluency, 99
 intervention, 39–40, 214, 217, 223, 230, 234, 244
 labels, 4–5
 listener reactions, 105
 overt behaviors, 99–105
 parent information handout, 301–302
 phonemes, 105, 242
 rating scales, 76–77
 sampling techniques, 67
 self-perception, 98
 speech rate, 104, 242
 support groups, 222, 223
Summers, P. A., 19
Swindell, C. S., 140

Templin, M. C., 86
Terkel, S., 19, 29
Tests. *See* Diagnostic tests
Taylor, O., 15, 24, 29
Therapy
 dyadic, 1, 210, 212
 group, 207–227
Traumatic brain injury, 134
 general behavioral problems, 134
 intervention, 216, 232
 speech and language behaviors, 134
 types of head injuries, 134
Triden, K. A., 105
Tulving, E., 243
Tyack, D., 64
Type token ratio, 73, 75

Values, 44
 clinical, 47–49
 personal, 45–47
 training program orientation, 49
Van Pelt, D., 6, 8
Van Riper, C., 22, 37, 104
Variables, 38
Verbal association, 175
Videotapes. *See* Data collection, videotapes
Voice and voice disorders, 105–110
 changing behaviors, 214
 data collection, 218
 diagnostic procedures, 251
 disorders of duration, 109
 disorders of loudness, 108–109, 218–219
 disorders of pitch, 107–108
 disorders of quality, 109–110
 disorders of resonance, 110
 intervention program, 235

Voice and voice disorders, *continued*
    parent information handout, 299–300
    support groups, 222
Vygotsky, L. S., 230

Wager, W. W., 203
Walker, H. M., 213
Warner, R., 222, 223
Waters, H. S., 242
Watts, A. W., 36, 49
Webb, E. J., 64, 77
Weber, M., 18
Webster, R., 242
Wepman, J., 6, 8
Wertz, R. T., 251
West, R. W., 109
Whitman, T. L., 243
Whorf, B., 23
Whorfian hypothesis, 23–24
Wiederholt, J., 17
Williams, D. E., 99
Wilson, G. T., 217

Winch, R., 27
Winnicott, D. W., 239, 247
Wolf, A., 217
Wood, D., 230, 231
Woolf, G., 17
Work settings
    community centers, 209–210
    preschools, 209
    public schools, 208–209
    senior centers, 209
Written forms
    data collection, 68, 70, 71
    fluency checklist, 100–101
    importance of, 67
    type token ratio, 73, 75
Wulf, 42, 51, 130–132, 140

Yetman, N. R., 14
Yorkston, K. M., 140

Zeskind, P. S., 21

ISBN 0-675-22160-9